Care of the acutely ill adult

Care of the acutely ill adult

An essential guide for nurses

Second Edition

Edited by

Fiona Creed

Academic Programme Lead,
Oxford University Hospitals NHS Foundation Trust,
Oxford, UK

Christine Spiers

Honorary Senior Lecturer, University of Brighton,
Brighton, UK

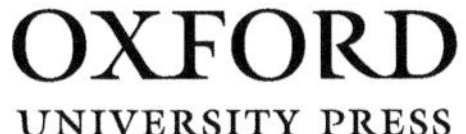

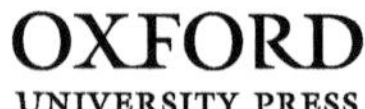

Great Clarendon Street, Oxford, OX2 6DP,
United Kingdom

Oxford University Press is a department of the University of Oxford. It furthers the University's objective of excellence in research, scholarship, and education by publishing worldwide. Oxford is a registered trade mark of Oxford University Press in the UK and in certain other countries

First Edition published in 2010
Second Edition published in 2020

Published in the United States of America by Oxford University Press
198 Madison Avenue, New York, NY 10016, United States of America

British Library Cataloguing in Publication Data

Data available

Library of Congress Control Number: 2019957200

ISBN 978–0–19–879345–8

Printed and bound by
CPI Group (UK) Ltd, Croydon, CR0 4YY

We dedicate this book to Isabel, Harry, and Jacob Creed, and to Tim and Emily Spiers.

Foreword

It is no surprise that Creed and Spiers have published a second edition of their very popular and highly respected *Care of the Acutely Ill Adult*. Nurses are expected and will continue to be expected to offer care to more acutely ill people. This new, updated, and revised edition of *Care of the Acutely Ill Adult* has responded to changes that have occurred in contemporary practice. The contents have been restructured but the new edition retains its user-friendly approach, and the format and the layout are provided in such a way that the reader can navigate the sometimes complex key concepts with ease and confidence.

Those patients who have been admitted to hospital are of the belief that they are entering a place of safety, and the patient, their families, and carers have a right to believe that they will be in receipt of the best possible care. They should be able to feel confident that if their condition should deteriorate, then they are in the best place to receive prompt and effective treatment. The second edition of *Care of the Acutely Ill Adult* will help provide nurses with the confidence and competence so that they can offer people safe and effective care. The nurse is professionally obliged to ensure that the people they have the privilege to care for are prioritized, that they practice in such a way that they are effective in what they do, they preserve patient safety, and they promote professionalism and trust. *Care of the Acutely Ill Adult* reinforces these four underpinning pillars of the Code (Nursing and Midwifery Council (NMC) 2015).

Those patients who are, or who become acutely unwell in hospital should not be receiving suboptimal care. Recognition of the deteriorating patient and taking action quickly whilst utilizing underpinning knowledge and understanding can significantly prevent inappropriate and unsafe care. Throughout *Care of the Acutely Ill Adult* there is a focus on the deteriorating patient and the actions that the nurse must take in order to prevent further clinical deterioration with an emphasis on effective communication and avoidance of any delay in admission to a critical care unit.

Creed and Spiers' second edition is timely as the National Early Warning Score 2 (NEWS2) is rolled out across care areas in the United Kingdom and beyond. The updated NEWS2 (Royal College of Physicians 2017) is evident throughout this book, enabling the reader to base care provision on reliable and contemporary materials as the nurse makes a standardized approach to the assessment of acute illness severity. Whilst the need for a comprehensive assessment is clearly evident in each of the chapters, Chapter 10 is concerned with systematic assessment and the escalation of concerns.

There is much emphasis in the book on nurses responding to patients' needs and preferences and each step of the patient journey sees the patient at the centre of all that is done. Chapter 1 sets the scene as acute care is introduced, stressing the need to treat the patient as a person who is in need of highly skilled, safe, and effective compassionate care. Treatment and care should take into account patients' needs and preferences. Those with an acute illness should, if appropriate, have the opportunity to make informed decisions about the care and treatment they are being offered and this should always be done in partnership with those who are providing care. Caring for the acutely ill patient will very often throw up a number of ethical and moral dilemmas that can be very difficult to grasp and deal with even for the most experienced senior nurse, the final Chapter 13 looks at ethics and offers an insight into this potential minefield.

This book aims to help nurses to develop knowledge and skills as they strive to make appropriate clinical decisions and responses to care needs in fast-changing and dynamic care environments. The editors and contributors of this second edition are well versed and respected in their sphere of practice ensuring that the theoretical components are closely aligned to the real world of care provision that is evidence-based.

The book covers the key topics and is aligned to a number of curricular frameworks, for example, the Standards of Proficiency for Registered Nurses (NMC 2018). This detailed text will become an essential study aid, particularly for those new to the acute care setting. Each chapter addresses important issues along with the knowledge and skills needed—from ethics to pain control—linking theory and practice. The central importance of holistic, patient-centred care has been duly recognized throughout.

I am delighted to have been invited to provide a Foreword for this second edition. Whether you are a student of nursing or healthcare or a registered healthcare practitioner you will find the support and guidance you need in this book to excel in care provision. I wholeheartedly recommend this book to you as it will provoke in you a sense of curiosity and a keen desire to delve deeper.

Professor Ian Peate
Editor in Chief, *British Journal of Nursing*
Head of School
School of Health Studies
Gibraltar

References

Nursing and Midwifery Council (2015) 'The Code: Professional Standards of Practice and Behaviour for Nurses and Midwives'. Available at: https://www.nmc.org.uk/globalassets/sitedocuments/nmc-publications/nmc-code.pdf; accessed 16 December 2019.

Nursing and Midwifery Council (2018) 'Standards of Proficiency for Registered Nurses'. Available at: https://www.nmc.org.uk/globalassets/sitedocuments/education-standards/future-nurse-proficiencies.pdf; accessed 16 December 2019.

Royal College of Physicians (2017) National Early Warning Score (NEWS) 2: Standardising the Assessment of Acute-illness Severity in the NHS. Updated Report of a Working Party. London: Royal College of Physicians.

Acknowledgements

We acknowledge the immense support that we have received from all our friends and colleagues during the production of this second edition. The generosity of our contributors cannot be underestimated, and we thank them unreservedly.

Contents

Glossary of terms and abbreviations

5HT	5-hydroxytryptamine
AI	Angiotensin I
AII	Angiotensin II
A&E	Accident and Emergency
AAGBI	Association of Anaesthetists of Great Britain and Ireland
ABC	airway, breathing, circulation (assessment tool)
ABCDE	Airway, Breathing, Circulation, Disability, and Exposure
ABG	arterial blood gas
AC	alternating current
ACE	angiotensin-converting enzyme
ACP	Advance Care Plan
ACS	acute coronary syndrome
ACVPU	Alert, Confused, responds to Voice, responds to Pain, Unresponsive
ADH	antidiuretic hormone
ADHF	acute decompensated heart failure
ADP	adenosine diphosphate
AED	anti-epileptic drugs
AED	automated external defibrillators
AF	atrial fibrillation
AHP	allied health professional
AHRF	Acute Hypercapnic Respiratory Failure
AKI	acute kidney injury
AKIN	Acute Kidney Injury Network
ALERT	Acute Life-Threatening Events Recognition and Treatment
ALS	advanced life support
AMI	acute myocardial infarction
ANS	autonomic nervous system
ANTT	aseptic non-touch technique
ANZCA	Australian and New Zealand College of Anaesthetists
A/P	anterior posterior
ATN	acute tubular necrosis
ATP	adenosine triphosphate
AV	Atrioventricular
AVPU	Alert, Verbal, Pain, Unresponsive
BAPEN	British Association for Parenteral and Enteral Nutrition
BE	base excess
BiPaP	Bi-phasic Positive airway Pressure
BLS	basic life support
BP	blood pressure
bpm	beats per minute
BTS	British Thoracic Society
BVM	bag valve mask

CAP	community-acquired pneumonia
CCI	chronic critical illness
CCOT	Critical Care Outreach team
CKD	chronic kidney disease
CNPI	Checklist of Non-Verbal Pain Indicators
CNS	central nervous system
COPD	chronic obstructive pulmonary disease
COX	cyclooxygenase
CPAP	continuous positive airway pressure
CPNB	continuous perineural blockade
CPP	cerebral perfusion pressure
CPR	cardiopulmonary resuscitation
CRP	C-reactive protein
CSF	cerebrospinal fluid
CT	computerized tomography
CTZ	chemoreceptor trigger zone
CURB	Confusion, Urea elevation, Respiratory rate, Blood pressure
CVP	central venous pressure
Cx	circumflex
DAPT	dual anti-platelet therapy
DC	direct current
DIC	disseminated intravascular coagulopathy
DKA	diabetic ketoacidosis
DNACPR	Do Not Attempt Cardio-Pulmonary Resuscitation
DNAR	do not attempt resuscitation
D/S	dextrose-saline
DVT	deep vein thrombosis
ECF	extracellular fluid
ECG	electrocardiogram
ED	Emergency Department
EDH	extradural haematoma
EEG	electroencephalogram
eGFR	estimated glomerular filtration rate
EPAP	expiratory positive airway pressure
ERAS	enhanced recovery after surgery
ESR	erythrocyte sedimentation rate
ESRF	end-stage renal failure
ET	endotracheal
ETT	endotracheal tube
FAST	Facial weakness, Arm weakness, Speech disturbance, Time to seek help
FEV	forced expiratory volume
FIO2	fraction of inspired oxygen
FPM	Faculty of Pain Medicine
FRIII	fixed rate intravenous insulin infusion
FTR-N	failure to rescue nursing
FVC	forced vital capacity
FY1	foundation-year doctor
GA	general anaesthetic
GCS	Glasgow Coma Scale
GFR	glomerular filtration rate

GI	gastrointestinal
GP	General Practitioner
GRACE	Global Registry of Acute Coronary Events
h	hour
Hb	haemoglobin
HCA	healthcare assistant
HCP	healthcare professional
HCT	healthcare team
HCl	hydrochloric acid
HDL	high-density lipoproteins
HDU	high dependency unit
HFpEF	heart failure with preserved ejection fraction
HFrEF	heart failure with reduced ejection fraction
HHS	hyperglycaemic hyperosmolar syndrome
HME	heat moisture exchangers
HRA	Human Rights Act
IABP	intra-aortic balloon pump
ICD	Implantable cardiac defibrillators
ICF	intracellular fluid
ICP	intra-cranial pressure
ICS	Intensive Care Society
I:E	inspiratory:expiratory
Ig	immunoglobulin
IM	intramuscular
IMCA	independent mental capacity advocate
INR	international normalized ratio
IO	intraosseous
IPAP	inspiratory positive airway pressure
ITU	intensive treatment unit
IV	intravenous
IVT	intravenous thrombolysis
J	joule
JVD	jugular venous distension
JVP	jugular venous pressure
LA	local anaesthetic
LABA	long-acting short-acting βeta_2-adrenergic agonists
LAD	left anterior descending
LAMA	long-acting muscarinic antagonists
LBBB	Left bundle branch block
LPA	Lasting Power of Attorney
LTRA	Leukotriene receptor antagonists
LV	left ventricle
LVSD	left ventricular systolic dysfunction
LMWH	low-molecular-weight heparin
min	minute
MAP	mean arterial pressure
MCA	Mental Capacity Act
MCA	middle cerebral artery
MC&S	microbiological culture and sensitivity testing
MDRD	Modified Diet Renal Disease

MDT	multidisciplinary team
MELD	Model for End-stage Liver Disease
MET	medical emergency team
MEWS	modified early warning score
MRI	magnetic resonance imaging
MRSA	Methicillin-resistant Staphylococcus aureus
MUST	Malnutrition Universal Screening Tool
NCAA	National Cardiac Arrest Audit
NCEPOD	National Confidential Enquiry into Patient Outcome and Death
NEWS	National Early Warning Score
NICE	National Institute of Health and Care Excellence
NIHSS	National Institute for Health Stroke Score
NIPPV	non-invasive positive pressure ventilation
NIV	non-invasive ventilation
NHS	National Health Service
NMDA	*N*-methyl-D-aspartate
NPPEoLC	National Partnership for Palliative and End of Life Care
NRAD	National Review of Asthma Deaths
NSAIDs	non-steroidal anti-inflammatory drugs
n-STEMI	non-ST-segment elevation myocardial infarction
OD	overdose
ODP	operating department practitioner
ONS	Office for National Statistics
PaO2	partial pressure of oxygen
PAINAD	Pain Assessment in Advanced Dementia
PART	Patient at Risk Team
PCA	Patient-Controlled Analgesia
PCI	percutaneous coronary intervention
PE	pulmonary embolus
PEA	pulseless electrical activity
PEARL	pupils equal and reactive to light
PECT	Plan for Emergency Care and Treatment
PEEP	positive end expiratory pressure
PEFRA	Peak expiratory flow rate
PONV	post-operative nausea and vomiting
p-PCI	primary percutaneous coronary intervention
PREPARE	Patient track and trigger; Rapid response; Education, training, and support; Patient safety and clinical governance; Audit and evaluation; monitoring of patient outcome and continuing quality care; Rehabilitation after critical illness; Enhancing service delivery
qSOFA	quick Sequential Organ Failure Assessment
RAAS	renin–angiotensin–aldosterone system
RAG	red, amber, green
RAS	reticular activating system
RBBB	Right bundle branch block
RCA	right coronary artery
RCoA	Royal College of Anaesthetists
RIFLE	Risk, Injury, Failure, Loss, End-stage
ROSC	return of spontaneous circulation
RR	respiratory rate

RRT	renal replacement therapy
RTA	road traffic accident
s	seconds
SA	Sino-atrial
SABA	short-acting βeta$_2$-adrenergic agonists
SAH	subarachnoid haemorrhage
SALT	speech and language team
SBAR	Situation, Background, Assessment, and Recommendation
SBP	systolic blood pressure
SC	subcutaneously
SDH	subdural haematoma
SE	status epilepticus
SEND	System of Electronic Notification and Documentation
SIGN	Scottish Intercollegiate Guidelines Network
SIRS	Systemic Inflammatory Response Syndrome
SNRI	serotonin norepinephrine reuptake inhibitor drug
SNS	sympathetic nervous system
SOCRATES	Site, Onset, Character, Radiation, Associated symptoms, Timing, Exacerbating factors, Severity
SOFA	Sequential Organ Failure Assessment
SPICT	supportive and palliative indicators care tool
SpO_2`	peripheral capillary oxygen saturation
S/T	spontaneous/timed
STEMI	ST-segment elevation myocardial infarction
SVR	systemic vascular resistance
SVT	supraventricular tachycardia
TACO	transfusion-associated circulatory overload
TBI	traumatic brain injury
TENS	Trans electrical nerve stimulation
TIA	transient ischaemic attack
TRALI	transfusion-related acute lung injury
UA	unstable angina
UTI	urinary tract infections
VF	ventricular fibrillation
VLDL	very low-density lipoproteins
VRS	Verbal Rating Scale
VT	ventricular tachycardia
VTE	venous thromboembolism
WCC	white cell count
WPW	Wolff–Parkinson–White
y	year

Contributors

Heather Baid
Senior Lecturer, School of Health Sciences
University of Brighton, Brighton,
UK

Kevin Barrett
Senior Lecturer, School of Health Sciences,
University of Brighton, Brighton, UK

Daren Briscoe
Senior Lecturer, School of Health Sciences,
University of Brighton, Brighton, UK

Wendy Caddye
Nurse Consultant in Pain Management,
Anaesthetic Department,
Brighton & Sussex Universities NHS Trust,
Brighton, UK

Fiona Creed
Academic Programme Lead, Oxford University
NHS Foundation Trust Oxford, UK

Lorna East
Heart Failure Nurse Specialist, Western Sussex
University Hospital NHS Foundation Trust,
Worthing, UK

Theofanis Fotis
Principal Lecturer, School of Health Sciences,
University of Brighton, Brighton, UK

Emma Gardner
Community Matron, Dorset Healthcare
University NHS Foundation Trust, Poole, UK

Kate Kemsley
Respiratory Clinical Nurse Specialist,
Cardio-Respiratory Department,
Guernsey Health & Social Care,
St Martins, Guernsey

Katharine Martyn
Principal Lecturer Nutrition, School of Health
Sciences University of Brighton, Brighton, UK

Cristina Osorio
Directorate lead Nurse for Renal,
Cardiac & Vascular services,
Specialist Division, Brighton & Sussex University
Hospitals NHS Trust, Brighton, UK

Christine Spiers
Honorary Senior Lecturer, School of Health
Sciences, University of Brighton, Brighton, UK

1

Acute care and failure to rescue

Setting the scene

Fiona Creed

Chapter contents

Changes to the delivery of acute healthcare, increasing technological advances and an ageing population with complex comorbidities have led to increased levels of acuity in hospital and acute community environments (MacIntosh and Sandall 2016). This, coupled with increasing evidence of failure to rescue acutely ill patients (NCEPOD 2012; NHS improvement 2016), has meant an increased focus on patient safety in acute care environments and the need for healthcare practitioners to have a better understanding of acute care delivery. In order to understand the complexities of issues involved in acute care delivery, failure to rescue, and the impact this may have on patient safety, this chapter will focus upon:

- changes to patient acuity levels in the United Kingdom
- reduced clinical exposure to acuity
- the concept of failure to rescue
- the complexities associated with failure to rescue
- factors relating to failure to rescue
- the impact of human factors on failure to rescue
- advances in care to reduce failure to rescue
- failure to rescue in the community
- how this book can help

Learning outcomes

This chapter will enable you to:

- understand the rationale for changes in patient acuity levels
- understand concepts of suboptimal care and failure to rescue
- explore the issues related to failure to rescue
- understand the impact of human factors on patient safety
- analyse the importance of patient safety frameworks
- explore advances in acute care delivery

Changes impacting on acute care

It is undisputed that the average age of the patient treated in acute care environments has gradually increased over the past two decades. A recent study (Cornell 2012) has identified that there are currently 3 million people aged over 80 in the United Kingdom, with current trends suggesting that this number will double by 2030. The majority of patients in hospital are over the age of 75 and the average age of the ward patient is now 82 years. Whilst over 50% of the ageing population reports good 'health', a significant percentage has one or more comorbidities and/or complex medical conditions that often lead to patient admission. This group represents a vulnerable patient population of individuals who are more likely to become unwell and rapidly deteriorate.

Alongside this there is an increasing demand for patient beds which impacts on patient bed turnover rates and therefore acuity levels. There is a greater number of emergency admissions and increased demand upon a smaller level of inpatient beds in acute hospitals. Statistical analysis of National Health Service (NHS) data highlights that in one month (November 2016) 1.25 million patients attended Accident and Emergency departments (A&E) in the United Kingdom with 500,000 of these requiring an acute hospital admission. Bed occupancy has been shown to be at a record high and in December 2016, 12 UK hospital trusts did not have a single bed available and another 30 had fewer than 10 beds free for patients (NHS Support Federation 2016).

Current acute care provision is therefore clearly impacted by an ageing population with complex care needs, and a decreasing number of acute hospital beds and increased demand. Recently implemented integrated care pathways may impact upon this situation as more acute beds are closed and care shifted to community settings, arguably transferring the issue of increasing patient acuity to these community settings as well.

Reduction in clinical exposure for novice practitioners

Paradoxically, as the level of acuity in the hospital ward areas increases, it is noted that acute clinical placements during nursing and medical education programmes have been reduced (Adam *et al.* 2010). Recent changes to undergraduate preparation of nurses and doctors have reduced hours worked in clinical placements and the drive towards integrated primary care has necessitated the need for an increased focus on community-based care. The five-year forward plan (NHS England 2014) clearly articulates the need for changes to service development and location of care and therefore the need for increased exposure to community-focused and integrated care. However, it could be argued that an increased focus on community placements may further add to a reduction in exposure to assessment and management of acutely ill patients. It is therefore vitally important that we strive to teach novice practitioners the importance of recognizing and effectively managing acutely ill patients.

Patient deterioration and suboptimal care: An ongoing issue

Within the United Kingdom, the concept of suboptimal care was first identified by McQuillain and colleagues (1998). The term 'suboptimal care' is used to relate to the multifactorial issues regarding the significance of clinical changes in patients causing potential misdiagnosis, inappropriate management, or lack of timely escalation and appropriate care delivery. McQuillain and colleagues (1998) identified that approximately 54% of patients had received 'suboptimal' care prior to admission to the intensive treatment unit (ITU). The study identified several potential problems, including:

- lack of knowledge/experience of staff
- failure to appreciate the urgency of the patient's changing condition
- failure to seek advice about the patient's condition
- lack of medical staff/supervision of medical staff
- organizational failings that prevented appropriate assessment and treatment of the patient who was deteriorating

Worryingly, the study highlighted a fundamental problem related to inadequate assessment of patients' breathing and circulation, which could quickly lead to untimely death if not treated appropriately.

A similar study (McGloin *et al.* 1999) also acknowledged that patients had shown clinical signs of deterioration that had not been recognized and had received inappropriate treatment. They concluded that patients with obvious clinical indicators of acute deterioration were sometimes overlooked and may have received inappropriate treatment.

Following these studies, several changes to healthcare practice have been implemented in an attempt to improve patient safety. These include the development of:

- acuity patient scoring tools
- critical care outreach services
- medical emergency teams/Patient at risk teams
- National Institute for Health and Care Excellence Guidance (NICE, 2007)
- track-and-trigger scoring systems
- electronic patient tracking systems
- escalation and communication tools
- national competency frameworks
- NHS data collection tools
- NHS patient safety initiatives

However, despite these developments, avoidable harm related to failure to recognize and appropriately treat deterioration remains high. In 2012, Hogan and colleagues found that 26% of preventable deaths were related to either failure to set up correct systems, failure to respond adequately to clinical deterioration, and failure to act upon patients' test results. Similarly, in 2015 the National Reporting and Learning Systems (NRLS) identified a 7% incidence of severe harm or death associated with failure to recognize or appropriately respond to patient deterioration. These studies suggest a continuing issue associated with recognition and management of the deteriorating patient that is leading to avoidable patient harm. Indeed, a study by the National Health Executive (2015) identified that avoidable deaths (for a number of reasons) were estimated to be in the region of 1,000 deaths per month. It is clear that failure to recognize deteriorating patients contributes to this figure (Waldie *et al.* 2016).

The concept of 'failure to rescue'

Failure to respond to deterioration is not isolated to the UK healthcare system and in the United States, Silber and colleagues (1992) initially conceptualized the notion of failure to rescue which is now used internationally to refer to incidences of suboptimal care. Initially 'failure to rescue' refers to a death after a treatable complication and was first developed as an indicator of patient safety by the US Agency for Healthcare Research. As with most concepts in healthcare there is no universal definition of failure to rescue and several different classifications, including failure to rescue nursing (FTR-N), are apparent in the literature (Silber 2007). More recently, failure to rescue has been taken as lack of recognition and response to acute patient deterioration leading to severe harm and/or death (Garvey 2015). Although a universal definition of failure to rescue is lacking, there is a consensus that failure to rescue is a complex multifactorial issue and as such will prove difficult to solve (NHS Improvement 2016).

Several factors have been identified that are commonly associated with failure to rescue. Moldenhauer and colleagues (2009) have suggested four main contributing factors to 'failure to rescue'. These included:

- failure to recognize signs of clinical deterioration
- failure to assess the patient physically in sufficient detail to identify signs of clinical deterioration
- failure to communicate and escalate professional concerns about clinical deterioration appropriately
- failure to diagnose signs of clinical deterioration and provide adequate treatment to the deteriorating patient

Similarly, analysis of UK research (Griffiths 2011) identified potential points of failure to rescue associated with:

- lack of taking patient observations appropriately
- lack of recording observations
- lack of recognition of early signs of deterioration
- lack of effective communication of concern about patients' observations

Whilst the nurse, by default, clearly has a fundamental role in detection of deterioration and therefore some of the issues may be related to problems with nursing care, other authors point to wider issues associated with failure to rescue. Alqanthani and Al Dorzi (2010) point to organizational failings. They suggest that factors that contribute to failure to rescue include:

- poor organizational structures and processes
- lack of adequate supervision of healthcare staff
- failure to get advice from other senior colleagues

This matches root cause analysis data from NHS Improvement data (2015). These data highlighted several organizational issues associated with failure including:

- poor team communication
- inaccurate patient diagnosis
- lack of clarity over senior clinician responsible for patient management plan
- lack of senior clinician review
- failure to evaluate treatment response
- lack of higher level facilities
- lack of equipment for recording observations

Unsurprisingly, root cause analysis identified staffing levels as a contributory factor in 16% of cases of failure to rescue.

Ghefari and Dimack (2015) explored reasons for failure to rescue in older patients. Their review of the literature identified three themes of resources, attitudes, and behaviours that appeared to impact upon failure to rescue statistics.

- *Resources*: A correlation was found between staffing levels, skills of staff and clinical expertise, and failure to rescue. Unsurprisingly, increased numbers of specialist staff with adequate knowledge decreases the frequency of failure to rescue deteriorating patients.
- *Attitudes*: The presence of a 'safety culture' in the ward environment such as a shared set of values, beliefs, behaviours, and norms has been shown to impact positively on failure to rescue statistics. Therefore, in environments where a safety culture is in place in relation to deterioration, there appears to be a drive towards minimizing patient harm.
- *Behaviours*: Communication or failure to escalate concern appears to be a significant contributory factor in failure to rescue. Communication breakdowns may occur at any point in the communication chain and may involve any member of the multidisciplinary team. Similarly, it is suggested where safety behaviour patterns are not embedded in clinical practice, there appear to be more issues around failure to rescue.

Human factors in failure to rescue

Initially, much of the focus on failure to rescue explored single issues in an endeavour perhaps to find the 'silver bullet' that would decrease failure to rescue rates. Researchers have analysed and implemented changes to physiological indicators of acute illness, track-and-trigger systems, systems of safer work, team work, critical care outreach systems, and education and communication systems. The continued incidence of failure to rescue therefore highlights the complex and multifaceted aspects of this phenomenon. Recent attention has focused upon human factors as a key component to failure to rescue.

Exploration of failure to rescue cases has identified the fundamental role that human behaviour plays. Acceptance that humans make mistakes is central to enabling development of safer systems of work, especially in healthcare where this fallibility can have devastating consequences on patient outcome. Working in a high-pressure environment is often a significant contributory factor in clinical practice. The common human factors identified in safety incidents and failure to rescue are:

- Psychological workload: work or personal stress and other factors such as fatigue can impact upon one's ability to concentrate or can lead to over-fixation upon one element of care to the detriment of the wider picture. In high-stress situations we sometimes see what we expect to see rather than what is really there. This is a psychological phenomenon known as involuntary automaticity.
- Distractions: these may include physical distractions such as noise or distractions such as interruption of thought during times that require concentration; this could be disruption by staff, other patients, or relatives.
- Physical tiredness: the impact of long shifts and physical tiredness can affect one's ability to make appropriate decisions.
- Team dynamics: evidence suggests that where teams work and communicate effectively together, risks to patients are minimized (Carthey 2009). However, where patient care is impacted by adherence to hierarchy and cultures that discourage challenge, clinical incidents are more likely to occur.

A recent study by Jones and Johnstone (2016) explored the impact of inattentional blindness on failure to rescue. This concept was developed by psychologists in the United States and is best demonstrated in the following video link showing 'the invisible gorilla': http://www.theinvisiblegorilla.com/videos.html

In practice, inattentional blindness may occur when attention is not fully focused on a given situation and a complex interaction of other issues may distort reality and prevent the nurse correctly focusing on that situation. These complex interactions can be linked to focusing on one task to the detriment of other aspects of the situation. Jones and Johnstone argue that this may limit attention on other factors or cause significant factors to be overlooked and enable them to go unnoticed. An example of this blindness is included in Box 1.1.

In exploring the incident in Box 1.1, we can see that inattention blindness of the nurse potentially led to this issue occurring but that other factors such as the doctor's inexperience and the busy nature of the ward played significant roles.

It is recognized that it is rare for factors relating to failure to be directly attributable to one person only and the complexities of human error have been widely noted. Woods (2010) highlights that error often involves a complex interplay of:

- context of the incident
- interaction of the humans involved in the incident
- organizational context/competing goals
- factors impacting upon human performance

A model that is often used as an analogy to the impact of human errors is the Swiss cheese model (Reason 2013). This model identifies that in most systems there are several different

Box 1.1 Inattentional blindness

Mr Hubert is an 85-year-old man admitted to your ward following surgery. Pre-operative assessment identified him at risk of falls and an appropriate 'at risk of falls' wristband was provided. The ward was very busy, and you are requested to see Mr Hubert following a fall or possible collapse. When you assess him, you find that his blood pressure (BP) is within normal limits, but the diastolic pressure has risen and Mr Jones is tachycardic. He is assessed by the foundation-year doctor (FY1) and the observed altered observations attributed to anxiety following the fall. Later, Mr Hubert is found collapsed again. He is found on the floor looking pale and clammy and has severe peripheral cyanosis. Physical assessment identifies hypotension, tachycardia, tachypnoea, and signs of decompensated shock. He has had a slow internal post-operative bleed.

On reflection, it becomes apparent that early warning signs of deterioration were missed as:

- The fall was attributed to his noted risk of falls from past medical history and not fully investigated.
- There was insufficient time to perform in-depth assessment after the initial fall.
- Initial early signs of deterioration (rising diastolic pulse) had been overlooked by the FY1.

layers of defence. Therefore, if a single minor error were to occur it would only bypass one layer of defence and the impact would be minimal. However, if several minor errors occurred then the impact could be more devastating as several layers of defence are breached. Therefore, visually, if all the holes in the Swiss cheese align, this allows a breach of a defence systems and a breach in patient safety (see Figure 1.1).

A hypothetical example of a clinical Swiss cheese model is included in Box 1.2.

Improving failure to rescue: A safety culture

As failure to rescue is a multifaceted complex issue it is clear that no single solution will solve this problem. A key driver within the contemporary NHS is to establish a safety culture that attempts to address safety issues, one of these being failure to rescue.

Reason (2013) argues that the impact of the Swiss cheese model is worsened if the organization:

- has a poor safety culture and is reluctant to invest in safe systems of practice.
- ignores operational hazards and/or supplies poor training/education relating to risks to its staff.
- is reluctant to deal proactively with barriers and safeguards that will enhance a safety culture.

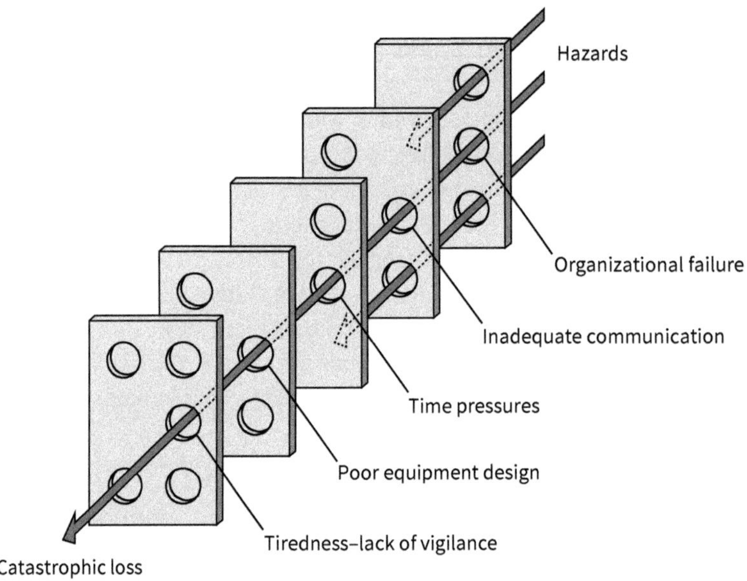

Figure 1.1 The Swiss cheese model

Reproduced from *BMJ*, Reason, J.T. Human error: models and management. 320(7237): 768–770. Copyright © 2000, British Medical Journal Publishing Group. With permission from BMJ Publishing Group Ltd doi: https://doi.org/10.1136/bmj.320.7237.768.

Modern NHS organizations therefore are striving towards implementing safety cultures to reduce the Swiss cheese model effect. Carthey (2009) highlights that a safety culture is effective within organizations when its culture is:

- open: enabling staff to feel confident to discuss safety issues.

Box 1.2 Clinical example

Mrs Jones is a 67-year-old lady admitted with pneumonia. The ward is short staffed (*organizational failure*) and the previous nurse caring for Mrs Jones did not identify that she had become sicker overnight (*communication failure*). The staff were busy with another patient (*time pressure*) and did not notice the deterioration in Mrs Jones' condition. Her observations were due at 08:00 but because this clashed with the medication round they were overlooked until 10:00 (*lack of vigilance*). At this time Mrs Jones condition had deteriorated significantly. A medical emergency call was put out and Mrs Jones was transferred to the critical care unit with severe respiratory failure and sepsis. Later that shift, Mrs Jones died. The inquest identified several areas where earlier deterioration could have been identified and treated. These included:

- Ineffective handover from day staff to night staff.
- Pressures which meant observation of the patient was delayed.
- Lack of vigilance of the patient in the ward environment.

- just: ensuring staff are treated fairly.
- reporting: incidents are reported, and a no blame culture adapted.
- learning: committed to learning and embeds learning in its culture.
- informed: Learns from previous incidents and implements safe systems of practice.

Improving failure to rescue: Implementing safe systems of practice

NHS improvement is working with NHS Trusts in the United Kingdom to establish safer patient care. Within NHS improvement there is a patient safety collaborative focusing upon recognition of deterioration with subgroups exploring high incident issues such as recognition of sepsis (see Chapter 8) and acute kidney injury (see Chapter 5). Alongside this, a number of initiatives have already been implemented to assist practitioners with recognizing and responding to acute deterioration.

Early warning scores and devices

The extensive use of track-and-trigger scoring systems has been implemented widely throughout the United Kingdom. This includes a National Early Warning score implemented by the Royal College of Physicians (2012 and 2017) which hopes to standardize assessment and escalation of acutely ill adults. Alongside this electronic scoring systems have been implemented including Patientrack© and other tools such as System of Electronic Notification and Documentation (SEND) currently being implemented at Oxford University NHS Trust (Wong *et al.* 2015). The advantage of electronic systems is the easier facilitation of data analysis that may be used to enhance future tools and potentially predict deterioration at an earlier stage (see Chapter 10 for more details on early warning systems).

Implementation of care bundles for high-risk events

Care bundles are being implemented widely throughout the United Kingdom. Simplistically put, a care bundle is a tool designed to enable a practitioner to deliver the best available care to improve patient outcome.

Care bundles are evidence-based quality improvement initiatives and they are normally based on Level 1 evidence. A care bundle offers a cohesive unit of steps that *must* be used if the tool is to improve patient outcome; generally, care bundles have three to five measurable patient outcomes. Within the United Kingdom, bundles are generally targeted at high-risk events and those relating to acute deterioration such as care bundles for Sepsis (Sepsis UK 2016), Acute Kidney Injury (NHS England 2015), Pneumonia and COPD (British Thoracic Society 2014), and end of life care/Amber Care bundle (Amber Care bundle 2014).

Development of safety huddles

A safety huddle is a multidisciplinary event that enables practitioners to review patient care and tackle potential local problems/issues. The aims of a safety huddle are to:

- reduce chance of avoidable harm and therefore optimize patient safety.
- ensure all staff feel empowered and accountable for care.
- enhance respect across divisions and foster collaborative decision-making and change.

A safety huddle is usually time limited and should include members of the multidisciplinary team. The overarching principle is to engender a collective situational awareness for the team and to enable shared decision-making.

Developing effective communication systems

Communication issues have been highlighted as being significant in several cases of failure to rescue, especially those pertaining to patient escalation. Simple tools such as the Situation Background Assessment and Recommendation (SBAR) initially developed for the US Navy submariners have been widely developed and internationally adopted. These communication tools are recommended to enhance escalation of patients throughout the United Kingdom. For further information see Chapter 10.

Acute care in the community

It would be remiss to ignore the impact that a changing focus on care delivery is having on acuity levels in the community. Earlier discussions highlighted the need for early discharge and therefore community-based professionals are facing increasing levels of acuity and an emphasis on admission avoidance and management of acutely ill patients in their own homes/care homes. Several initiatives including education programmes and community-focused protocols aimed at establishing acute care skills and patient management for community nurses are being implemented. However, the Royal College of Nursing (2014) stresses the need to invest in preparation of community nurses, highlighting the current lack of adequate investment despite increased acuity and complexity of issues faced in the community patient population.

Using this book to enhance caring for acutely ill patients

This book has been designed to help you enhance your care when nursing acutely ill and deteriorating patients. We hope this book will enable you to:

- revise knowledge associated with pathophysiology and therefore give you an enhanced understanding of the early presentation of acute illness and associated signs and symptoms.
- develop patient assessment skills and understand how accurate patient assessment when linked to prompt intervention improves patient outcome.
- understand the evidence base for current practice and explore National Guidance and Care bundles where they are applicable.
- acknowledge the importance of safe systems of practice and evaluate how you can use these in your current practice.
- apply theory to practice using the patient scenarios throughout the book
- develop the knowledge and skills to allow you to respond quickly and effectively to patient deterioration in a competent manner.

References

Adam, S., O'Dell, M., Welch, J. (2010) *Rapid Assessment of the Acutely Ill Patient.* Oxford: Wiley Blackwell.

Alqanthani, S., Al Dorzi, H. (2010) Rapid response systems in acute hospital care. *Annals Thorac Med*, 5:1–4.

Amber Care Bundle.org (2014) *The Amber Care Bundle.* Available at: http://www.ambercarebundle.org/homepage.aspx; accessed 8 December 2019.

British Thoracic Society (2014) *The British Thoracic Society Pilot Care Bundle Project: A Care Bundles-Based Approach to Improving Standards of Care in Chronic Obstructive Pulmonary Disease and Community Acquired Pneumonia.* London: British Thoracic Society.

Carthey, J. (2009) The 'how to guide' for implementing human factors in Healthcare. Available at: https://www.guysandstthomas.nhs.uk/resources/education-training/sail/reading/human-factors.pdf; accessed 8 December 2019.

Cornwell, J. (2012) *The Care of Frail Older People with Complex Needs: Time for a Revolution.* London: The Kings Fund.

Garvey, P.K. (2015) Failure to rescue: The nurses impact. *Med.Surg Nursing*, 24(3):145–9.

Ghefari, A., Dimick, J. (2015) Importance of teamwork, communication and culture on failure to rescue in the elderly. *Br J Surg*, 103(2):47–51.

Hogan, H., Healy, F., Neale, G. (2012) Preventable deaths due to problems in care in English acute hospitals: A retrospective case record review study. *BMJ Quality and Safety*, 21(9):735–41.

Jones, A., Johnstone, M.J. (2016) Inattentional blindness and failure to rescue the deteriorating patient in critical care, emergency and perioperative settings: Four case scenarios. *Australian Critical Care.* Available at: http://dx.doi.org/10.1016/j.aucc.2016.09.005; accessed 8 December 2019.

Mackintosh, N., Sandall, J. (2016) The social practice of rescue: The safety implications of acute illness trajectories and patient categorisation in medical and maternity settings. *Sociol Health Illn*, 38(2):257–69.

McGloin, H., Adam, S., Singer, M. (1999) Unexpected deaths and referrals of ITU of patients on wards. Are some cases avoidable? *Clin Med*, 33:255–9.

McQuillain, P., Pilkington, S., Allan, A., *et al.* (1998) Confidential inquiry into quality of care before admission to ITU. *BMJ*, 316:1853–58.

Moldenhauer, K., Sabel, *et al.* (2009). Clinical triggers: An alternative to a rapid response team. *Jt Comm J Qual Patient Saf*, 35(3):164–74.

National Health Executive (2015) Hunt orders annual review into avoidable deaths. Available at: http://www.nationalhealthexecutive.com/Health-Care-News/hunt-orders-annual-review-into-avoidable-deaths; accessed 8 December 2019.

NICE (2007) *Acutely Ill Patients in Hospital: Recognition of and Response to Acute Illness of Adults in Hospital* CG70. London: HMSO.

NHS England (2014) Five year forward view. Available at: https://www.england.nhs.uk/wp-content/uploads/2014/10/5yfv-web.pdf; accessed 8 December 2019.

NHS England (2015) Think Kidneys: Recommended minimum requirements for a care bundle for patients with AKI in Hospital. Available at: https://www.thinkkidneys.nhs.uk/aki/wp-content/uploads/sites/2/2015/12/AKI-care-bundle-requirements-FINAL-12.07.16.pdf; accessed 8 December 2019.

NHS England (2016) *Sustainability and Transformation Plans.* Available at: https://www.england.nhs.uk/stps/; accessed 8 December 2019.

Reason, J. (2013) *A Life in Error: From Little Slips to Big Disasters.* Surrey: Ashgate Publishing.

Royal College of Nursing (2014) *Moving Care to the Community: An International Perspective.* London: Royal College of Nursing.

Royal College of Physicians (2012) *National Early Warning Scores: Standardising the Assessment of Acute Illness Severity in the NHS.* London: Royal College of Physicians.

Royal College of Physicians (2017) *National Early Warning Scores 2: Standardising the Assessment of Acute Illness Severity in the NHS.* London: Royal College of Physicians.

Sepsis UK (2016) *Toolkit: Emergency Department Management of Sepsis in Adults and Young People over 12 Years.* Available at: Sepsis.Org.UK; accessed 8 December 2019.

Silber, J.H., Williams, S.V., Krakauer, H. (1992) Hospital and patient: Characteristics associated with death after surgery: A study of adverse occurrence and failure to rescue. *Medical Care*, 30(7): 615–29.

Silber, J.H., Romano, P.S., Rosen, A.K. (2007) Failure-to-Rescue: Comparing definitions to measure quality of care. *Medical Care*, 8(10):918–25.

Waldi, J., Day, T., *et al.* 2016 Patient safety in acute care: Are we going around in circles *Br J Nursing*, 25(3):747–51.

Wong, D., Bonnici, T., Knight, J. (2015) *SEND: A System for Electronic Notification and Documentation of Vital Sign Observations.* BMC: Medical Informatics and Decision Making 15(68):1–12.

Woods, D., Decker, S., Cook, R. (2010) *Behind Human Error.* Surrey, Ashgate Publishing.

2
Respiratory assessment and care

Daren Briscoe

Chapter contents

Respiratory disease affects one in five people and is the third largest cause of death in the United Kingdom, killing 80,000 people in 2012, not including lung cancer (35,500). It is responsible for around 1 million hospital admissions and costs the National Health Service (NHS) an estimated £4.7 billion a year (APPG on Respiratory Health, British Lung Foundation 2014). Timely evidence-based respiratory care in the community reduces hospital admissions and is cost effective, encompassing asthma action plans, smoking cessation strategies, and pulmonary rehabilitation. However, it is reported that these have been implemented inconsistently across the United Kingdom (APPG on Respiratory Health, British Lung Foundation 2014), potentially increasing emergency presentations of the acutely ill respiratory patient. This chapter will examine:

- the normal anatomy of the respiratory system
- physiological mechanisms which control the respiratory function
- respiratory assessment
- respiratory monitoring
- principles of arterial blood gas analysis
- respiratory management of the patient who is breathless, and:
    - on oxygen
    - requiring physiotherapy
    - on drug therapy
    - on non-invasive ventilation
    - has a chest drain
    - has a tracheostomy
- an overview of three common respiratory disorders

Learning outcomes

This chapter will enable you to:

- review the normal structure and function of the respiratory system
- develop an understanding of the physiological mechanisms which control respiratory function

- consider the assessment, diagnosis, and management of the patient with respiratory disorders
- identify the critically ill respiratory patient and know when to refer to senior/ medical staff
- understand the impact of respiratory problems on the patient and carers
- use a skills assessment tool to assess your clinical practice

Introduction

The respiratory system is designed to actively move oxygen (O_2) from the air during inspiration into the alveolar sacs as it flows into the lungs. This is called external respiration and diffuses oxygen across the alveolar membrane into the small capillaries that cover the alveolar sacs. This ensures that oxygen in the air enters the lungs by inspiration and the waste product of carbon dioxide (CO_2) is excreted from the body by expiration. The oxygen is then delivered by the circulation to tissues to enable cellular metabolism which is called internal respiration.

The anatomy of the lungs

The anatomy of the respiratory system consists of the lungs, which are contained in the thoracic cavity and protected by the spine, manubrium, sternum, ribs, costal cartilages, and the hemispherical dome of the diaphragm (see Figure 2.1). The upper airways extend from the nose, mouth, and oropharynx to the larynx. The lower airways consist of the cartilaginous rings of the trachea and bronchi, smooth muscle tubes called bronchioles, and delicate alveoli

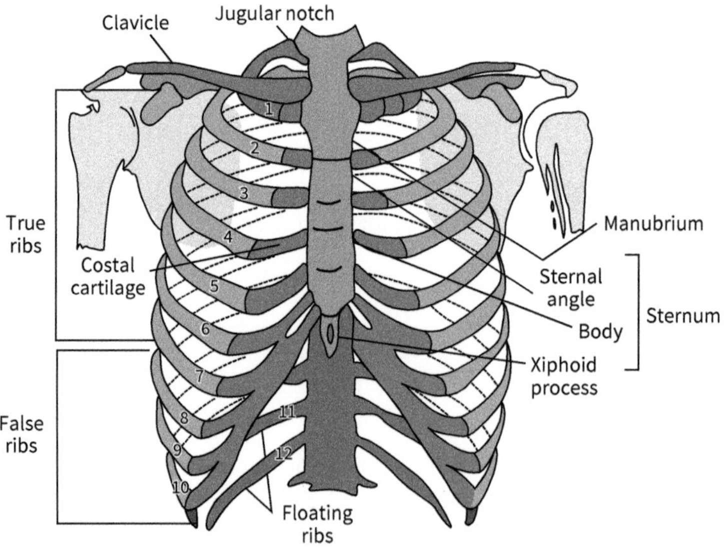

Figure 2.1 The bony thorax.

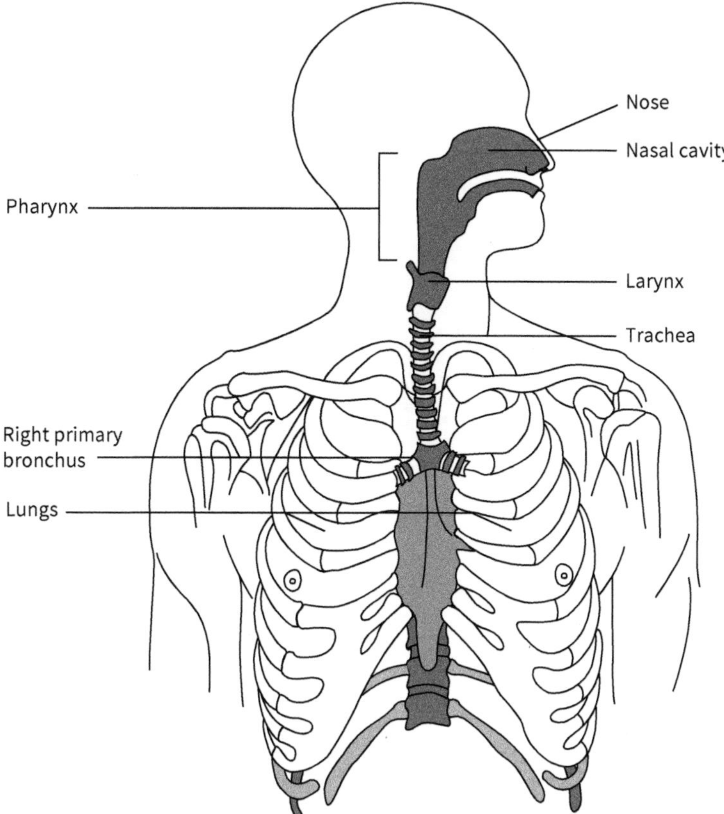

Figure 2.2 The anatomy of the respiratory system.

sacs. The trachea and bronchi are lined with a ciliated epithelium which produces a wave, resulting in an upward movement of the mucus thereby removing inhaled particles from the lungs (see Figure 2.2). The lungs are divided into lobes, with three on the right and two on the left to make room for the heart (see Figure 2.3). They are contained in the thorax by the pleurae. The parietal pleura adheres to the outer thorax, while the visceral pleura adheres to the lungs.

Physiological mechanisms of the respiratory function

Pulmonary ventilation

Pulmonary ventilation is where air is passed in and out of the lungs as the ribs and thoracic cage actively enlarges upwards and outwards in inspiration or passively retracts on expiration, forcing air out. In inspiration, the intercostal muscles move the ribs out and the diaphragm flattens (see Figure 2.4). As the thoracic cage enlarges, the volume of air drawn in increases, dropping the pressure and sucking in more air. In expiration, the intercostal muscles relax, the diaphragm rises, the ribs move back downwards and inwards, reducing the size of the thoracic cavity, enabling elastic recoil of the lungs so that air is exhaled.

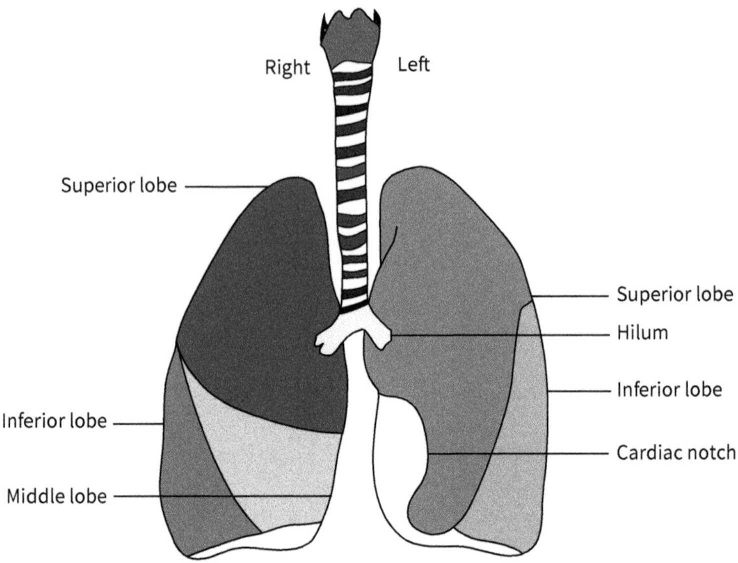

Figure 2.3 The lobes of the lungs.

Thoracic expansion is also determined by the normal elastic recoil of alveolar tissue, the resistance to airflow, which is dependent on the diameter of the bronchioles and the surface tension forces at the liquid/air interface (Gibson and Waters 2017).

Lung compliance refers to the distensibility (stretchiness) or elasticity of the lung tissue which is essential in allowing the chest to expand and draw in air. It is the difference between

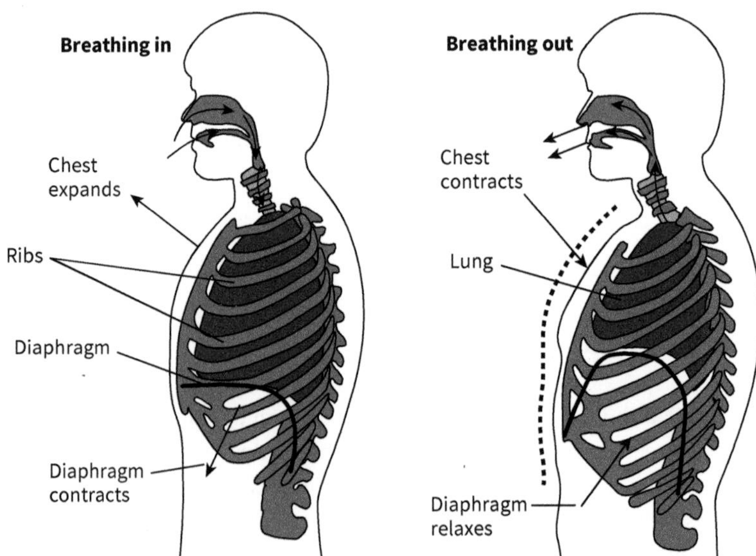

Figure 2.4 Inspiration and expiration.

the gaseous pressure/volume within the lungs and the outside atmospheric pressure that causes air to be drawn in (Boyle's Law), but it is the elasticity of the lungs that allows the chest to expand and alter the pressure. It therefore follows that abnormally stiff, non-compliant lungs cause a restriction of lung expansion (low compliance), giving rise to a ventilation deficit (reduced volume or breath size) and increased work of breathing to maintain oxygenation.

Airway resistance is the opposition to flow caused by the forces of friction and/or by abnormalities within the lung parenchyma (lung tissue). Resistance is inversely proportional to compliance and therefore a highly compliant lung will have low resistance (normal lung dynamics) and a highly resistant lung will have low compliance (abnormal lung dynamics). This can be seen in respiratory disease where there is an increase in the alveolar surface tension and/or increased bronchiole obstruction and mucous production, as in bronchitis, which increases resistance to flow and therefore lowers lung compliance (Gibson and Waters 2017).

Surfactant

Increased alveolar surface tension by either a lack of surfactant in the alveoli or inflammation increases resistance causing the work of breathing to increase. The higher the surface tension, the lower the compliance and resistance is increased.

Surfactant is a mixture of phospholipids that is produced by type II alveolar cells and reduces the surface tension (or maintains its homeostasis) within the alveoli making it easier to open the alveoli during inspiration. This also increases alveolar stability by inhibiting alveolar collapse as they shrink. Pulmonary disease associated with increased mucous production, which has a dilution effect on surfactant, plus inflammation causes increased surface tension and low compliance, giving rise to theories of surfactant dysfunction being associated with the pathophysiology of asthma, chronic obstructive pulmonary disease (COPD) and other acute respiratory diseases with bronchial obstruction (Calkovska *et al.* 2015).

Similarly, surface tension of serous fluid within the pleural membranes ensures that when the parietal pleura (attached to the chest wall) expands, the lungs (attached to the visceral pleura) also expand. Reduction in the surface tension of the serous fluid produces a pneumothorax or air within the pleural cavity (its potential space). Increased surface tension of the serous fluid (e.g. inflammation of the pleural membranes) increases resistance and reduces compliance of the lungs to ventilate.

External respiration

Gaseous exchange takes place as oxygen molecules move by diffusion from the alveoli to the capillaries and carbon dioxide moves in the opposite direction along a pressure gradient (the partial pressures (Dalton's Law) of oxygen and carbon dioxide). Carbon dioxide has the ability to diffuse more readily than oxygen because it is a more soluble gas (Henry's Law) (see Figure 2.5; Table 2.1).

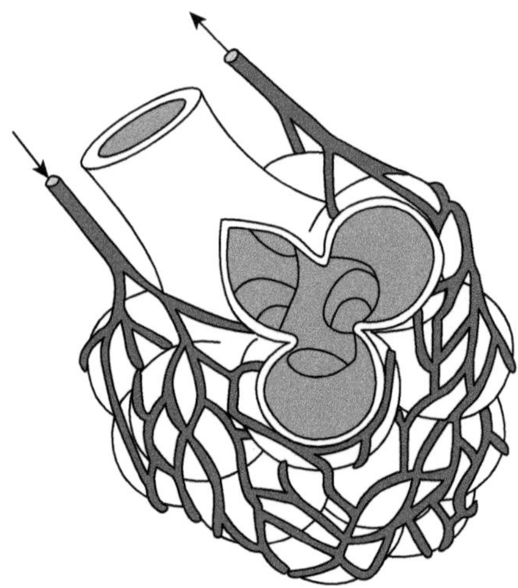

Figure 2.5 An alveolus and its blood supply.

Internal respiration

This exchange of gases in the tissues is referred to as internal respiration. Cells need oxygen and glucose to survive and are used in several key metabolic processes, for example Kreb's cycle and ATP production (energy) in the form of energy-rich phosphate bonds by converting adenosine diphosphate (ADP) to adenosine triphosphate (ATP) (see Figure 2.6). The waste products of cell metabolism are water and carbon dioxide (see Figure 2.7).

The transport of gases—oxygen

The transport of gases utilizing haemoglobin as the carrier is essential. The majority of oxygen (approx. 98%) is transported on the haemoglobin molecule, while a small amount is

Table 2.1 Respiratory gas laws

Name of law	Law states	Clinical application
Boyle's law	At a constant temperature, the volume of a gas varies inversely to the pressure acting on it.	On inspiration, the pressure in the lungs reduces as the volume increases.
Dalton's law	The total pressure of a mixture of gases is the sum of the partial pressures of the component gases. PTotal = Pgas1 + Pgas2 + Pgas3 …	The transfer of oxygen and carbon dioxide from the alveolar to the blood is dependent on the pressure gradient.
Henry's law	At a constant temperature the amount of gas that will dissolve in a liquid is proportional to the partial pressure of the gas in contact with the liquid.	The concentration of dissolved oxygen in blood is directly proportional to the partial pressure of oxygen and its solubility. Nitrogen is not very soluble and therefore there is very little dissolved in blood.

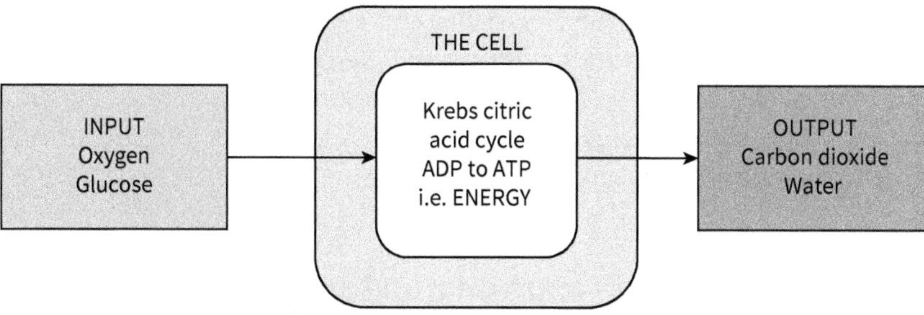

Figure 2.6 Cell metabolism.

dissolved in plasma (approx. 2%). The uptake of oxygen, either at the alveolar level or tissue level, is determined by several processes. This is represented by the oxyhaemoglobin dissociation curve which shows the affinity of oxygen for haemoglobin at both the alveolar and tissue level along the sigmoid shaped curve. The curve can shift either to the left or to the right depending on factors such as pH, temperature, increased $PaCO_2$, and exercise, amongst others. This change reduces or increases the affinity of oxygen to bind to haemoglobin.

Normally the main factor that affects oxygen affinity for haemoglobin is the concentration of oxygen at the alveoli level. If the concentration is high, oxygen will continue to bind with the haemoglobin until saturation occurs, and as the circulation reaches the anaerobic environment of the tissues, oxygen will be conserved until all the tissues have been reached when oxygen is readily made available and affinity is lost.

A number of chemical processes facilitate the release of oxygen at the tissue level before the oxygen dissociates from the haemoglobin molecule and enters into the cells. A number of factors, usually present when the cell is very active, will facilitate oxygen release earlier,

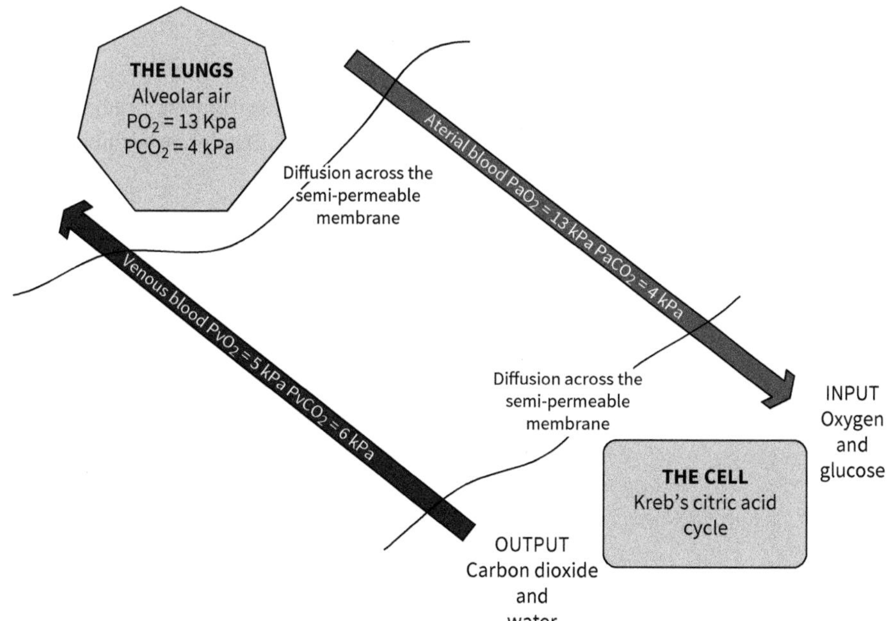

Figure 2.7 Partial pressures and gas exchange in external and internal respiration.

represented on the oxyhaemoglobin dissociation curve as a right shift. These factors include the presence of hydrogen ions, acidosis, pyrexia, and exercise; that is, a higher metabolic rate. These factors facilitate the release of oxygen from the haemoglobin molecule and ensure that cells that are actively metabolizing receive this increased demand for oxygen which will need to be matched by supply; that is supplementary oxygen.

The transport of gases—carbon dioxide

The transport of carbon dioxide, as a waste product of tissue metabolism, to the lungs is complex. Carbon dioxide is carried in three ways:

1 7% dissolved in plasma.
2 23% combines with haemoglobin.
3 70% is transported in plasma as bicarbonate ions.

Carbon dioxide can diffuse from the tissues into blood, where a small proportion is dissolved in the plasma. Carbon dioxide also diffuses into red blood cells where it combines with haemoglobin, forming carbaminohaemoglobin. However, most carbon dioxide is converted into bicarbonate and is transported in plasma.

Initially carbon dioxide binds with cellular water to form carbonic acid. This would potentially increase the acidity of the blood which is often detrimental to cellular function. Therefore it is important that carbon dioxide is 'buffered' to prevent abnormal changes in blood pH.

Carbon dioxide and water are rapidly converted to bicarbonate and hydrogen ions through the reaction with carbonic anhydrase, an enzyme in red blood cells. The equation for this is:

$$\mathbf{CO_2 + H_2O <--> HCO_3^- + H^+}$$
$$\text{carbon dioxide} + \text{water} \rightarrow \text{bicarbonate} + \text{hydrogen}$$

As this is a reversible reaction, bicarbonate can also diffuse from the plasma, where it is used to buffer the pH of blood, back to CO_2 in the red blood cells, and expired through the lungs.

Ventilation perfusion ratios

The two core components of respiratory function are ventilation and perfusion:

- ventilation (V) moving air/oxygen into the alveoli for gaseous exchange
- perfusion (Q) pulmonary circulation and deoxygenated capillary network surrounding the alveoli for the diffusion of oxygen into the blood.

An example of the ratio of ventilation to perfusion:

$$\frac{\text{alveolar ventilation (V)} = 4 \text{ litres per minute}}{\text{pulmonary perfusion (Q)} = 5 \text{ litres per minute}}, \text{V} : \text{Q ratio} = 0.8$$

This ratio varies due to the effects of gravity, with greater perfusion at the bases and greater ventilation at the apices. Changes in the V/Q ratio give rise to an increased physiological shunt or venous admixture, in which deoxygenated blood enters the arterial circulation and lowers the overall oxygen concentration of the blood. This might be because ventilation is reduced, giving a low ratio, or because perfusion is reduced, giving a high ratio, as illustrated in the following examples:

- If ventilation were reduced to 2 L but perfusion remained at 5 L, the V/Q ratio would be low at 0.4. A clinical example of a low V/Q ratio is atelectasis.
- If ventilation remained at 5 L but perfusion is reduced to 3 L, the V/Q ratio would be high at 1.7. A clinical example of a high V/Q ratio is pulmonary embolism.

The control of breathing

Breathing is controlled by the medulla and the pons in the brain. In the medulla, the dorsal respiratory group controls inspiration and the ventral respiratory group controls expiration by neural contraction of the muscles of respiration that change the rate, depth, and rhythm of breathing. There are several mechanisms that stimulate the brain:

- mechanical receptors
- the cerebral cortex
- central and peripheral chemoreceptors

Mechanical receptors are located in the upper airways, juxta-capillary (j receptors) in the alveoli, and stretch receptors in the lung tissue. These mechanisms ensure that the lungs are protected from over-inflation.

The *cerebral cortex* can act on the respiratory centre and increase the respiratory rate, rhythm, and depth. This is triggered by higher brain functions such as emotion/fear, etc.

Chemoreceptors in the medulla, aortic arch, and carotids are sensitive to changes in the pH, carbon dioxide, and oxygen levels in the blood and cerebral spinal fluid. As there is an increase in carbon dioxide in blood (causing a fall in pH) and/or the oxygen content of the blood falls, chemoreceptors stimulate the respiratory centres to contract the muscles of respiration, causing an increase in the rate and depth of breathing, giving rise to the sensation of breathlessness (Nair and Peate 2013). This is shown diagrammatically in Figure 2.8).

Respiratory assessment

The assessment of patients with acute respiratory failure requires the following:

- Evaluation of the presenting respiratory problem.
- Assessment and management of any life-threatening injuries or pathophysiology requiring an urgent medical review.
- A full health history including mental health, social, and drug history will be obtained once the patient is stabilized.

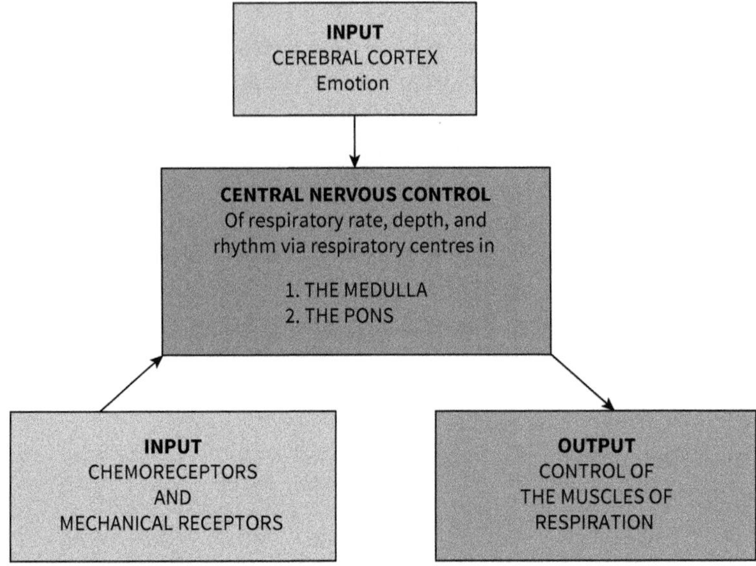

Figure 2.8 Central control of respiration.

- Assessment of respiratory rate, depth, rhythm, and use of accessory muscles.
- Inspection, palpation, percussion, and auscultation.
- Oxygen saturations and arterial blood gas to assess for hypoxia or hypercarbia.
- Physiological scoring—NEWS2 (RCP 2017).
- Severity of illness and chronic health scores (CURB—see in pneumonia revision).
- Mental health, safeguarding, and social assessments.

The respiratory presentation may range from slight breathlessness to acute breathlessness. Past medical history, particularly chronic respiratory disease, social factors, medication, and risk factors such as smoking or occupational history should be sought. Smoking is an important risk factor and may be calculated in pack years: the number of cigarettes smoked per day, multiplied by the number of years smoked, divided by 20. If the patient has smoked 10 cigarettes per day for 10 years, the number of pack years is 5. Employment history may also be significant, indicating risk of occupational respiratory disease (Gibson and Waters 2017). This is related to the inhalation of toxic chemicals or particles, which can cause fibrosis or lung cancer; for example, miners, bakers, carpenters, builders, and those who have worked in the printing or dyeing industries are susceptible. Other significant history includes anorexia and weight loss, which may indicate malignancy or chronic infection and sleep disturbance. The most common respiratory symptoms include:

- breathlessness
- fatigue
- peripheral and central cyanosis
- cough
- sputum production
- reduction in exercise tolerance

- abnormal or added (adventitious) respiratory sounds
- night sweats
- pain
- depression

Breathlessness—assessment of respiratory rate and pattern

Breathlessness can cause the patient to become frightened or anxious. An abnormal respiratory rate or tachypnoea is one of the most significant predictive indicators of both in-hospital serious illness and admission to critical care (Gibson and Waters 2017). It is an important component of the multiple parameter track-and-trigger systems such as the National Early Warning Score (NEWS2) used across the National Health Service (NHS) (RCP 2017). NEWS 2 is an adjunct to predict hospital mortality, discriminate patients at risk of cardiac arrest, unanticipated intensive care unit (ICU) admission, or death within 24 hours (Smith *et al.* 2013).

The respiratory rate should be counted for one full minute and the pattern and depth of respiration observed. Any irregular or asymmetrical patterns of respiration should be noted, for example see-saw (paradoxical movement), and these require an urgent medical review.

When the patient experiences breathlessness due to hypoxia, the work of breathing is increased by the use of accessory muscles, the sternocleidomastoid and scalene muscles. Additionally, other muscles can contribute such as the trapezius, pectoralis major, and abdominal muscles, as in exacerbations of COPD. In patients with splinting of the diaphragm, neuromuscular disorders, or restrictive lung disease there may be little or no chest movement. Hyperventilation may be caused by anxiety increasing pulmonary ventilation, being both deep and rapid, causing respiratory alkalosis in severe cases. The breathless patient may also have a high heart rate and be hypertensive as a result of the sympathetic stress response and adrenaline acting on the β_1-receptors in the heart.

Inspection of the patient's head, neck, thorax, and spine is necessary to identify any physical abnormalities that might restrict ventilation. Scars may indicate previous surgery and bruising of the thorax may suggest fractured ribs. Increased abdominal fat or pregnancy may also impact on respiratory function and should be noted.

Palpation is a technique used to assess the movement of the chest wall, diaphragmatic excursion and chest symmetry during inspiration. Tracheal deviation may indicate a mediastinal mass, pleural effusion, or pneumothorax. The trachea deviates toward the affected side in a collapsed lung and away from the affected side in a tension pneumothorax and large pleural effusion (Bickley *et al.* 2017).

Percussion can be used to determine areas of the lung that may contain fluid or that are collapsed or consolidated. The lung fields are normally tympanic (sound like a drum full of air) but when consolidated or collapsed become dull to percussion (Bickley *et al.* 2017).

Auscultation is a skill that requires practice and determines whether breath sounds are normal, abnormal, or added (adventitious). The normal breath sounds heard on auscultation, going from the apex to bases of the lungs, are bronchial, broncho-vesicular, and vesicular sounds. Bronchial breath sounds are hollow, harsh, tubular sounds that are low pitched and can be heard normally over the large airways in the upper central chest. Vesicular sounds are soft, low-pitched sounds during inspiration and expiration. These are normally heard

Table 2.2 Abnormal breath sounds

Crackles	signify fluid in the small airways and absent sounds may be a sign of lung collapse and/or consolidation of fluid or sputum.
Bronchial breathing	in the bases or more laterally is abnormal and associated with collapse and consolidation of lobes.
Wheeze	can sometimes be audible without a stethoscope and is a high-pitched whistling sound caused by reduced airflow through narrowed bronchial tubes.

over the small peripheral airways of the lateral chest. Bronchovesicular are a mixture of both between these areas. Abnormal sounds are described in Table 2.2.

Peripheral and central cyanosis

Central cyanosis of the oral mucosa, lips, tongue, or upper chest is a sign of severe deoxygenated haemoglobin and usually suggests hypoxia. Peripheral cyanosis may indicate poor peripheral perfusion rather than hypoxia. In black or dark-skinned patients, cyanosis may not appear in the skin and the oral mucosa should be examined. In severe anaemia, cyanosis may be absent because of the lack of haemoglobin in the presence of acute hypoxia (Gibson and Waters 2017).

Cough

If the patient is able to give a full history you should enquire about coughing to include precipitating or relieving factors and whether dry or productive.

Sputum production

Sputum can be described as normally clear with a normal consistency. The amount, frequency, colour, and consistency are also sought. Abnormal sputum is described in Table 2.3.

Table 2.3 Abnormal sputum production

Viscous	thick and tenacious
Green or yellow	infected
Pink or red	signs of bleeding in the mouth, sinuses, pharynx, trachea or lung tissue (haemoptysis)
Watery, pink, and frothy	pulmonary oedema

Exercise tolerance

Exercise tolerance in terms of metres that the patient can comfortably walk should be included in the history, along with any other limitations to activities of daily living.

Pain

Breathlessness is sometimes accompanied by chest pain which should be assessed using a pain scoring system. Cardiac pain should be ruled out as this is a 'red flag' for acute coronary syndrome (ACS). It should be established where the pain is, its nature, intensity, and duration; relieving and precipitating factors; on inspiration or expiration; and whether it is pleural or lung parenchymal from assessment.

Respiratory monitoring

Type I and Type II respiratory failure

Type 1 respiratory failure is lower than normal arterial oxygen concentration as measured by an arterial blood gas: the partial pressure of oxygen (PaO_2). This is defined as a normal pH and arterial carbon dioxide ($PaCO_2$), but low arterial oxygen (PaO_2). A normal response to hypoxaemia is an increased respiratory rate and expired carbon dioxide (CO_2). This compensation cannot be maintained indefinitely and, left untreated, will lead to alveolar hypoventilation as the patient tires, the $PaCO_2$ rises, and therefore the pH falls. Type II respiratory failure is a low pH, high $PaCO_2$, normal or low PaO_2 (respiratory acidosis).

The principles of arterial blood gas analysis

Arterial and venous blood gas measurement

The parameters on an arterial and venous blood gas (ABG/VBG), used to assess the levels of oxygen (O_2) and carbon dioxide (CO_2), do not correlate and therefore to determine the adequacy of ventilation and gas exchange accurately, the arterial (PaO_2 and $PaCO_2$) blood gas should be used, particularly in the critically ill patient (see Table 2.4). However, for acutely ill patients, venous blood gas CO_2 can be used as a guide (e.g. for CO_2 levels in COPD), although there should be caution with assessing CO_2 in shock as correlation deteriorates. Peripheral oxygen saturations and end tidal CO_2 monitoring can also be used to assess for hypoxia and hypo/hypercarbia.

The parameters used to assess metabolic disorders have small differences (correlate) and are comparable for acutely ill patients and these are the bicarbonate (HCO_3), base excess (BE), and blood pH which are used to determine alterations to acid–base balance.

An arterial sample is normally taken from the radial artery unless the patient is very poorly peripherally perfused, in which case one of the femoral arteries may be used. Arterial

Table 2.4 Comparisons between arterial and venous blood gas measurements

	Arterial (ABG)	Venous (VBG)	Correlate?
PO_2 (kpa)	10.6–13.3	4.0–5.3	no, use O_2 sats or ABG (if critically ill)
PCO_2 (kpa)	4.5–6.0	5.5–6.8	no, can use VBG as a guide in COPD, caution shock, use end tidal CO_2
pH	7.35–7.45	7.33–7.43	yes, use in acutely ill
Bicarbonate (mmol/L)	22–28	23–29	yes, use in acutely ill
Base excess (BE)	$^-2$–$^+2$	$^-2$–$^+2$	yes, use in acutely ill

sampling is painful and a local anaesthetic should normally be used (O'Driscoll *et al.* 2017). Venous samples are usually taken peripherally as a stab or via a central venous catheter (broader reflection of systemic pH and CO_2).

What is the pH?

The pH is a scale that measures the relative acidity or alkalinity of a substance, ranging from 0 (most acidic) to 14 (most alkaline). It is a measurement of hydrogen ion concentration and the higher the hydrogen ion concentration, the lower the pH. A normal blood pH is 7.35–7.45. The pH matters because a change in pH will alter the structure and function of protein. An altered hydrogen ion concentration will 'denature' or change a protein's structure. Enzymes are proteins and the body's cell chemistry depends on enzymes as biological catalysts. Enzymes cannot function physiologically outside this narrow pH range.

Acids, bases, and buffers

An acid is a substance that has the ability to donate a hydrogen ion. A base is a substance that has the ability to accept a hydrogen ion and remove it from the circulation. Acids and bases are carefully regulated but in acute illness may move out of the normal pH range. In health, irregularities are corrected by the lungs, kidneys, and buffer systems to maintain the pH within normal limits. The principal buffers are:

- plasma proteins, such as haemoglobin
- bicarbonate buffer system
- phosphate buffer system (H^+ combines with phosphate in renal tubules)

Plasma proteins enable hydrogen ions (from cell metabolism) to be transported to the lungs and kidneys, for example haemoglobin. At the lungs, the haemoglobin gives up the hydrogen as it takes on oxygen and carbon dioxide is excreted into the alveoli. The end products of cellular metabolism are water and carbon dioxide. When these combine in the plasma they form carbonic acid (H_2CO_3) which then splits one hydrogen ion (buffered by plasma proteins, e.g. haemoglobin) leaving bicarbonate circulating in the blood and allowing safe transport to the organs of excretion.

$$CO_2 + H_2O \rightarrow H_2CO_3 + HCO_3^- + H^+$$
$$\text{carbon dioxide} + \text{water} \rightarrow \text{carbonic acid} + \text{bicarbonate} + \text{hydrogen}$$

Acid–base disturbances

This may be from a respiratory or metabolic cause or both. The patient will present with either an acidosis or an alkalosis.

Respiratory acidosis

Respiratory acidosis is a high arterial carbon dioxide concentration ($pCO_2 > 6.0$) and a low pH ($pH < 7.35$). This occurs when there is an accumulation of carbon dioxide in the blood which then combines with water in the plasma to form carbonic acid. Respiratory acidosis commonly occurs as a result of decreased alveolar ventilation and prevention of carbon dioxide removal by the lungs. It may be caused by a number of respiratory disturbances, such as atelectasis, lung infection, neuromuscular dysfunction, or COPD. It may also be seen post-operatively in patients whose breathing is shallow due to pain, analgesic, or anaesthetic drugs.

Respiratory alkalosis

Respiratory alkalosis is a low arterial carbon dioxide concentration ($pCO_2 < 4.5$) and a high pH ($pH > 7.45$). If the respiratory rate or depth increase, excessive amounts of carbon dioxide will be removed, making the blood alkaline. Respiratory alkalosis is commonly seen in states that may cause the patient to hyperventilate such as pain or fear.

Metabolic acidosis

Metabolic acidosis is a low arterial bicarbonate level ($HCO_3 < 22$) and a low pH ($pH < 7.35$). Metabolic acidosis occurs if there is an excessive build-up of acid-based waste products from metabolism in the blood or failure of the kidney to excrete or regulate acid and bases. Examples of these are lactic acid (lactate) and ketones in acute illness. Lactate is produced by anaerobic metabolism caused by poor perfusion to tissues and cells where a lack of blood flow means that demand for oxygen exceeds supply, for example sepsis and shock. Bicarbonate will be used up to buffer the acids which is why the bicarbonate is low. The lungs are unable to excrete ketones and lactate as these are not gases and require excretion via the kidneys.

Ketones are produced as an end product of fat metabolism in place of glucose and, for example, uncontrolled diabetes mellitus. In this example, lack of insulin prevents the normal metabolism of glucose by cells and fat is broken down to provide energy.

Patients with acute kidney injury (AKI) may be unable to produce sufficient amounts of bicarbonate, buffer acids, or excrete hydrogen ions, causing the pH to fall.

Metabolic alkalosis

Metabolic alkalosis is a high arterial bicarbonate (HCO_3 > 28) and a high pH (pH > 7.45). This is usually due to a large amount of hydrogen loss from the body (e.g. vomiting, nasogastric aspiration, or the excessive use of diuretics) or excess amounts of base substances with the circulation (e.g. ingestion of large amounts of antacids).

Compensation

Respiratory compensation is through increased ventilation to remove arterial carbon dioxide. Metabolic compensation occurs in the plasma (buffer systems) or in the kidneys by the regulation and excretion of hydrogen ions. An increase in respiratory rate and/or depth will compensate for a metabolic cause and only partially compensate for a respiratory cause due to the respiratory nature of the cause.

Assessing a patient's arterial blood gas

ABG analysis takes time to learn and become familiar with normal variants (see Table 2.5). ABGs should be interpreted in the context of the individual patient and their presenting symptoms. It is useful to use a systematic tool to assess blood gases to ensure each element of the gas is given consideration.

A systematic method

There are many tools available to assist ABG interpretation. Typically, they use a stepwise process that may include:

1. Assess oxygenation—need for additional oxygen?
2. Determine pH—acidosis or alkalosis?
3. Assess carbon dioxide—PCO_2
4. Assess bicarbonate—HCO_3

Table 2.5 Arterial blood gas values

Value	Function	Normal values
pH	a measure of hydrogen ion concentration	7.35–7.45
PaO_2	partial pressure of oxygen dissolved in plasma	10.6–13.3 kPa
$PaCO_2$	partial pressure of carbon dioxide dissolved in plasma	4.5–6.0 kPa
HCO_3	amount of bicarbonate in plasma	22–26 mmol/L
BE	the base excess, preceded by a $^+$ (indicating alkalosis) or a$^-$ (indicating acidosis)	−2 to +2
SaO_2	the amount of oxygen bound to the haemoglobin molecule	>95%

5. Assess whether a respiratory or metabolic cause—direction of two values (either pH and PCO_2 or pH and HCO_3)
6. Assess for compensation—HCO_3 or PaCO2

1. Assess oxygenation

The PaO_2 should be examined for signs of hypoxia. This value should be considered alongside the inspired oxygen concentration. If the PaO_2 is low, supplemental oxygen may be required but titrated to the patient's oxygen saturations. High oxygen levels usually require a reduction in oxygen administration as it is preferable to keep inspired oxygen concentrations as low as possible to minimize any adverse consequences of oxygen (O'Driscoll *et al.* 2017).

2. Assess pH

The pH should be checked to see if it is in the normal range or whether there is an acidosis (< than 7.35) or an alkalosis (> 7.45). A normal pH may also indicate problems that have been corrected by compensation, so it is essential to examine the rest of the arterial blood gas result as either the HCO_3 or the $PaCO_2$ will be deranged if compensation has occurred.

3. Assess carbon dioxide ($PaCO_2$)

The $PaCO_2$ should be checked to see if it is high, low, or within normal range. A high $PaCO_2$ indicates a respiratory problem and is usually accompanied by an acidic pH unless renal compensation has occurred. A low $PaCO_2$ indicates either a respiratory alkalosis (high pH) or partial or full compensation for a metabolic acidosis (low or normal pH).

4. Assess bicarbonate (HCO_3)

The bicarbonate level should be assessed to see if it is high, low, or normal. If a metabolic acidosis is present, the bicarbonate level will be low. If a metabolic alkalosis is present, the bicarbonate will be high. The bicarbonate may also be high if there is chronic compensation for a respiratory problem; in this example the high bicarbonate will be accompanied by a high $PaCO_2$ level.

5. Assess whether a respiratory or metabolic cause

To determine whether the ABG has a respiratory or metabolic component you can apply the following rules: in a respiratory cause the pH and $PaCO_2$ will usually move in the opposite direction and in a metabolic cause the pH and HCO_3 will usually move in the same direction. Acutely ill patients may present with a mixed (respiratory/metabolic) acidosis or alkalosis. For example, a patient with severe sepsis who is tiring may present with a low bicarbonate level because of the sepsis (compensation for a metabolic acidosis) and a high $PaCO_2$ because they are becoming increasing tired (respiratory acidosis). These patients require urgent medical intervention.

6. Assess for compensation

A patient's ABG results may be:

- uncompensated—abnormal pH, a low or high $PaCO_2$ or HCO_3 (and the other will be normal). Go to Step 5 for respiratory or metabolic cause.

- partially compensated—abnormal pH, a low or high $PaCO_2$ and HCO_3 (move in same direction). Go to Step 5 for respiratory or metabolic cause.
- fully compensated—normal pH, a low or high $PaCO_2$ or HCO_3 (move in same direction). *Go to Step 5 for respiratory or metabolic cause. A low or high pH is determined by whether the value is < 7.40 (low) or > 7.40 (high).*

Practice analysing ABGs alongside an expert practitioner, and further reading is recommended. Some clinical examples are included below in the Clinical links 2.1a and 2.1b. The answers to these scenarios are given in the Appendix.

Clinical link 2.1a (see Appendix for answers)

Patient A is a 56-year-old lady admitted to your ward post-operatively. She has been given some intravenous morphine and she is quite sleepy. Analyse the blood gas results and discuss further management.

- pH: 7.30
- PaO_2: 10 kPa
- $PaCO_2$: 6.5 kPa
- HCO_3: 24
- BE: −3
- SaO_2: 94%

Clinical link 2.1b (see Appendix for answers)

Patient C is a 65-year-old admitted to a medical ward with an acute exacerbation of COPD. She is complaining of severe breathlessness and is expectorating green sputum. Analyse her blood gas result and discuss further management:

- pH: 7.32
- PaO_2: 8 kPa
- $PaCO_2$: 8.5 kPa
- HCO_3: 31
- BE: −4
- SaO_2: 88%

Peak expiratory flow rate

Peak expiratory flow rate (PEFR) is the maximum flow rate achieved in rapid forced expiration following maximum inspiration. It depends on patient effort and technique but is widely used in acute care as a measure of the effectiveness of inhaled bronchodilators by pre and post testing. The PEFR varies with gender and age and it is generally the trend that is significant.

Measures of lung volume using spirometry are used clinically to assess respiratory function and find causes of common respiratory pathologies. In acute care the vital capacity (i.e. the maximum volume that can be inhaled and exhaled) and the tidal volume (i.e. the volume breathed in and out in one normal breath) are the most useful. The forced expiratory volume 1 (FEV1), that is the forced expiratory volume in 1 second, should be about 80% of the forced vital capacity (FVC), and the ratio of the FEV1 to the vital capacity is used as an indicator of severity in obstructive lung disease. The ratio normally declines with age and so actual and predicted measures are used in assessment.

Pulse oximetry

Pulse oximetry is a simple non-invasive method of monitoring the percentage of haemoglobin (Hb) that is saturated with oxygen. The pulse oximeter consists of a probe attached to the patient's finger or earlobe (which is preferable in acute illness), and findings should be recorded on the patient's chart along with the level of inspired oxygen.

It is important to remember that there are situations when the pulse oximeter will be inaccurate, for example poor peripheral perfusion (as in shock or hypovolaemia), cold peripheries, nail varnish, different forms of haemoglobin (as in carboxyhaemoglobin when there is a high level of carbon monoxide in the blood), or vasoconstriction. In the acutely ill patient, a central measurement of capillary refill time is preferred.

Fatigue

Respiratory fatigue is caused by an increased respiratory effort over time with the prolonged use of accessory muscles. Shallow, rapid breathing may indicate fatigue, and/or the transition from type I to type II respiratory failure showing a deterioration in the patient's condition.

Respiratory management

Oxygen therapy

The administration of oxygen to the hypoxaemic patient, whether type 1 or type II, leads to an increase in PaO_2, preventing cell death and respiratory failure. Hypoxia can cause breathlessness but not all breathless patients are hypoxic and oxygen is not always needed and could have negative physiologic effects, for example in COPD, acute coronary syndrome (Stub *et al.* 2012).

The British Thoracic Society guidelines (O'Driscoll *et al.* 2017) suggest initial oxygen therapy is delivered at low flow rates via nasal cannulae at 2–6 L/min or a simple face mask at 5–10 L/min to a target saturation level (ensure flow rates are set to at least 5 L/min as there is a risk of rebreathing carbon dioxide when set below the manufacturer's recommended minimum flow rate). Higher flow rates are delivered via fixed percentage systems (e.g. 24%) or a reservoir mask at 10–15 L/min.

Oxygen should be prescribed to achieve a target saturation of 94–98% for most acutely ill patients or 88–92% in COPD (or patient-specific target range for those at risk of hypercapnic respiratory failure). If the target range cannot be achieved with nasal cannulae or simple face mask, change to a reservoir mask or fixed percentage system and ensure medical review. Humidification may not be required for low-flow or short-term oxygen administration (< 24 h) but may be useful in loosening viscous sputum. High-flow humidified nasal oxygen should be considered in patients with acute respiratory failure without hypercapnia. The flow rate of oxygen and inspired oxygen percentage, along with oxygen saturations should be recorded.

Physiotherapy

Physiotherapy can enhance the overall treatment and play a part in the prevention of deterioration of the breathless patient. Physiotherapy treatment aims to optimize tidal volume and clearance of secretions, thus improving gas exchange. Positioning the patient in an upright position, and regular repositioning enables the mobilization of secretions, encourages cough, and reduces atelectasis (O'Driscoll *et al.* 2017). Full discussion of physiotherapy intervention is beyond the scope of this chapter but treatment may include:

- effective positioning and repositioning in bed or a chair to prevent atelectasis
- mobilizing the patient
- deep breathing and coughing exercises to clear secretions and prevent atelectasis
- suctioning of artificial airway if appropriate to clear secretions

Oral hygiene

A high respiratory rate, pyrexia, and mouth breathing will increase the risk of dehydration and careful monitoring of fluid balance is essential. Oral hygiene is important and patients may need frequent help with mouth care when weak and dehydrated.

Drug therapy

The main treatment for obstructive lung disease is the inhaled bronchodilator medication. Bronchodilators are commonly used in conjunction with steroids (systemic or inhaled). Lower doses can be administered directly into the lungs as opposed to oral or intravenous administration giving unwanted systemic effects.

β_2-adrenergic agonists

β_2-adrenergic agonists are the most widely used bronchodilators (e.g. salbutamol). Their action is sympathomimetic (i.e. they act like adrenaline, stimulating the sympathetic nervous system) and cause relaxation of the smooth muscle in the airways which improves symptoms. They are delivered by hand-held, metred-dose inhalers, or by nebulization. They may be short acting (SABAs) or long acting (LABAs) and the long-acting drugs are used in primary care in the maintenance of symptom control (Gibson and Waters 2017). Technique is crucial, particularly in the very young and elderly patients who may need a spacer device, which requires less coordination, and is seen as best practice. In the acutely ill, nebulizers use high pressure gas (air or oxygen) to vaporize liquid into a fine spray, which is inhaled into small bronchioles. They have an effect within a few minutes and the duration of action is 4–6 h. Oxygen or air is used to drive nebulizers in asthmatic patients and air is used in patients with COPD who retain carbon dioxide.

Anti-muscarinic bronchodilators

Anti-muscarinic bronchodilators such as ipratropium have an effect on the neuromuscular junction. They work by inhibiting the acetylcholine-mediated transmission of the nervous impulse across the neuromuscular junction. As they block the muscarinic receptors in the respiratory tract, smooth muscle in the airways is relaxed, relieving bronchoconstriction. Long-acting muscarinic antagonists (LAMAs) such as tiotropium or glycopyrronium last at least 24 hours. Dual bronchodilator (LAMA/LABA) combinations are available (BTS/SIGN 2016).

Inhaled corticosteroids (ICS)

In patients with asthma or COPD, inhaled corticosteroids (ICS) will help to reduce exacerbations and hospital admissions. ICS/LABA combinations are used to give maximum benefit (BTS/SIGN 2016).

Leukotriene receptor antagonists (LTRA)

Cysteinyl leukotrienes are released from mast cells and basophils as a mediator of an allergic response to an allergen, stimulating smooth muscle which in turn causes bronchoconstriction. Leukotriene receptor antagonists (LTRA) block this action, causing bronchodilation (Rang *et al.* 2003) and are recommended by the NICE (2017) asthma guidelines to add after low-dose inhaled corticosteroids (ICS) have not completely resolved symptoms. This is contrary to BTS/SIGN (2016) who advocate LABA after low-dose ICS.

Theophylline

Theophylline has an anti-inflammatory effect similar to corticosteroids and inhibits the enzyme phosphodiesterase in the smooth muscle wall of the airways, resulting in relaxation and the relief of bronchospasm.

Non-invasive ventilation

Non-invasive ventilation (NIV) is now commonly used to provide support to patients who are experiencing type I or type II respiratory failure. There are two methods of delivery: Continuous Positive Airway Pressure (CPAP) which is usually the mode preferred to treat type 1 respiratory failure such as pneumonia, and Bi-phasic Positive airway Pressure (BiPaP) which is synonymous with NIV and used to treat type II respiratory failure, as in COPD.

There are only two ways to increase the PaO_2 in patients with type I respiratory impairment:

1. Increase the inspired oxygen
2. Increase the expiratory positive airway pressure (EPAP) with continuous positive airways pressure (CPAP) in spontaneously ventilated patients or positive end expiratory pressure (PEEP) in ventilated patients.

CPAP entrains a mixture of air and oxygen, which can be titrated to a percentage while 'forcing oxygen onto the haemoglobin by increasing the pressure gradient across the alveolar/capillary interface of the alveolar units'. CPAP is maintained by a 'closed circuit' that requires a tightly fitting mask ('0 cm H_2O leak') that is held in place with head straps or nasal masks can be used if there is minimal rather than excessive mouth breathing. End expiratory pressure holds open the alveolar membranes on full end expiration increasing the gas exchange time, reducing respiratory effort (work of breathing) on the next inspiratory breath. Alveolar collapse is prevented by the end expiratory pressure and collapsed alveoli are recruited, leading to an increase in alveolar ventilation and gaseous exchange. The increase in pressure can also be used as a treatment for pulmonary oedema by forcing fluid away from the alveolar/capillary interface (interstitial space) and thus encouraging gas exchange (see Figure 2.9).

There are only two ways to decrease the $PaCO_2$ in patients with type II respiratory impairment:

1. Increase the tidal volume so that more carbon dioxide is exhaled.
2. Increase the rate in patients who are ventilated, but this is obviously not an option in spontaneously ventilating patients in whom a rapid respiratory rate is already initiated as a normal physiological response.

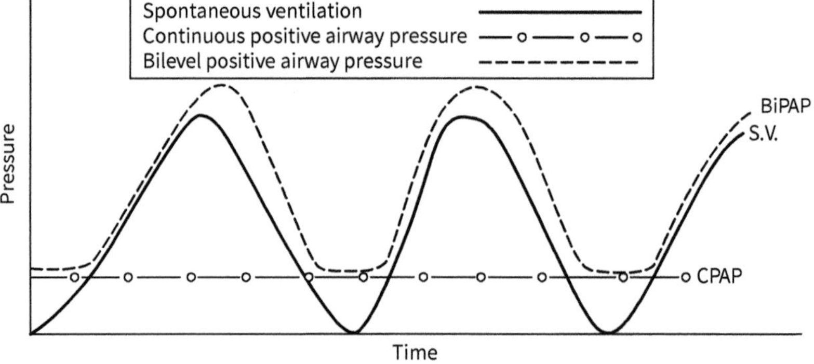

Figure 2.9 Differences between CPAP and normal ventilation.

The inspiratory positive airway pressure (IPAP) is set on the machine in order to increase the tidal volume and is delivered with oxygen via a face mask. The increased inspiratory pressure will increase the tidal volume or breath size (to a set pressure on the machine, e.g. IPAP 15 cm H_2O). EPAP is less important without hypoxia, hence a leak is not detrimental (normally between 10–30 litres per minute) and facilitates patient synchrony and comfort. EPAP is usually set at around 4 cm H_2O, which will increase oxygenation but because of the leak is not as effective as CPAP. Therefore, its use is not to increase PaO_2, although it will have an effect, but to ensure the alveolar do not completely collapse, which in turn reduces the work of breathing.

Although each machine varies, they are sensitive to slight changes in flow and pressure, which means that a very slight inspiratory effort by the patient is used to trigger the machine. The flow is increased to produce a breath at the preset inspiratory pressure. The machine can usually be set to deliver the preset pressure very rapidly or in a slower, gentler *rise* (0.1–0.6 s). In patients with high airway resistance such as asthma or COPD the rapid pressure rise may be less effective than a slower rise because the resistance will mean that the preset pressure is achieved too quickly to increase the tidal volume.

It is the responsibility of nurses who care for patients using NIV to ensure that they are familiar with the machines and adhere to local policies. Guidelines for the Ventilatory Management of Acute Hypercapnic Respiratory Failure (AHRF) in Adults have been produced by the British Thoracic Society (BTS) and Intensive Care Society (ICS) (Davidson *et al.* 2016).

Indications for NIV in AHRF

According to the BTS and ICS (Davidson *et al.* 2016) guidelines, the indication for NIV in AHRF varies according to the underlying cause, severity of illness, and associated complicating factors. Indications for NIV include the diagnoses of COPD, pH < 7.35, $pCO_2 > 6.5$, respiratory rate > 23, if persistent after bronchodilators and oxygen therapy. Broad criteria can be applied for both absolute and relative contra-indications. Absolute contra-indications include severe facial deformity, facial burns, and fixed upper airway obstruction. Relative contra-indications include: pH < 7.15, pH < 7.24 plus additional adverse features, Glasgow Coma Scale (GCS) < 8, confusion/agitation, and cognitive impairment when intubation and ventilation may be more appropriate. Criteria for neuromuscular disease and chest wall disease are also covered in the guidelines.

It is important that the medical team responsible for the patient make an anticipatory treatment plan around the time of a new diagnosis or when increasing frailty is recognized. Exploring the potential path of a condition to enable an awareness of benchmarks of deterioration can pre-empt decisions in an emergency. If admission to intensive care is indicated, anaesthetic review will be necessary because anaesthetists are responsible for the admission and discharge of intensive care patients and they will coordinate the transfer of patients.

The BTS and ICS (Davidson *et al.* 2016) guidelines recommend the following:

- A variety of masks should be available, including nasal masks for patient comfort.
- In the spontaneous/timed (S/T) mode (also known as assist control), a backup rate is set by the operator, usually between 16 and 20. If the patient's respiratory rate (RR) is slower than the backup rate, machine-determined breaths will be delivered (i.e. controlled ventilation) and will show as 'timed' breaths.

- Set inspiratory time (0.8–1.2 s) and inspiratory:expiratory (I:E) ratio (1:2–1:3) in COPD, 1:1 in neuromuscular disease and chest wall disease; see guidelines.
- An initial IPAP of 15 cm H_2O (20 cm H_2O if pH < 7.25) and EPAP of 3 cm H_2O (or higher if known obstructive sleep apnoea and patient uses higher pressures at home) but no more than 8 cm H_2O.
- IPAP should be increased over 10–30 mins to a pressure target of 20–30 cm H_2O (but no more than 30 cm H_2O) to achieve adequate augmentation of chest/abdomen movement and slow respiratory rate or until patient tolerability has been reached.
- Oxygen, when required, should be entrained into the circuit and the flow adjusted to achieve the target saturation, usually 88–92% in COPD.
- Bronchodilators, although preferably administered off NIV, should as necessary be entrained between the expiration port and face mask.

Nursing considerations

NIV can be difficult to tolerate due to high pressures and the constant and sometimes asynchronous nature of the flow of gases. Poor-fitting masks can result in leaks that cause rapid drying of the eyes and is uncomfortable. The breathless patient will feel like they are suffocating and require skillful reassurance and patience to initiate NIV. This includes low initial pressures, short trials of the mask without the airflow from the machine, and feeling the flow of gas against the skin of the arm can also help the patient to prepare for a brief initial trial. It is extremely important that the patient retains control throughout this therapy. Regular monitoring of its effectiveness is required, including respiratory assessment, ABGs, and pulse oximetry recording. The following nursing considerations should also be addressed:

- Monitoring and recording vital signs, including pulse oximetry and respiratory rate over a minute is essential.
- Oral intake should be encouraged during rest periods including meals.
- Nurses must keep the medical team informed of progress and ensure that arterial blood gas analysis is carried out in accordance with local guidelines to monitor the effectiveness of NIV.
- Nurses should ensure that they receive appropriate education and training to maintain their knowledge and skills in the use of NIV including how to troubleshoot and signs of NIV failure.
- Local protocols for the clinical management of NIV should be followed to ensure patient safety and optimal care.
- Above all, nurses should support and encourage the patient to relieve their anxiety and in doing so, promote patient cooperation and the consequent effectiveness of NIV.

Management of patients with chest drains

Chest drains are tubes inserted into the pleural space to drain air, blood, or pus (empyema) and facilitate re-expansion of the lung. Indications for a chest drain are:

- primary pneumothorax (air) or haemothorax (blood)
- large secondary spontaneous pneumothorax in patients aged > 50 years

- malignant pleural effusion
- empyema (infection and pus)
- traumatic haemo-pneumothorax
- post-operatively following thoracotomy

In a primary spontaneous pneumothorax small-bore (< 14F) chest drain insertion is recommended. It is probable that small-bore 'Seldinger' (catheter over guide wire) chest drains are used more widely than large-bore due their ease of use (MacDuff *et al.* 2010).

A wide bore tube may be preferred when draining an empyema or haemothorax as blockage is a common complication of small-bore drains. Regular flushing of the drains with either saline or a fibrinolytic drug is often helpful.

Pleural aspirations and chest drains should be inserted in a clean area using full aseptic technique normally by a trained medical doctor (Havelock *et al.* 2010). To reduce pain associated with chest drains, analgesia and local anaesthesia should be considered as premedication and should be prescribed for all patients with a chest drain in place.

There are many drainage systems available that have a one-way valve mechanism. The most common is the underwater seal bottle (although flutter bags and 'Heimlich valves' have been successfully used). The end of the drain is placed below the surface of water in a bottle to create an underwater seal and so ensure that there is a one-way flow of air or fluid out, while preventing air from flowing back into the pleural space (see Figure 2.10). The end of the drain should be immersed by no more than 3 cm to minimize resistance to drainage as per local chest drain policy.

The drain may be positioned apically to drain air or basally to drain fluid. The drain is secured by two sutures, one to close the incision and one to secure the drain. A chest X-ray is performed after insertion to confirm position of the drain. A transparent dressing allows the wound site to be inspected by nursing staff for leakage or infection.

Bubbling in the bottle will occur while air is draining from a pneumothorax in the pleural space and the drain will stay in place until the bubbling has ceased. It is very important that the bottle should remain below the level of the patient's chest and remain upright at all times to prevent backflow into the pleural space or breaking the seal. Either would cause collapse of the lung and rapid desaturation. The water in the tubing should swing with respiration and

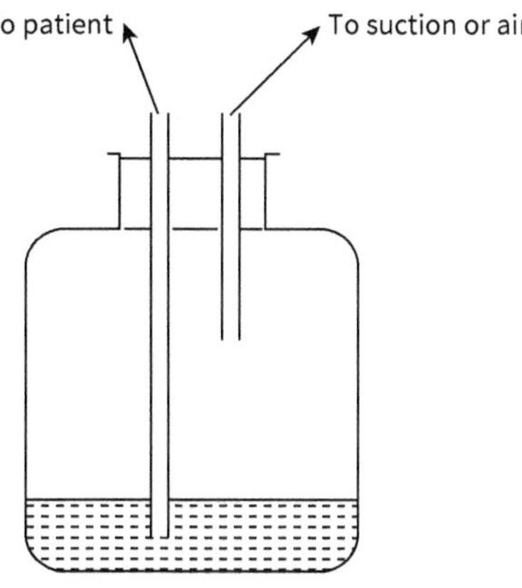

Figure 2.10 Underwater seal chest drain.

bubbling and drainage should be recorded. A chest drain should never be clamped especially if it is bubbling. No more than 1.5 litres of fluid is removed in the first hour after insertion. Large-bore chest drains may be clamped when the bottle is being changed, when two clamps should be used, one above and one below the junction between the drain in the patient and the tubing leading to the bottle or as per local chest drain policy. Low-pressure suction is not recommended but if required may be used at 10–20 cm H_2O and this requires a special low suction unit, normal wall suction cannot be used (MacDuff *et al.* 2010). Complications of chest drains include:

- infection
- surgical emphysema at the insertion site
- damage to internal structures
- accidental breaking of the underwater seal by knocking the bottle over

Removal is with a brisk, firm, pulling movement while an assistant ties the previously placed suture. Clamping of the drain prior to removal is generally unnecessary. If using suction pressure, a period of water-seal only drainage prior to removal may reduce the possibility of recurrence of the pneumothorax.

Patients should be managed in specialist wards where nursing staff have appropriate training and care should follow the local Trust procedures or policy.

Overview of three common respiratory disorders

The causes of breathlessness

The causes of breathlessness are numerous and include the following:

- primary lung conditions
- neurological causes
- musculoskeletal conditions
- cardiovascular conditions
- metabolic causes

Lung disorders are in two categories. *Obstructive lung diseases* are those in which there is increased resistance caused by an obstruction with the bronchus or bronchioles to inspired airflow such as mucus in bronchitis or bronchospasm in asthma. *Restrictive lung diseases* are diseases of the alveolar sacs or outer functions of the lung itself in which lung volume is reduced without reduction of flow in the airways, often characterized by a reduced vital capacity and impaired gas exchange.

Asthma

Asthma is diagnosed on the basis of clinical assessment and history, as there is no single diagnostic test. Spirometry and PEFR seek to demonstrate airflow obstruction and are useful.

Asthma is triggered by a stimulus that causes airway inflammation, bronchospasm and a variable narrowing of the airways. Symptoms of asthma include a wheeze, cough, breathlessness, and chest tightness that vary over time (BTS/SIGN 2016).

The aetiology is complex and research continues to develop knowledge in this area. There is evidence that environmental, genetic factors, and a history of atopic conditions such as eczema and rhinitis increases the probability of childhood asthma. House dust mite and cat allergen exposures in early life may increase the risk of immunoglobulin E (IgE) sensitization and asthma (BTS 2016).

Mature-onset asthma may be triggered by pollution, exercise, viral infections, or some drugs, such as aspirin and βeta-blockers. Hyper-responsiveness and airway inflammation are the dominant features and these are initiated by the release of mediators such as leukotrienes, histamine, cytokines, prostaglandin, and platelet-activating factor. Eosinophils, mast cells, neutrophils, and macrophages have all been implicated in the complex pathology of asthma. Patients may be asymptomatic between attacks because the airway obstruction/bronchoconstriction is reversible and variable in presentation producing false negative diagnosis and spirometry testing (BTS/SIGN 2016). Re-modelling of the airways occurs with hypertrophy of smooth muscle and mucous glands, resulting in abnormally thick mucus and fixed narrowing (see Figure 2.11).

The BTS and SIGN (2016) provide a comprehensive national guideline on all aspects of asthma care, both in the community and acute hospitals. NICE (2017) has produced slightly different guidelines on diagnosis, monitoring, and chronic asthma management. The differences are in the diagnosis and management of asthma including inhaler use and drugs to prevent exacerbations.

Assessment is based on the clinical presentation, history, FEV1 and PEFR ($<$ 70% indicates airway limitation), pulse oximetry and saturations, ABG analysis, and response to β_2-agonist bronchodilators. ICS should be considered for patients with any of the following asthma-related features:

- asthma attack in the last two years
- using inhaled β2-agonist bronchodilators three times a week or more
- symptomatic three times a week or more
- waking one night a week

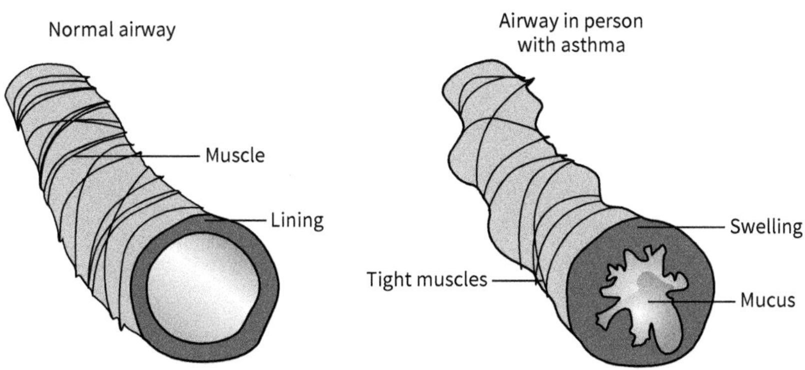

Figure 2.11 Airway changes in asthma.

Acute severe asthma has been associated with a high mortality rate, particularly before admission to hospital. The report of the UK-wide National Review of Asthma Deaths (NRAD) in 2014 reaffirmed the multifactorial nature of the disease and associated factors leading to death, including the medical management and the patient's behaviour or psychosocial status. The NRAD report highlighted an increased risk of death within one month of discharge from hospital following an acute attack and therefore follow-up in primary care is essential (RCP 2014).

There are many risk factors associated with death including inadequate treatment with ICS or steroid tablets and/or inadequate objective monitoring of their asthma; heavy or increasing use of inhaled β_2-agonist therapy; inappropriate prescription of β-blockers and non-steroidal anti-inflammatory drugs (NSAIDs), and adverse psychosocial and behavioural factors.

Acute severe asthma is characterized by the following:

- PEFR 33–50% best or predicted
- respiratory rate ≥ 25/min
- heart rate ≥ 110/min
- inability to complete sentences in one breath

Life-threatening asthma is also characterized by the following:

- altered conscious level
- exhaustion/poor respiratory effort
- arrhythmias or hypotension
- PEFR < 33% best or predicted
- $SpO_2 < 92\%$

Near-fatal asthma is also characterized by the following:

- silent chest
- raised $PaCO_2$

Patients with an acute asthma attack should not be sedated unless this is to allow for anaesthetic or intensive care procedures.

The BTS/SIGN (2016) recommendations for the management of acute asthma include:

- Give controlled supplementary oxygen to all hypoxaemic patients with acute severe asthma, titrated to maintain an SpO_2 level of 94–98%.
- Use high-dose inhaled β2-agonists as first-line agents in patients with acute asthma and administer as early as possible. Reserve intravenous β_2-agonists for those patients in whom inhaled therapy cannot be used reliably.
- Nebulized β_2-agonist bronchodilators should be driven by oxygen and consider continuous nebulization for the poorly responsive patient.
- Give steroids in adequate doses in all cases of acute asthma.

- Add nebulized ipratropium bromide (0.5 mg, 4–6 hourly) to β_2-agonist treatment for patients with acute, severe, or life-threatening asthma or those with a poor initial response to β_2-agonist therapy.
- Intravenous magnesium sulphate (1.2–2 g IV infusion over 20 minutes) may also be prescribed if the patient fails to respond to normal therapy or is having a life-threatening exacerbation of their asthma.
- Use IV aminophylline only after consultation with senior medical staff.
- Evidence to support the use of NIV in adults is limited and inconclusive.

Clinical link 2.2 (see Appendix for answers)

This is a 45-year-old female admitted from the accident and emergency (A&E) department into the medical assessment unit with breathlessness. She wants you to phone her husband at work because she is very anxious about not being able to pick up the children from school. She came to hospital following an asthma attack while doing some cleaning at home. Nebulized β_2-agonist was given in A&E with nebulized ipatropium.

She is distressed and frightened and peripherally cyanosed. There is an audible respiratory wheeze and she is using the accessory muscles of respiration. She is on oxygen at 35%. She is unable to give a history but her medical notes state that she is a known asthmatic with an allergy to dust and house mites. She is prescribed salbutomol and ipatroprium via nebulizers, which are in progress, but she keeps removing the mask and asking you to get her the phone. There is no evidence of thoracic abnormality or finger clubbing, and her vital signs are as follows:

- respiratory rate: 36
- temperature: 37.0°C
- peripheral pulse: 110
- blood pressure: 145/90
- SpO_2: 85%

Her chest X-ray is clear and her arterial blood gas analysis taken in A&E 1 h ago shows:

- pH: 7.35
- PaO_2: 9.8 kPa
- $PaCO_2$: 3.5 kPa
- SBC: 26 mmol/L
- BE: $^{+}2$ mmol/L

Consider the following questions:

- What type of respiratory failure does this patient have and what is the most likely cause?
- What are your main priorities and why?
- What clinical actions should you take and why?

Chronic obstructive pulmonary disease (COPD) revision

COPD is a generic term describing the effects of two main conditions with which it is associated: emphysema and chronic bronchitis. It means that the patient is suffering from chronic and poorly reversible airway obstruction. Patients experience increasing breathlessness, poor exercise tolerance, chronic cough with sputum production, over-inflated lungs, and impaired gas exchange (NICE 2010). Pursed-lip breathing may be present in which the patient closes the lips on expiration to increase the pressure in the airways and by splinting, prevent their collapse. The principal cause of COPD is smoking, which accounts for 95% of cases in the United Kingdom. COPD is a slowly progressive disease, characterized by airway obstruction and increasing breathlessness, initially on exertion and then at rest. Acute intermittent exacerbations that may be infective occur. Structural changes arising from emphysema result in reduced compliance and collapse of the small airways on expiration, which causes air trapping and hyperinflation. The PEFR, FEV1, and FEV1/FVC ratio are reduced, hence the diagnosis of COPD is made by the assessment of symptoms and post-bronchodilator spirometry (NICE 2010).

The FEV1 as a percentage of the predicted value is used to classify the severity of the disease as mild, moderate, severe, or very severe (see Table 2.6).

In chronic bronchitis there is an increased number of goblet cells in the larger airways, resulting in increased sputum production and a productive cough for most days over three months in more than two successive years. There is also a loss of elastic tissue in the smaller airways, with diffuse airway narrowing and fibrosis. In emphysema there is destruction of the alveolar wall and dilation of the airspaces in the lungs, with loss of alveolar capillary surface area. Elastic recoil is reduced and the airways are more prone to collapse and increase the work of inspiration. Emphysema may also be associated with an inherited deficiency of α_1-antitrypsin.

Persistently high carbon dioxide levels lead to a reduced responsiveness and hypoxia becomes the dominant respiratory drive so that the administration of oxygen can worsen respiratory failure and increase the level of carbon dioxide (O'Driscoll *et al.* 2017). The key aspects of management are:

Table 2.6 Classification of chronic obstructive pulmonary disease (NICE 2018)

Chronic obstructive pulmonary disease category	FEV1 (% of predicted value)	FEV1/FVC
Severity of airflow obstruction post bronchodilator		
Stage 1: Mild*	≥ 80%	< 0.7
Stage 2: Moderate	50–79%	< 0.7
Stage 3: Severe	30–49%	< 0.7
Stage 4: Very severe**	< 30%	< 0.7

FEV1, forced expiratory volume 1. *Symptoms are present in mild airflow obstruction. **Or FEV1 < 50% with respiratory failure.

- diagnosis
- smoking cessation
- effective inhaler therapy, determined by < or > 50% predicted FEV1
- short-acting bronchodilators as required, the use of long-acting β_2-agonist (LABA) or long-acting muscarinic antagonist (LAMA), inhaled corticosteroids (ICS) in a combination inhaler (see section on inhaler therapy)
- oral corticosteroids
- pulmonary rehabilitation for all who need it
- use of non-invasive ventilation (see section on the principles of non-invasive ventilation)
- management of exacerbations to minimize impact
- multidisciplinary working

Differentiation between asthma and COPD is not always clear and some of the guidelines are shown in Table 2.7.

In hospital management of acute exacerbations, the following investigations are required:

- chest X-ray and electrocardiogram (ECG) to exclude comorbidities
- arterial blood gas analysis and inspired oxygen concentration recorded
- full blood count urea and electrolytes
- theophylline level if appropriate
- sputum culture and sensitivity if sputum purulent.
- blood cultures taken if patient pyrexial

Treatment is with oxygen so as to maintain saturations at 88–92% or within an individualized target range (see section on oxygen therapy), bronchodilators, oral antibiotics as indicated, and oral steroids (30 mg prednisolone daily for 7–14 days). If a patient is hypercapnic or acidotic the nebulizer should be driven by compressed air, not oxygen (to avoid worsening

Table 2.7 NICE (2018) summary of differentiating features between chronic obstructive pulmonary disease and asthma

Feature	Chronic obstructive pulmonary disease	Asthma
Smoker or ex-smoker	Nearly all patients	Possibly
Symptoms began under 35 years of age	Rare	Often
Chronic and productive cough	Common	Uncommon
Patient is breathless	Persistent and progressive	Variable
Night waking/wheeze	Uncommon	Common
Day-to-day variability	Uncommon	Common

hypercapnia). If oxygen therapy during nebulization is needed it should be administered simultaneously by nasal cannulae. NICE (2010) guidelines recognize the possibility of depression and anxiety for patients with COPD, which should be treated. Restricted activity, social isolation, and the fear of dying with each exacerbation and admission to acute care are aspects of this disease that require sensitive and compassionate nursing care. Multidisciplinary care, including physiotherapists, dietitians, and primary care practitioners, is essential and discharge planning should include consideration of patient education and the involvement of the primary care team for future management of acute exacerbations (NICE 2010).

Pneumonia revision

It is estimated that between 5–12% of adults who present to their General Practitioners (GPs) with symptoms of lower respiratory tract infection are diagnosed with pneumonia and of these 22–42% are admitted to hospital. Those admitted to hospital with community-acquired pneumonia (CAP) have a mortality rate of between 5–14%, the majority in older people, and between 1.2%–10% will be admitted to the ICU, where the risk of dying is > 30% (NICE 2014).

Pneumonia is an acute lower respiratory tract infective illness causing alveolar inflammation and a build-up of exudate. Risk factors include age, chronic disease of heart, lungs or kidneys, immunological suppression, aspiration, and environmental factors such as recent travel, exposure to birds, and farm animals. Clinically significant factors are the age of the patient, their previous health, the causative organism, and the severity. Pneumonia presents with breathlessness, cough, pleuritic chest pain, and pyrexia. Fever may be severe with rigors, anorexia, and vomiting may also be present. Cyanosis may occur, chest expansion may be reduced on the affected side, and chest X-ray usually shows signs of consolidation (Bickley *et al.* 2017). The severity of illness and prognostic indicators are indicated by the CURB score, which allocates 1 point for each of the following features:

- confusion
- urea elevation
- respiratory rate > 30
- blood pressure < 90 systolic

Lim W. et al. Defining community acquired pneumonia severity on presentation to hospital: an international derivation and validation study. *Thorax*. 2003; 58(5): 377–382. doi: 10.1136/thorax.58.5.377.

Investigation is by chest X-ray, sputum and blood culture to identify the causative organism, full blood count, urea, and electrolytes. Arterial blood gas analysis to determine a type I or type II respiratory failure or a mixture of both (e.g. respiratory tiredness can show hypoxia and hypercapnia); degree of hypoxia which may be severe, and acid–base balance. Treatment is with oxygen, analgesia, and antibiotics, in accordance with local policy, consideration of sepsis protocols until the culture and sensitivity findings identify the causative organism. Hospital-acquired (nosocomial) pneumonia is caused by different organisms. Gram-negative bacteria are more prevalent in hospital infections, while in the community, droplet infection in winter of previously well patients is most commonly caused by *streptococcus pneumoniae*, mycoplasma, *legionella*, and *chlamydia*. Hospital-acquired pneumonia includes that caused by aspiration as well as by opportunistic pathogens, including *escherichia, pseudomonas, klebsiella*, and multi-drug resistant *staphylococcus aureus* (Gibson and Waters 2017). In severe cases it may be complicated by empyema or lung abscesses (Kumar and Clarke 2017).

Clinical link 2.3 (see Appendix for answers)

Patient 2 is a 74-year-old male, admitted to a medical ward from A&E yesterday. He is very thin, with a marked barrel chest. He uses oxygen at home and since his wife died six months ago he has needed help with shopping and housework from his daughter, who lives nearby. He has had three admissions in the last year for acute exacerbation of his COPD. He is peripherally and centrally cyanosed and his fingers are clubbed. His speech is wheezy and staccato, and he is breathing through his mouth, which is dry. His tongue is coated. He looks ill and tired and, although he is not using the accessory muscles, he is clearly having to make an effort to breathe. He is sitting slumped in the bed and he says he is fed up and can't be bothered with anything. His fluid chart indicates a poor oral intake and low urine output for that six hours. He has been catheterized and the urine in the bag appears dark in colour. His vital signs are:

- respiratory rate: 28
- temperature: 37.8°C
- peripheral pulse: 110
- blood pressure: 180/95
- SpO_2: 85%

He is on oxygen at 2 L via nasal specs and is producing viscous green sputum. His chest X-ray shows consolidation of the left base and his arterial blood gas analysis shows:

- pH: 7.2
- PaO_2: 8.7 kPa
- $PaCO_2$: 6.3 kPa
- HCO_3: 32 mmol/L
- BE: $^+$7 mmol/L

Consider the following questions:

- What type of respiratory failure does this patient have and what is the cause?
- What are your main priorities and why? What clinical actions should you take and why?

Tracheostomy care

It is vital that the patency of the tracheostomy is maintained at all times to prevent respiratory compromise and potential respiratory arrest. Suctioning of tracheostomies is an essential skill required of healthcare professionals caring for patients with tracheostomy tubes. The most common emergencies related to tracheostomy tubes are tube blockage and accidental decannulation (Dawson 2014). It is vital that nurses who accept patients from ICU understand how to manage tracheostomy care appropriately to avoid potential life-threatening problems (ICS 2014).

This section will explore:

- the rationale for tracheostomy
- preparing to receive a patient with a tracheostomy
- the need for humidification
- the need for removal of secretions
- maintenance of airway patency/changing inner tubes
- prevention of infection
- emergency procedures for blocked tracheostomy tubes
- removal of tracheostomy tubes

Rationale

Early insertion of the tracheostomy tube in critical care is routinely performed as it can reduce sedation requirements and promotes earlier weaning and mobilization. On admission to the ward the patient may still be weak and therefore the tracheostomy is left *in situ*. This helps to reduce the workload of breathing and facilitate suctioning, particularly if the patient has copious secretions or they are unable to clear secretions because of physical frailty/inability to cough sufficiently (ICS 2014).

Preparing to receive a patient with a tracheostomy

A checklist of equipment for transfer and information about the tracheostomy, for example type and size of the tracheostomy the patient has *in situ*, how long the patient has had the tracheostomy in, frequency of suctioning, communication methods (speaking valve) should be available prior to transfer. It is vital that sufficient space is available for the following equipment and that a safety checklist is available for each shift to check for any missing equipment. The following equipment should be available:

- tracheostomy tubes (same size and one size smaller)
- face mask and oxygen source
- scissors (to cut tapes if tracheostomy holder not being used)
- 10 mL syringe (to deflate tracheostomy cuffed tube if required)
- inner tubes for tracheostomy and appropriate cleaning equipment
- wall suction (portable if wall suction not available) and appropriate equipment
- suction catheters (sized correctly as per Table 2.8)
- gloves, apron, and protective eyewear
- tracheostomy disconnection wedge
- equipment to allow emergency replacement of tracheostomy tube if required

Table 2.8 Tracheostomy tube suctioning

Action	Rationale
Gain consent if patient is able and explain suctioning procedure to patient	To ensure that informed consent is gained
Hands should be decontaminated before suction. Personal protective equipment (aprons, goggles, visor) should be worn	To reduce risk of infection to the patient and nurse
Ensure that all equipment is working correctly: • a working suction unit (preferably wall-mounted), set correct pressure • suction catheter (catheter size should be calculated using the formula: size of tracheostomy tube (–2 ×2) • fluid to flush suction tubing • each suction catheter should only be passed once	It is important that the suction catheter is not too large as this will increase the hypoxic effects of suction Maintain tube patency To prevent bacterial contamination
A non-touch technique should be used and clean disposable gloves applied	To prevent bacterial contamination
The suction catheter should be passed in to just above the carina (about a third of catheter length, the patient should begin to cough)	To minimize the hypoxic effects of suctioning and prevent trauma to tracheal mucosa and to prevent infection
The catheter should be withdrawn whilst suction is applied. The total duration of this procedure should be not more than 10–15s	To prevent sputum being aspirated
The patient's oxygen should be reapplied immediately	To maintain oxygenation
The patient should be reassessed throughout the procedure to ensure that: • secretions have been cleared • respiratory assessment is now satisfactory • the patient is comfortable • there are no sign of respiratory distress	It is important to evaluate the effectiveness of suctioning
• reassurance should be provided to the patient	To reduce the anxiety of the patient if needed
Suctioning and sputum appearance should be documented in patient's notes • colour, consistency, and amount of sputum should be documented • excessive sputum production may indicate the need for more frequent suctioning/referral to a physiotherapist	To ensure accurate documentation and appropriate future interventions
Wash hands following suctioning procedure	To reduce risk of cross-infection

Humidification

The tracheostomy will bypass the nasopharynx and the oropharynx and as a result bypass the normal functions of warming, humidifying, and filtering air before it reaches the alveoli. It is important that some sort of humidification device is used to prevent dry, sticky, mucous plugs, which may lead to atelectasis (areas where there is alveolar collapse). It is important to ensure that the patient remains well-hydrated to ensure moist mucosal membranes and thinner secretions. Patients who are receiving oxygen via their tracheostomy will increase the potential for mucus plug formation and atelectasis as it further dries the airways and may lead to inflammation and ulceration (ICS 2014).

Various methods of humidification exist and the type selected will be dependent on the concentration of oxygen required and the patient's need for removal of secretions. The ICS (2014) Standards provide a guide to humidification in terms of 'the humidification ladder', for example heat moisture exchangers (HME) such as the Buchanon bib or Swedish nose; cold/heated water bath; additional use of saline nebulizers or mucolytics to ensure adequate hydration if secretions are still difficult to clear.

Heat moisture exchangers

These are plastic devices that have two 'sponges' either side. Inspired air passes through the sponges, which are warm and moist (from patient's expired air), and this enables air to be warmed and humidified. Some of these devices allow the delivery of a low concentration of oxygen through an additional side port. They are not useful if the patient is requiring more than 4 L of oxygen or if the patient has excessive secretions and in such cases wet humidification should be used instead. Nurses should ensure that these are changed as per manufacturers guidelines (usually every 24 h) as they may become a source for bacterial growth and infection. Care should also be taken to assess the suitability of these for patients with excessive loose secretions that they are able to cough out. Excessive secretions may block the device and necessitate increased frequency of changing. In this situation a water system may be better for the patient and more cost-effective.

Water humidification

In this system oxygen flows through a water reservoir. As the oxygen flows through the water, droplets humidify the oxygen. Different types of humidification systems are available which either use a droplet or nebulizer effect to humidify the oxygen. The net effect is moistened/humidified oxygen delivery to the patient. Again, manufacturer's recommendations should be followed regarding frequency of humidification/tubing change. Staff should be aware that water vapour may return to its normal state and water may collect in the tubing. Care should be taken with tubing so that it does not allow a flow of water vapour collection into the patients' lungs or the connection of a water trap to collect excess water can be used.

Removal of secretions

It may be necessary to suction the patient's tracheostomy to enable removal of secretions. This should only be carried out if necessary and if the patient is unable to cough the secretions out of the tube themselves. It should be remembered that suctioning is an invasive procedure, which may be uncomfortable and frightening for the patient (ICS 2014). It should only be carried out following careful assessment of the need for suctioning and should only be undertaken by practitioners who are competent. Patient indications for suctioning may include:

- visible or audible secretions that patient are unable to clear
- patient distress
- increased workload of breathing
- clammy skin or sweating
- increased heart rate/respiratory rate
- reduced oxygen saturations
- reduced airflow at stoma site

When suctioning, the nurse should ensure that their technique results in a maximum removal of secretions and minimum complications of suctioning. Complications related to suctioning include:

- hypoxia
- laryngospasm
- trauma to tracheal tissue
- mucosal damage
- cardiac arrhythmias/bradycardia/vasovagal stimulation
- infection
- hypertension
- raised intracranial pressure
- death (from hypoxia or a dangerous dysrhythmia)

Patients have also reported feelings of pain, suffocation, pressure, choking, and gagging, especially if an unskilled practitioner is undertaking this technique. The technique for suctioning is included in Table 2.8. Practitioners should ensure that they are familiar with suctioning equipment as a variety of equipment is available.

Alongside coughing and suctioning it is important to remember that other factors will contribute to the effective removal of secretions, including:

- effective patient positioning to facilitate mobilization of secretions
- regular chest physiotherapy to provide enhanced techniques to mobilize and clear secretions
- deep breathing exercises to minimize atelectasis and mobilization of secretions
- appropriate humidification and use of nebulizer therapy

Maintenance of tube patency/changing inner tubes

Although suctioning and effective clearance of secretions will contribute to the maintenance of tube patency, other areas need consideration. The patient should be transferred to the ward with a tracheostomy tube that has a removable inner tube (St George's University Hospitals Trust 2019 or local tracheostomy policy). The inner tube can then be removed and cleaned to reduce the likelihood of tracheostomy obstruction. 'Uncuffed' tracheostomy tubes are used for patients who can protect their own airway, have an adequate cough reflex, and, most importantly, can manage their own secretions. They help to re-establish a normal swallow reflex and the patient's voice can be heard with the concomitant use of a speaking valve. Note: a speaking valve can only be used in patients who have airflow through their pharynx into their nose and mouth (St George's University Hospitals Trust 2019).

There are several general recommendations:

- The inner tube should be inspected and cleaned every 4 h. It may be appropriate to reduce this frequency overnight, but careful patient assessment is vital.
- Non-disposable inner cannulae should be cleaned according to the manufacturers' instructions or with sterile water and air-dried thoroughly before replacing.
- Brushes are not recommended for the cleaning of inner tubes as they may scratch the surface and increase the colonization of bacteria.
- The inner tubes should never be soaked or left in any type of fluid as this will increase the likelihood of infection.
- If a temporary inner tube has been used this should be cleaned and stored in a dry, clean covering (St George's University Hospitals Trust 2019).

Care should be taken when removing the inner tube as this may cause the patient to cough excessively.

In addition to changing the inner tube, the tracheostomy tube will require periodic changing every 30 days or to the manufacturer's recommendations. The need for this should be assessed individually as a more frequent change may be necessary. It is usual to wait 7–10 days post tube insertion to allow the stoma to form before attempting to change the tube. Practitioners who undertake this role should ensure an adequate level of competence (St George's University Hospitals Trust 2019).

Prevention of infection/stoma dressings

The tracheostomy stoma breaches the body's natural defences to bacteria and allows direct entry to the trachea. In addition, the use of humidification and suction has the potential to increase the risk of infection. It is vital that adequate procedures are in place to minimize the risk of infection.

Effective cleaning and dressing of the stoma site is required to prevent the development of localized infection. The tracheostomy should be redressed as required. The stoma site should be checked for signs of infection and cleaned with appropriate solution and a clean dressing applied (see in equipment list above). The dressing and tube should be held in place using a specially designed tracheostomy tube holder. It is essential to have two nurses when dressing a tracheostomy to ensure that accidental displacement does not occur. The patient may cough during dressing changes so adequate assessment of need for suction before dressing change is required (St George's University Hospitals Trust 2019).

If a chest infection is suspected a sputum specimen should be obtained by either encouraging the patient to expectorate or by using a sputum trap when suctioning. If the stoma site appears to be infected, then swabs should be taken.

Emergency procedure for blocked tracheostomy tubes

Tracheostomy tubes may become blocked if the patient has thick, tenacious secretions or if aspects of management of the tracheostomy have been inadequate. Signs of blockage will include:

- respiratory distress
- increased workload of breathing
- use of accessory muscles, typically abdominal muscles
- possible stridor or no air sounds from tracheostomy
- cyanosis of patient or extreme pallor
- profuse sweating of patient and tachycardia
- no respiratory movement, if completely blocked

In the initial stages the patient may appear panicked and will require treatment and reassurance to facilitate removal of the obstruction. In later stages the patient's consciousness may be impaired. If the patient is not breathing or does not have a cardiac output, then cardiac arrest procedures should be referred to.

If some respiratory effort is present and the patient has a cardiac output, then simple procedures such as removal of the inner cannula or suctioning may resolve the problem. The emergency tracheostomy management for patients with a tracheostomy and patent upper airway or tracheostomy/laryngectomy with no patent upper airway are described in flowcharts cited by the St George's University Hospitals Trust (2019) and adapted from the National Tracheostomy Safety Project: http://www.tracheostomy.org.uk. These should be available by the patient's bedside.

Removal of tracheostomy tubes

Most patients will recover sufficiently to allow removal of tracheostomy. Indicators for tracheostomy removal are:

- the patient is able to cough effectively and maintain their own airway;
- the patient has been assessed by the medical staff to ensure that they are free of infection;
- the patient's respiratory status is stable and they are receiving less than 40% oxygen.

Once the tube has been removed the tracheostomy stoma should be covered with an occlusive dressing and this should be re-dressed to check for signs of healing (most tracheostomy stomas will heal without further intervention). Occasionally, it may be necessary to suture the site.

Laryngectomy patients

A total laryngectomy is sometimes performed in patients with advanced laryngeal cancer. This is the removal of the entire larynx and a permanent stoma created on the lower neck and tracheotomy (opening of the trachea) with loss of airflow from the mouth and nose to the lungs. Post surgery, total laryngectomy patients can never be ventilated via their mouth and nose and therefore it is important for critical care teams such as medical emergency and resuscitation teams to be made aware of these patients as per local policy and procedures on the emergency laryngectomy patient.

End of chapter test

It is important that you understand both the theory related to respiratory care and the practice of specific respiratory skills to care safely for patients with respiratory problems. To test your knowledge and apply this knowledge to clinical practice you should undertake the following assessment with an appropriately trained member of staff in clinical practice. If you are unable to answer any question it may be helpful to revisit the relevant section in this chapter.

Knowledge assessment

Work with your mentor/supervisor in practice and ask them to test your knowledge in relation to the following areas. Incorrect answers/lack of knowledge will require further reading of this chapter.

- Discuss altered physiology of the acutely ill respiratory patient including chronic conditions and vulnerable groups at risk of deterioration.
- Critically discuss methods of respiratory assessment including PEFR and FEV1.
- Critically discuss causes and treatments of breathlessness in the acutely ill patient.
- Discuss indications for oxygen and the titration of oxygen in critically ill patients.
- Critically examine the value of oxygen saturation monitoring and highlight the limitation of saturation recording.
- Discuss pharmacological actions of bronchodilators.
- Critically evaluate the role of arterial blood gas measurement in patient assessment and interpret ABGs accurately.
- Distinguish between type I and type II respiratory failure.
- Discuss indications/contraindications for CPAP and BiPaP.
- Discuss advantages and disadvantages of NIV.

Patient with a tracheostomy tube

- Discuss rationale for patient's tracheostomy insertion.
- Analyse the need for two-part tracheostomy tube (inner tube).
- Describe the essential equipment that is needed when caring for a patient with a tracheostomy.
- Discuss a respiratory assessment of a patient with a tracheostomy.
- Examine the need for appropriate humidification and discuss rationale.
- Analyse rationale for clearance of secretion, discussing potential complications that can occur during suctioning.
- Describe when it is appropriate to use endotracheal suctioning technique and describe how suctioning should be performed.
- Explains how tracheostomy blockage may present and discusses management of a patient with a blocked tube.
- Describe how the stoma should be cared for (to include redressing/types of dressing and infection prevention).
- Evaluate the communication problems faced by the patient and examines how these may be overcome.
- Examine the swallowing difficulties of the patient with a tracheostomy.

Skills assessment

Work with your mentor/supervisor in practice and ask them to assess your ability to care for patients with respiratory impairment using the following criteria where appropriate. Note that you may not be able to demonstrate all these skills. Ask your mentor/supervisor to give you feedback on areas where you did well and areas that may require improving.

- Observes for signs of respiratory distress and reports appropriately.
- Monitors respiratory rate and utilizes the NEWS2 trigger system to facilitate reporting of concerns.
- Increases rate of respiratory monitoring as per trigger score.
- Auscultates chest if appropriately trained and reports changes.
- Ensures patient positioned appropriately.
- Monitors oxygen saturation, explaining potential limitations.
- Identifies any potential causes of hypoxia and takes appropriate action.
- Administers oxygen as prescribed, selecting appropriate delivery system and concentration.
- Administers medication, for example nebulizers, as prescribed and monitors this.
- Refers to physiotherapist as appropriate.
- Recognizes the need for arterial blood sampling and demonstrates ability to interpret blood gas result accurately.
- Evaluates patient's response to changes made and communicates concerns to medical staff or the critical care outreach team.
- Assists with implementation of NIV where local policy allows.

- Monitors effectiveness of NIV (if used).
- Documents changes and hands over plan of care appropriately.

Patient with a tracheostomy tube

- Ensures all equipment required for caring for patient with tracheostomy tube is available including emergency equipment.
- If required, ensures that humidification system is set up and changed as per manufacturer's guidelines.
- Prevents any condensate from humidification system from entering the patient's airways.
- Ensures suctioning equipment is in working order.
- Takes appropriate infection control precautions when carrying out tracheal suctioning.
- Assesses the need for clearance of secretion and evaluates need for suctioning.
- Performs suction technique as per local guidelines and assesses patient for complications associated with suctioning.
- Reassesses patient following suctioning and evaluates need for further intervention.
- Cleans suction equipment and stores appropriately, ensuring suctioning equipment is readily available for next patient suctioning episode.
- Provides psychological support to the patient during suctioning.
- Observes for signs of respiratory distress that may indicate tube blockage and takes appropriate action.
- Changes inner tube as per trust guidelines, ensuring that inner tube is cleaned and stored in a dry, clean container.
- Redresses tracheostomy stoma site as per Trust guidelines.

References

APPG on Respiratory Health, British Lung Foundation. Report on Respiratory Health. Available at: https://publications.parliament.uk/pa/cm/cmallparty/170329/respiratory-health.htm accessed 12 January 2010.

Bickley, L.S., Szilagyi, P.G., Hoffman, R.M. (2017) *Bates' Guide to Physical Examination and History Taking*. Philadelphia, PA: Wolters Kluwer.

BTS/SIGN (British Thoracic Society, Scottish Intercollegiate Guidelines Network) (2016) *British Guideline on the Management of Asthma*. A national clinical guideline. Revised 2016.

St. George's Healthcare NHS Trust (2019). Tracheostomy Guidelines. Available at: https://www.stgeorges.nhs.uk/gps-and-clinicians/clinical-resources/tracheostomy-guidelines/, accessed 20 January 2020.

Calkovska, A.B., Uhliarova, M., Joskova, S. *et al.* (2015) Pulmonary surfactant in the airway physiology: A direct relaxing effect on the smooth muscle. *Respir Physiol Neurobiol*, 209:95–105.

Davidson, A.C., Banham, S., Elliott, M., *et al.* (2016) British Thoracic Society, Intensive Care Society (BTS and ICS) guideline for the ventilatory management of acute hypercapnic respiratory failure in adults. *Thorax*, 71(Suppl 2): ii1–ii35.

Dawson, D. (2014) Essential principles: Tracheostomy care in the adult patient. *Nurs Crit Care*, 19(2): 63–72.

Gibson, V., Waters, D. (2017) *Respiratory Care*. Boca Raton, FL: CRC Press/Taylor & Francis Group.

Havelock, T., Teoh, R., Laws, D., *et al.* (2010) Pleural procedures and thoracic ultrasound: British Thoracic Society pleural disease guideline 2010. *Thorax*, 65:i61–i76.

ICS (2014) Standards for the care of adult patients with a temporary tracheostomy; Standards and Guidelines. Intensive Care Society Standards 2014 Tracheostomy Care. Available at: https://www.ics.ac.uk/ICS/ICS/GuidelinesAndStandards/ICSGuidelines.aspx, accessed 20 January 2020.

Kumar, P., Clark, M. (2017) *Clinical Medicine* 9th edn. London: Elsevier.

MacDuff, A., Arnold, A., Harvey, J. (2010) Management of spontaneous pneumothorax: British Thoracic Society pleural disease guideline 2010. *Thorax*, 65:ii18–ii31.

Nair, M., Peate, I. (2013), *Fundamentals of Applied Pathophysiology: An Essential Guide for Nursing and Healthcare Students* 2nd edn. Chichester:Wiley-Blackwell.

NICE (2010) *Chronic Obstructive Pulmonary Disease in Over 16s: Diagnosis and Management 2010.* CG101. London: National Institute for Health and Care Excellence.

NICE (2014) *Pneumonia in Adults: Diagnosis and Management 2014.* CG191. London: National Institute for Health and Care Excellence.

NICE (2017) *Asthma: Diagnosis, Monitoring and Chronic Asthma Management 2017.* NG80. London: National Institute for Health and Care Excellence.

O'Driscoll, B.R., Howard, L.S., Earis, J., *et al.* (2017) British Thoracic Society (BTS) guideline for oxygen use in adults in healthcare and emergency settings. *Thorax*, 72(Suppl 1):ii1–ii90.

Rang, H.P., Dale, M.M., Ritter, J.M., *et al.* (2003) *Pharmocology*. London: Elsevier.

RCP (2017). National Early Warning Score (NEWS) 2: Standardising the assessment of acute-illness severity in the NHS. Updated report of a working party. London: Royal College of Physicians.

RCP (2014) Why asthma still kills: The national review of asthma deaths (NRAD). Confidential enquiry report. London: Royal College of Physicians.

Smith, G., Prytherch, D., Meredith, P., *et al.* (2013) The ability of the National Early Warning Score (NEWS) to discriminate patients at risk of early cardiac arrest, unanticipated intensive care unit admission, and death. *Resuscitation*, 84(4):465–70.

Stub, D., Smith, K., Bernard, S., *et al.* (2012). A randomized controlled trial of oxygen therapy in acute myocardial infarction. Air Verses Oxygen In myocarDial infarction (AVOID Study). *Am Heart J*, 163(3):339–45.

3
Cardiovascular assessment and care

Christine Spiers

Chapter contents

Cardiovascular disease remains the main cause of death worldwide (Bhatnagar *et al.* 2016). An understanding of cardiovascular anatomy and physiology is essential in understanding how to assess and manage patients with potential cardiovascular problems and complications. This chapter will examine:

- the normal anatomy of the heart and vascular system
- physiological mechanisms which control the cardiovascular function
- normal compensatory mechanisms that regulate blood pressure
- cardiovascular assessment
- cardiovascular monitoring
- cardiovascular management of the patient with:
    - chest pain
    - acute coronary syndromes
    - heart failure
    - cardiogenic shock

Learning outcomes

This chapter will enable you to:

- review the normal structure and function of the cardiovascular system
- develop an understanding of the physiological mechanisms which control cardiovascular function
- consider the assessment, diagnosis, and management of the patient with cardiovascular disorders
- identify the critically ill cardiac patient and know when to refer to senior/medical staff
- understand the impact of cardiovascular problems on the patient and carers
- use a skills assessment tool to assess your clinical practice

Introduction

The cardiovascular system is a sophisticated transport system that serves to distribute essential substances to the cells of the body and to remove unwanted by-products of metabolism for elimination from the body. The cardiovascular system that completes this function is made up of a pump (the heart), a collection of distribution and collecting tubes (the arteries and veins), and a series of extensive, thin-walled vessels that permit interchange between the vascular system and the tissues of the body (the capillaries).

The closed transport circuit that achieves this action comprises a vascular system and two pumps in series. The heart itself is described as a double-sided muscle pump, comprising a low- and a high-pressure system. The low-pressure output from the right ventricle sends blood into the pulmonary vasculature, where gaseous exchange between the blood and the alveoli in the lungs occurs. Oxygenated blood returns to the left side of the heart via the pulmonary veins. The relatively high pressure generated by the left ventricle propels blood into the systemic circulation and a series of arterial vessels distributes the blood to the tissues of the body. Exchange of nutrients and metabolic by-products takes place at the capillary level and deoxygenated blood then drains back into small venules and veins and eventually back into the major veins (superior and inferior vena cava), which drain into the right atrium of the heart (Figure 3.1).

To understand the care and management of patients with cardiovascular problems fully, knowledge of the anatomy and blood flow through the heart is essential.

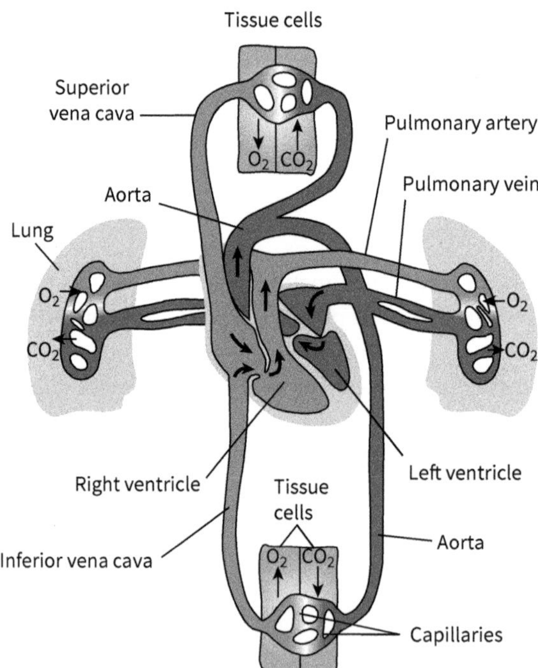

Figure 3.1 Systemic and pulmonic circulations.

The anatomy of the heart

The adult heart is cone-shaped and lies between the lungs in the mediastinum. It is approximately the size of a person's fist, weighing between 220 g and 350 g. The top of the heart referred to as the base lies beneath the sternum and the pointed lower section, the apex is located to the left of the sternum. The base of the heart is aligned with the second intercostal space and the apex can be located in the fifth intercostal space in the mid-clavicular line. This can be palpated in a healthy adult and is known as the 'apex beat'. The location of the apex beat is an important clinical assessment and if the apex beat is displaced leftwards this can be an indication of cardiac enlargement.

Functionally the heart comprises the right heart and the left heart separated by a septum. Vessels bring blood into the upper two chambers, the atria, and leave the heart via outflow tracts from the lower ventricular chambers. The two sets of valves (atrioventricular and semilunar) ensure directional flow of blood through the heart.

Deoxygenated blood returns to the right side of the heart via the large superior and inferior vena cava veins. This is referred to as the venous return. Blood flows passively through the tricuspid valve into the right ventricle. The right ventricle pumps the blood into the pulmonary artery via the pulmonary valve. The pulmonary artery takes the blood to the lungs, where gaseous exchange takes place. The oxygenated blood then returns to the left atrium via the four pulmonary veins (two from each lung). The blood flows through the mitral valve into the left ventricle where it is then ejected from the heart via the aortic valve into the aorta and the systemic circulation (Figure 3.1).

The heart is afforded protection by the pericardium, a tough sac surrounding the heart with attachments to adjacent structures. The two layers of pericardial tissues (parietal and visceral) have a narrow space between the two layers filled with pericardial fluid. The pericardium allows the heart to contract smoothly within the thorax.

The myocardium comprises two types of cardiac cells; myocardial and electrical. The majority of the heart comprises of myocytes, which are striated involuntary muscle cells that have the capacity to contract due to specialized contractile proteins. The electrical cells or automatic cells form the specialized conduction system discussed later in this chapter.

Cardiac muscle cells contain cross-striated myofibrils, which have contractile properties and extensive numbers of mitochondria for the production of the energy source adenosine triphosphate (ATP); the contractile units are known as sarcomeres.

The endocardium is composed of endothelial cells and provides a smooth lining for the chambers of the heart which is continuous with the lining of the blood vessels (tunica intima). The endothelial cells ensure smooth blood flow through the heart. The four heart valves are created from folds of endocardium thickened by fibrous tissue. The tricuspid and pulmonary valves are on the right side and the mitral and aortic valves on the left side. The two atrioventricular valves separate the atria from the ventricles (tricuspid and mitral valves) and the two semilunar valves are situated at the exit point of both ventricles (aortic and pulmonary valves). The atrioventricular valves have chordae tendineae, which are strong cord-like structures attached to papillary muscles within the ventricular chambers. The chordae tendineae prevent inversion and incompetence of the valves during ventricular systole.

At the junction of the upper third of the heart, a deep oblique atrioventricular groove separates the atria from the ventricles. Two other grooves, the anterior and posterior interventricular grooves, run towards the apex of the heart. These grooves mark the position of the interventricular septum, which separates the right and left ventricles and the grooves also form a route for the coronary artery circulation.

Physiological mechanisms of the cardiovascular function

The coronary circulation

The heart receives its blood supply from the coronary arteries, which arise from the sinuses of Valsalva, just above the semilunar cusps of the aortic valve. The right coronary artery arises from the right aortic sinus and the left coronary artery from the left aortic sinus (see Figure 3.2).

The left coronary artery comprises the left main stem which rapidly divides into two components: the left anterior descending coronary (LAD) artery and the left circumflex (Cx). The LAD coronary artery travels anteriorly and downwards within the interventricular groove towards the apex of the heart and ends in the inferior portion of the heart. The LAD provides septal and diagonal branches. The diagonal branches of the LAD supply the anterior, apical, and lateral walls of the left ventricle. The septal branches supply the interventricular septum and the right bundle branch and part of the left bundle branch. The Cx runs posteriorly along the atrioventricular groove to supply the posterolateral aspect of the left ventricle (LV). The right coronary artery (RCA) runs down the anterior atrioventricular groove, supplying the right side of the heart, the inferior and posterior surface of the heart, the sino-atrial (SA) node, and the atrioventricular node.

The venous drainage of the heart is via the great, middle, and small cardiac veins which drain blood into the coronary sinus, which is situated on the posterior wall of the left ventricle. The coronary sinus drains into the right atrium. Venous blood from the anterior cardiac veins drains directly into the right atrium and the remaining blood drains directly from the Thebesian veins into the cardiac chambers.

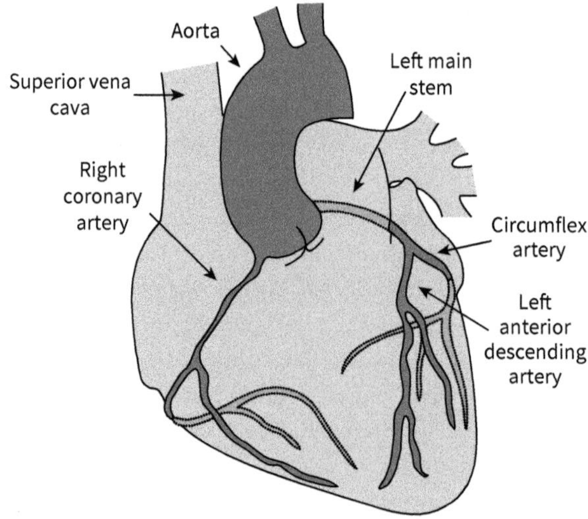

Figure 3.2 Coronary artery circulation.

The heart is therefore a double-sided pump, which maintains a constant circulation of blood to the body. At rest, the heart pumps at approximately 70 beats per minute and maintains a cardiac output of 5 L/min. The cycle of blood flow through the heart is referred to as the cardiac cycle.

The conduction system

An understanding of the conduction system and the association with the electrocardiogram (ECG) is essential for any practitioner working with acutely ill patients. Most acute units have facilities to monitor the patient's cardiac rate and rhythm, and technology also makes the continuous recording of 12-lead ECGs a possibility.

The cardiac conduction system consists of specialized electrical or 'automatic' cells, which contain specific properties that allow the generation, propagation, and conduction of electrical impulses from the atria and into the ventricles to produce myocardial contraction (Figure 3.3).

The cardiac conduction system comprises the:

- Sino-atrial (SA) or sinus node
- Atrioventricular (AV) node or junction
- Bundle of His
- Right bundle branch
- Left bundle branches (anterior and posterior fascicles)
- Purkinje fibres.

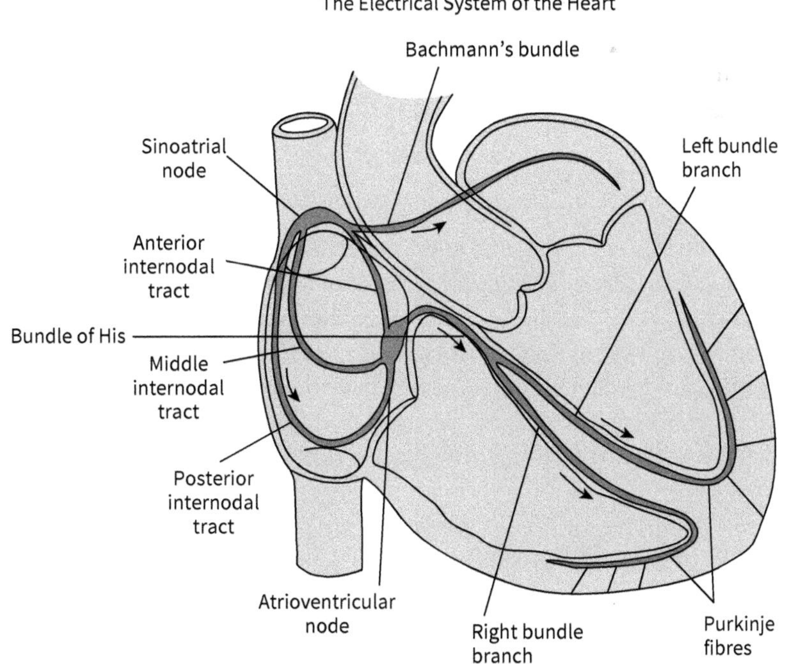

Figure 3.3 Electrical conduction system.

The sino-atrial node

The SA node, sometimes referred to as the cardiac pacemaker, is located on the posterior wall at the junction of the right atrium with the superior vena cava. It is heavily innervated with autonomic nerve fibres and the predominant influence on the SA node is the parasympathetic branches of the right vagus nerve.

The SA node has the property of *intrinsic automaticity*, which means that the SA node spontaneously depolarizes at a rate determined by the autonomic nervous system in order to cause atrial contraction. The coordination and transmission of right and left atrial activity is by specialized conducting pathways, the most well-defined of these being Bachmann's bundle, which links the right and left atria. The blood supply to the SA node is from the nodal artery, which arises from the right coronary artery in 60% of adults and the left coronary artery in the remaining 40%.

The atrioventricular node

In health, the AV node is the only electrical connection between the atria and the ventricles. The annulus fibrosus (atrioventricular fibrous ring) creates an electrical insulator between the atria and the ventricles. The AV node is situated at the junction between the interatrial septum and the tricuspid valve annulus. The AV node creates a delay in transmission of electrical stimuli to the ventricles and this allows for atrial systole to occur, which allows the atrial contents to be expelled into the ventricles prior to ventricular systole. The AV node is richly innervated by parasympathetic branches from the left vagus nerve and it receives its blood supply from the AV nodal artery, derived in 90% of cases from the RCA and in 10% of cases from the Cx. Reduction in blood flow to the AV node, as occurs in inferior wall infarction (RCA infarction), sometimes results in AV block (or heart block).

The His–Purkinje system

The transmission of electrical stimuli to the ventricular tissue is via the bundle of His, right and left bundle branches, and Purkinje fibres. Failure of conduction through the bundle branches is referred to as bundle branch block and this may affect either the right or the left bundle branch. Right bundle branch block (RBBB) is relatively common and may occur in a structurally normal heart as well as secondary to pathological processes. Left bundle branch block (LBBB) is never normal and is generally the result of severe cardiac disease such as myocardial infarction, hypertensive heart disease, or cardiomyopathy (Wesley 2017).

Autonomic nervous system

Whilst the heart has the intrinsic nervous system described above, the conduction system itself is regulated by the autonomic nervous system. Control of the autonomic nerves is via the cardiac centre in the medulla oblongata. The sympathetic nerve supply to the heart is to the SA node, AV node, His–Purkinje system, and the atrial and ventricular myocardium. The parasympathetic nerves to the heart (the vagus nerve) supply mainly the SA and AV nodes and, to a much lesser extent, the atrial and ventricular myocardium. Sympathetic nerve activity is mediated via adrenaline and nor-adrenaline and the β-receptors. Increased sympathetic activity increases heart rate and stroke volume. Stroke volume is defined as the amount of blood ejected from the ventricle per beat. In health the heart is principally influenced by the parasympathetic nervous system which slows the heart rate. In situations where there is enhanced parasympathetic stimulation mediated via acetylcholine, the heart rate and myocardial contractility decreases.

Cardiac cycle

The cardiac cycle can be defined in terms of the mechanical events which occur from the beginning of one heart beat to the beginning of the next. This cycle is characterized by a series of pressure changes, which results in blood flowing from areas of high pressure to areas of low pressure. The cyclical contraction (systole) and relaxation of the heart (diastole) of the cardiac cycle is divided into four phases.

Ventricular filling

During early to mid diastole the pressures in the heart are low and blood returns passively to the atria and into the ventricles via the open atrioventricular valves; this is known as *passive ventricular filling* and 70–80% of ventricular filling occurs at this stage. The semilunar valves are closed at this stage due to the pressure in the pulmonary artery and aorta being higher than the pressure in the respective ventricles. Towards the end of diastole, *active ventricular filling* occurs as a result of atrial contraction initiated by stimulation from the SA node (P wave on the ECG). Atrial contraction (systole) forces the remaining 25% of blood into the ventricles. In atrial fibrillation (AF) there is loss of synchronized atrial contraction and thus patients in AF may experience up to 25% reduction in cardiac output as a result of diminished ventricular filling.

Ventricular contraction

Atrial relaxation occurs next and the ventricles are depolarized (QRS complex on the ECG), resulting in ventricular contraction. As the ventricles start to contract, the pressure within the ventricles starts to rise, causing the atrioventricular valves to close. At this stage the volume of blood in the ventricles is constant, all four heart valves are closed, and the ventricles contract causing the pressure within the ventricular chambers to rise; this is known as *isovolumetric contraction.*

Ventricular ejection

As the pressure in the ventricles continues to rise, the pressure in the ventricles exceeds the pressure in the major arteries and the semilunar valves are forced open; this is the *ventricular ejection phase.* During the ejection phase blood is ejected into the pulmonary artery and aorta.

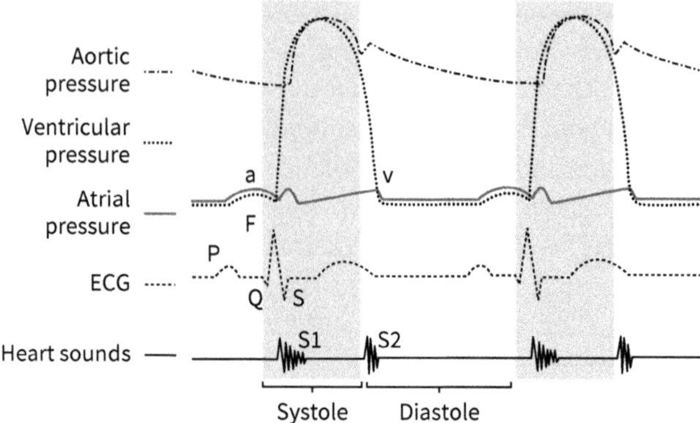

Figure 3.4 Cardiac cycle, including ECG waveforms and heart sounds.

Isovolumetric relaxation

Repolarization of the ventricles occurs resulting in relaxation (diastole) of the ventricles (T wave on the ECG). The pressure falls in the ventricles allowing the aortic and pulmonary valves to close again. Once again, the ventricles are closed chambers; all four valves are closed. During this time the atria are filling with blood (passive venous return) and once the pressure within the atria is higher than the pressure in the ventricles, the AV valves open and blood flows into the ventricles again (*ventricular filling phase*). The pressure changes in the ventricles, and corresponding ECG waveforms and heart sounds are indicated in Figure 3.4.

Heart sounds

The normal heart sounds (lub-dup) arise from the closure of the heart valves during the cardiac cycle. The first heart sound (S_1) is principally the sound of the simultaneous closure of the mitral and tricuspid valves at the onset of ventricular systole (lub). The sound is loudest at the apex and may also be heard at the lower left sternal border. The second heart sound (S_2) is due to closure of the aortic and pulmonary valves at the end of ventricular systole and it forms the 'dup' component of lub-dup. It is heard at the upper left sternal border and both sounds are best heard with the diaphragm of the stethoscope. Familiarizing yourself with normal heart sounds is a useful skill as once you are used to recognizing normal heart sounds you are more likely to be able to identify added sounds and murmurs. Added sounds and murmurs are usually due to turbulent blood flow through the heart, across the valves or the great vessels. There are many causes of murmurs that are beyond the scope of this chapter.

Cardiac output

Cardiac output is defined as the total volume of blood ejected by the heart into the systemic circulation in L/min. This is normally calculated as:

$$\text{cardiac output (CO)} = \text{heart rate (HR)} \times \text{stroke volume (SV)}$$

The stroke volume is the amount of blood ejected from the ventricles per beat. In the resting adult, the cardiac output is approximately 5 L/min. The average heart rate (70 beats per minute) multiplied by an average stroke volume (70 mL of blood) is equal to 4.9 L/min. Cardiac output can vary between at-rest values of 4.5 L/min and 25 L/min during vigorous exercise. Increases in heart rate or stroke volume or both can increase the cardiac output, whereas profound bradycardia or reduced stroke volume can decrease the cardiac output.

Cardiac output is therefore dependent on the relationship between the stroke volume and the heart rate.

Heart rate

In normal circumstances the heart rate is regulated by the activity of the SA node and its innervation from the autonomic nervous system (ANS) described above. Impulses from the sympathetic branches of the ANS have a *positive chronotropic* effect, which increases the heart rate; a similar chronotropic effect is produced by drugs such as β-adrenergic stimulants, such as salbutamol, and caffeine or nicotine.

The parasympathetic innervation to the SA node is via the vagus nerve and this acts as a 'brake' on the heart rate, causing it to slow. *Negatively chronotropic* effects may be caused by increased vagal stimulation as seen in extreme, intense visceral pain or stimulation of baroreceptors in the carotid sinus or aortic arch. Negatively chronotropic medications include β-blockers and digoxin.

Stroke volume

Three significant factors affect stroke volume and thus cardiac output; 'preload', 'myocardial contractility', and 'afterload'.

Preload

Preload can be defined as the tension exerted on the cardiac muscle at the end of diastole. The principle determinant of preload is the venous return, and this is often referred to as 'ventricular filling'. The heart can adapt to varying loads of inflowing blood and it is partly this capacity which alters the cardiac output. In situations where there is reduced blood volume such as hypovolaemia, cardiac output and hence blood pressure will fall (see explanation of blood pressure).

Myocardial contractility

Contractility is a property of myocardial fibres and essential for the effective pumping action of the heart; the strength of myocardial contraction is influenced by many factors. Sympathetic nervous stimulation, adrenaline (epinephrine) and nor-adrenaline (norepinephrine), and cardiac stimulants (such as caffeine) may increase the speed and strength of myocardial contraction. This is a *positive inotropic effect* and can be augmented by positive inotropic drugs such as dobutamine and digoxin. *Negative inotropic* effects (reduced contraction) may be induced by myocardial hypoxia or ischaemia or negatively inotropic drugs such as β-blockers.

Within physiological limits, cardiac muscle may be stretched to achieve increases in stroke volume and this is the Frank–Starling mechanism. Starling's law of the heart states that the myocardial fibres respond with a more forceful contraction when they are stretched. An example of this is to consider how an elastic band can be stretched to increase the elastic recoil when the elastic band is released. If an elastic band is continually overstretched, it will eventually lose its recoil and elasticity. Pathological processes such as cardiomyopathy and uncontrolled hypertension over a period of time may result in overstretching of the myofibrils and a subsequent reduction in cardiac stretch and hence reduced stroke volume. Reduction in the effectiveness of the contraction results in heart failure.

Afterload

Afterload is the force opposing the ejection of blood from the ventricles, and is a function of the resistance offered by peripheral (systemic) blood vessels and the size of the left ventricle. Pathologic conditions which increase afterload are either those which increase peripheral resistance (systemic or pulmonary hypertension) or conditions which obstruct outflow from the ventricles (aortic stenosis, pulmonary stenosis, or coarctation of the aorta), for example if the patient has high blood pressure this puts additional strain on the left ventricle (increased afterload) and this may eventually cause left ventricular failure and a reduction in cardiac output.

Blood pressure

Blood pressure is defined as the force or the pressure the blood exerts upon the vessel walls and it is a function of cardiac output and systemic vascular resistance, hence the equation below is sometimes used:

$$\text{blood pressure (BP)} = \text{cardiac output} \times \text{systemic vascular resistance}$$

Clinically, however, the blood pressure is essentially the arterial pressure in the systemic circulation and the systolic pressure occurs as a result of systole and the diastolic pressure results from diastole in the cardiac cycle. The *pulse pressure* is the difference between systolic and diastolic blood pressure and the *mean arterial pressure* is the pressure in the large arteries averaged over time. The mean blood pressure depends on the mean blood volume in the system and on the compliance of the arterial vessels. Mean arterial pressure, whilst not directly measured in acute care settings, is a useful value given on the automated blood pressure machines in practice. Generally, a mean arterial pressure of 60 mmHg is needed to sustain perfusion pressure to vital organs.

Blood pressure is maintained by many factors, including:

- cardiac output
- blood volume
- elasticity and tone of the blood vessels

Blood volume

Blood pressure is also affected by the volume of blood in the circulation and this is dependent on fluid and electrolyte balances and their controls (see Chapter 7).

Elasticity and tone of blood vessels

The arteries distribute blood to the cells and tissues of the body. Arteries are elastic vessels that help to maintain the forward (driving) pressure in the circulation. They also offer a variable resistance to blood flow. Arteries branch to become smaller arteries and eventually arterioles. Small arteries and arterioles have a greater proportion of elastic tissue within their walls and this enables them to alter their internal diameter. *Vasoconstriction* reduces the internal diameter of the vessel and *vasodilation* increases the vessel diameter. Normally the vessels are in a state of partial constriction and are said to have *tone*. Vasoactive substances such as neurotransmitters, hormones, and local factors can alter the arterial tone and these are listed in Table 3.1.

Arterial pressure needs to be maintained at a regular level and autoregulation of blood pressure can occur in the brain and kidneys up to a certain point. However, when blood pressure is significantly lowered, reduced blood flow to the brain and heart may result in loss of consciousness. Conversely, consistently raised blood pressure can cause irrevocable damage to internal organs and tissues.

Blood pressure is monitored and regulated by:

- neural mechanisms (baroreceptors, reflexes, and control centre)
- hormonal factors
- renal controls

Table 3.1 Vasoactive substances in the control of blood pressure

Vasoactive substance	Vasoconstriction	Vasodilation
Neurotransmitters		
Noradrenaline	Yes (α-receptors)	
Acetylcholine		Yes
Adrenaline	Yes (α-receptors)	Yes (β-receptors)
Hormones		
Angiotensin	Yes	
Serotonin	Yes	
Bradykinin		Yes
Local metabolites		
Carbon dioxide		Yes
Hypoxia	Yes	

Neural mechanisms

Pressure sensors (baroreceptors) situated in the aortic arch and carotid sinus monitor changes to blood pressure and send afferent impulses to the cardiovascular centre in the brain stem. Baroreceptors are excited by stretch; impulses are transmitted from the receptors along the sensory nerve fibres to the spinal cord.

Neural responses

A fall in blood pressure is sensed by the baroreceptors; this stimulus acts via the control centres in the medulla oblongata to increase cardiac output and arterial resistance to blood flow. This is mediated via the sympathetic nervous system. Adrenaline released by the adrenal gland acts via the α-receptor sites in the blood vessel walls to cause vasoconstriction. In addition, adrenaline mediates an increase in heart rate via the SA node and an increase in cardiac contractility by direct effect on the myocardium. The subsequent increase in heart rate and contractility contributes to an increase in cardiac output.

Hormonal factors

Although baroreceptor-mediated autonomic nervous activity can maintain sudden changes in blood pressure within seconds, other hormones released by endocrine glands are also vasoactive. Catecholamines (adrenaline and noradrenaline) released from the adrenal medulla should maintain blood pressure by increasing heart rate, myocardial contractility, and arterial vasoconstriction to increase cardiac output. Other hormones such as bradykinin act as local regulators of blood flow in the circulation.

Local metabolites

Many local metabolites, such as carbon dioxide, hydrogen ions, and low levels of oxygen, may act as vasodilators. The vasodilation activity of the metabolites counteracts the vasoconstriction effects of the sympathetic nervous system. This therefore allows local blood flow to active tissue to be maintained, despite increased activity by the sympathetic nervous system.

Renal controls

Changes in baroreceptor activity also controls the synthesis and release of the renin–angiotensin–aldosterone cascade which is a more elaborate mechanism for maintaining blood pressure. If blood pressure or blood flow falls abruptly to the kidneys there is increased sympathetic nervous system (SNS) output and SNS stimulation at the kidney promotes the synthesis and release of renin. Renin is an enzyme synthesized by the kidney that converts angiotensinogen (a pro-hormone) to angiotensin I. Angiotensin I is converted to angiotensin II (AII) in the lungs by angiotensin-converting enzyme (ACE). AII exerts its effect on angiotensin receptors in blood vessels resulting in vasoconstriction and a rise in blood pressure. AII also promotes the synthesis and release of aldosterone from the adrenal gland. Aldosterone acts on the renal tubules to cause sodium and fluid reabsorption. Anti-diuretic hormone further influences fluid balance. The use of ACE inhibitors such as ramipril for the management of long-term hypertension manipulates the renin–angiotensin–aldosterone system (RAAS) and is effective in disrupting this pathway (Chaterjee and Topol 2015). Further discussion of renal mechanisms of blood pressure control are included in Chapter 5.

Pathophysiology of atherosclerosis

Atherosclerosis is a chronic progressive inflammatory process affecting the intimal layer of artery walls. It evolves from the complex interaction of the blood elements, vessel wall changes, and alterations in blood flow. It is characterized by the proliferation of smooth muscle cells and the accumulation of elevated white lesions known as plaques which, when established, are encased in a hard fibrous cap.

Atherosclerosis may cause coronary heart disease (acute coronary syndrome), cerebrovascular disease (transient ischaemic attack or stroke), or peripheral vascular disease (limb claudication or acute limb ischaemia). For a discussion of cerebrovascular disease see Chapter 4.

The extent of arterial plaques does increase with advancing age but may occur in earlier age groups related to a number of risk factors. The role and importance of risk factors for coronary heart disease has been well demonstrated in epidemiological and interventional trials and many key factors have emerged (Public Health England 2016). Non-modifiable risk factors include age, gender, ethnicity, and familial history. Many modifiable risk factors are identified including:

- smoking
- hypertension
- lipid levels
- diabetes mellitus
- lack of exercise
- abdominal obesity
- psychological factors
- alcohol intake

These risk factors are synergistic, and the number of risk factors significantly increases the risk of developing atherosclerotic disease. Other factors have also emerged that are referred to as protective factors and appear to confer some degree of risk protection for individuals. These include:

- physical activity (moderate exercise five times per week);
- diet rich in antioxidants (particularly onions and garlic) and the inclusion of five to seven portions of fruit and/or vegetables daily;
- diet rich in omega-3 rich fish oils (two to three portions of oily fish weekly);
- vitamin C- and vitamin E-rich foods.

The reader is referred to the British Heart Foundation for useful health promotional literature.

Nursing assessment management of cardiovascular disorders

Cardiac conditions often present acutely, and this requires urgent assessment and intervention by the nursing staff. Care should be aimed at:

- accurate and timely cardiovascular assessment;
- relief of immediate life-threatening and distressing symptoms (this will prevent further deterioration and is of course essential for ensuring patient comfort);
- timely nursing/medical intervention.

A comprehensive systematic approach to patient assessment is required in the acutely ill adult. This may uncover concerns about red flags, identify other unsuspected problems, and provide information to guide investigations and treatment.

Cardiovascular assessment

History taking

The history-taking process is fundamental and should not be omitted unless the patient is in a critical state and requires an ABCDE assessment (see Chapter 10). The aim of history taking is to enable the patient to give a clear description of the presenting symptoms, to uncover any precipitating or relieving factors, and to identify any pattern to symptom episodes. Past medical history, medications, and risk factor identification, social factors, and occupational status enhances the assessment. The most common cardiovascular symptoms include:

- breathlessness
- palpitations
- dizziness and syncope
- claudication
- fatigue
- chest pain

Breathlessness

Breathlessness is a common and distressing symptom in cardiac and respiratory disease (see Chapter 2). Breathlessness is a common symptom for patients with cardiac arrhythmias, heart failure, and low cardiac output states.

Breathlessness may be a chronic symptom (as in biventricular heart failure), may occur with an acute exacerbation of a chronic problem (ventricular tachycardia in cardiomyopathy), or may present as the principal symptom in an acute illness (acute pulmonary oedema secondary to myocardial infarction). Whatever the cause, the patient will be extremely anxious and distressed and will require urgent intervention. Some patients may only experience breathlessness when lying down (*orthopnoea*) or may be woken during the night with sudden episodes of breathlessness relieved by sitting upright (*paroxysmal nocturnal dyspnoea*). The symptoms of orthopnoea and paroxysmal nocturnal dyspnoea are often an indication of heart failure.

Palpitations

Palpitations are a common, but distressing, symptom. Palpitations can be defined as an abnormally perceived heartbeat. Palpitations may represent an increased awareness of a slow, rapid, or irregular heart rhythm and it is useful to ask patients to tap out the rhythm of the palpitations with their hand (Bunce and Ray 2017).

An irregular heart beat may be caused by atrial or ventricular ectopic beats and periods of palpitations may be commonly experienced during periods of stress or anxiety. Ectopics or 'extra beats' may be triggered by caffeine, alcohol, or cocaine. Atrial fibrillation, which is less benign, commonly presents with irregular and chaotic bouts of tachycardia and may be associated with episodes of breathlessness and syncope. It is a serious arrhythmia requiring urgent intervention to control the rate and protect the patient against thromboembolic risks (NICE, 2014a).

Occasionally, a pounding or forceful heart beat at a moderate rate (90–120/min) may reflect normal cardiac function in the presence of exercise, stress, anxiety, or a hyperdynamic state such as pregnancy or hyperthyroidism.

Syncope

Syncope is a transient loss of consciousness due to inadequate cerebral blood flow and it has many neurological and cardiac causes (Bunce and Ray 2017). Neurological causes include epilepsy, cerebrovascular ischaemia, and neoplasms (see Chapter 4).

The most common cause of syncope or a simple faint is *vasovagal* attack. These episodes are usually preceded by dizziness, nausea, and sweating, and recovery normal occurs quickly if the patient assumes a supine position. More serious causes include cardiac arrhythmias (bradycardia and tachycardia), left ventricular outflow obstruction (aortic stenosis or hypertrophic cardiomyopathy), and postural hypotension (associated with autonomic dysfunction or induced by cardiac drugs such as vasodilators and diuretics). Cardiac syncope requires further investigation, which may include 12-lead ECG, ambulatory ECG and event recording, ambulatory blood pressure recording, echocardiography, tilt testing, and electrophysiological studies.

Claudication

Claudication, or ischaemic pain affecting the calf and other leg muscles, is described as peripheral vascular disease and is generally due to widespread atherosclerosis. Pain occurs on exercise and is relieved by rest. The best treatment is to reduce exacerbating risk factors, such as smoking cessation, management of lipid disorders, and the institution of antiplatelet therapy. Regular exercise may relieve the symptoms of claudication due to the development of collateral circulation.

Fatigue

Fatigue and lethargy may be an indication of reduced systemic perfusion in heart failure. It is a debilitating symptom in chronic heart failure and it may be further exacerbated by skeletal muscle atrophy due to immobility. Anaemia is also seen in patients with chronic heart failure and can trigger anginal-type chest pain. Fatigue can lead to depression and social isolation (NICE 2016a).

Chest pain

Chest pain is one of the most common reasons for a consultation at the General Practitioner (GP) and in addition it is a leading cause of emergency hospital admission. It is one of the most frightening symptoms experienced by patients, many of whom will know that it may herald an acute cardiac event such as a 'heart attack' or 'cardiac arrest'. The SOCRATES tool is commonly used to assess symptoms:

S—Site
O—Onset
C—Character
R—Radiation
A—Associated symptoms
T—Timing
E—Exacerbating factors
S—Severity

There are many causes of chest pain, some of which are life-threatening and many others which are less serious. The causes of chest pain from non-cardiac causes are considered in Table 3.2.

The causes of chest pain are therefore many and varied and the underlying problem may be life-threatening or trivial. A strategy of caution is, however, always adopted in assessing and managing chest pain to rule out life-threatening causes and to investigate possible cardiac causes.

Cardiac causes of chest pain include:

- acute coronary syndromes (angina, unstable angina, non-ST-segment elevation myocardial infarction and ST-segment elevation myocardial infarction)
- myocarditis, pericarditis, and endocarditis
- acute aortic dissection
- aortic stenosis
- cardiac arrhythmias
- hypertrophic obstructive cardiomyopathy
- Takotsubo cardiomyopathy 'broken heart syndrome'

Takotsubo cardiomyopathy is a rare cause of chest pain which has the same presentation as acute coronary syndrome but is not caused by coronary artery disease. Research suggests that the sudden release of adrenaline following a significant emotional or physical stress such as a bereavement stuns the heart, leading to changes in myocardial contractility and perfusion. It is more likely to occur in female middle-aged patients (Kato *et al.* 2017). The importance of history taking is thus highlighted here as Takotsubo should be a consideration in the differential diagnoses for a middle-aged lady who is presenting with sudden onset of chest pain after the sudden death of a loved one. When assessing chest pain, patients should be encouraged to give the history of their symptom in their own words. Assessment of the characteristics of cardiac chest pain caused by myocardial infarction is demonstrated using the SOCRATES tool (see Table 3.3). The management of chest pain will be explored later in this chapter.

Monitoring of the vital signs, respiratory rate and character, heart rate and rhythm, and blood pressure are a fundamental part of cardiac care.

The assessment may raise concern about red flags and used in conjunction with NEWS2 may identify unsuspected problems, enable early identification, and a timely and competent clinical intervention (RCP 2017).

Table 3.2 Differentiation of chest pain from non-cardiac causes

Cause of chest pain	Nature of pain	Other symptoms
Pulmonary		
Pneumonia	Sharp, stabbing	Cough
Chest infection		Wheeze
Pleurisy		Breathlessness
Pneumothorax		Sputum production
Pleural effusion		Haemoptysis
		Circulatory collapse
Musculoskeletal		
Blunt injury acquired from: contact sport, road traffic accident, physical assault	Sharp, diffuse, or stabbing	Pain is often positional and exacerbated by deep breathing, turning or arm movement
Inflammatory, or autoimmune conditions; costochondritis, ankylosing spondylitis	Widespread and diffuse	Pain is associated with localized tenderness and/or swelling
Acute oesophagogastric disorders		
Oesophageal rupture	Severe, burning	Excruciating retrosternal pain radiating to the back, chest, or abdomen
		Associated symptoms include breathlessness, hypotension, poor peripheral perfusion, and peripheral cyanosis
Gastro-oesophageal reflux	Upper or lower retrosternal, burning	Pain may be related to dietary intake, intermittent dysphagia or pain on bending forwards
Chest pain due to pulmonary embolism	Substernal, may be pleuritic in nature	Pain is not the major presenting feature; sudden onset of breathlessness is common. Massive PE presents clinically with shock, hypotension, gallop rhythm (tachycardia with an added S_3), and raised JVP.

JVP, jugular venous pressure; S_3, third heart sound.

Vital signs

Respiratory rate

A raised respiratory rate is an important physiological indicator in identifying the critically ill patient. An increased respiratory rate may indicate acute hypoxia secondary to sudden-onset pulmonary oedema, reduced myocardial perfusion, or reduced cardiac output. It may also indicate sepsis, metabolic acidosis, central nervous system (CNS) impairment, and be a

Table 3.3 Description of myocardial chest pain using SOCRATES tool

SOCRATES	
Site	Central chest
	Retrosternal
	Back
	Jaw
Onset	Exercise
	Emotion
	Cold weather
	Rest
Character	Heavy
	Dull
	Gripping
	Constricting
Radiation	Arms
	Neck and jaw
	Back
	Upper epigastrium
Associated symptoms	Dyspnoea
	Diaphoresis
	Nausea
	Syncope
	Extreme anxiety
Timing	Sudden onset
	Pain lasts longer than 20 minutes without relief
Exacerbation	Exercise
	Emotion
	Following meals
	Extreme weather temperatures
Severity	Can be scored using a numerical rating tool
	Pain is usually at high end of scale, although patients with diabetes and elderly patients may experience less pain

Adapted with permission from *MEDSURG Nursing*, 2000, Clayton HA et al. A novel program to assess and manage pain. Volume 9, Number 6, pp. 318–321, 317.

sign of acute pain and distress. Monitoring and tracking the respiratory rate is thus vital in assessing all patients and a respiratory rate of < 12 or > 20 should trigger further investigations from the nurse.

Heart rate

Heart rate may be estimated by measuring and recording radial or carotid pulses. A heart rate of < 51 or > 90 triggers further investigation using NEWS2. If an irregular pulse is identified, listening at the apex beat (fifth intercostal space, midclavicular line) whilst counting the radial pulse may identify atrial fibrillation or ventricular ectopics. A 12-lead ECG should be recorded which will assess heart rate, cardiac rhythm, and possible causes of the arrhythmia such as myocardial ischaemia.

Blood pressure

Blood pressure is the force exerted by the volume of blood on the arterial walls and is a function of cardiac output and systemic vascular resistance. It is a dynamic and constantly changing pressure and varies by up to 30 mmHg throughout the day. It can be influenced by blood volume, time of the day, anxiety, pain, and various drugs.

Measurement of blood pressure using a sphygmomanometer involves the occlusion of an artery using a cuff and either detection of Korotkoff sounds (auscultatory method) or monitoring by using oscillometry. The most common method employed in acute areas is the oscillometric method (automated method) although automated machines are less reliable in the event of tachycardia and irregular rhythms such as AF.

Systolic blood pressure (SBP) is given greater credence in NEWS2 than diastolic blood pressure, although both should be recorded. In NEWS2 SBP of ≤ 111 or ≥ 219 mmHg should alert the acute care practitioner to early intervention. A low or falling SBP may indicate sepsis, a reduced blood volume, or heart failure. Many patients with cardiac disorders do have relatively low blood pressure, due to their reduced cardiac output and also related to commonly used cardiac drugs such as β-blockers ACE inhibitors, which lower the blood pressure. It is important to note that the blood pressure (BP) will remain stable during the initial stages of deterioration because of the compensatory mechanisms previously described. Generally, the SBP will not reduce until approximately one-third of the circulating blood volume has depleted and the heart begins to fail. It is important to monitor the diastolic blood pressure as this will start to rise with the vasoconstriction brought about by the compensatory measures. The pulse pressure is often overlooked in acute clinical practice. Pulse pressure is a simple calculated value:

$$\text{Pulse pressure} = \text{Systolic pressure} - \text{Diastolic pressure}$$

If the pulse pressure is narrowing or decreasing, it may be an indication of vasoconstriction and be suggestive of hypovolaemic or cardiogenic shock. A widening pulse pressure indicates vasodilation and may suggest sepsis or the early stages of anaphylactic shock. A widened pulse pressure such as 160/40 mmHg is often seen in patients with aortic valve regurgitation.

Finally, mean arterial pressure (MAP) is another important indicator and it reflects perfusion of major organs. Whilst electronic sphygmomanometers will display MAP, this is not generally documented onto NEWS2 forms. Most patients require a MAP of 60 mmHg to maintain adequate organ perfusion to avoid deterioration (such as acute kidney injury). Elderly patients and those with known (or untreated) hypertension may require a higher MAP to maintain organ perfusion.

Oxygen saturation

Oxygen saturation indicates how much arterial oxygen is combined with haemoglobin and is expressed as a percentage. Pulse oximetry is a simple and widely available tool which enables integrated assessment of cardiopulmonary function. Oxygen saturation levels $\leq 94\%$ trigger further investigation and may indicate pulmonary oedema, heart failure, myocardial infarction, or cardiogenic shock. There is, however, concern that there is heavy over-reliance on the use of oxygen saturation, with Mok and colleagues (2015) identifying that many nurses incorrectly felt that oxygen saturation can effectively replace respiratory observations. In the early stages of deterioration, compensatory mechanisms will normalize saturation recordings. It is also important to note that many factors will affect the accuracy of saturation recordings such as poor perfusion, anaemia, arrhythmias, skin colouration, and reduced temperature.

Peripheral perfusion

Peripheral fingers and toes should be examined for evidence of pallor and cyanosis; removal of nail varnish enables clear visualization of the nail beds. The capillary refill is measured by placing the patient's hand at heart level and compressing the nail bed of a finger for 5 seconds (s). In some patients it may be preferable to record a central capillary refill time using a similar technique but pressing on the sternum instead of the peripheries. Pressure is released and the time to regain normal colour is measured. The normal capillary refill time should be 2 s although 2–3 s is considered acceptable in the elderly. Capillary refill estimation is an important parameter in assessing patients undergoing fluid resuscitation for septic shock (Bridges 2017).

Cardiac monitoring

Most acute-care settings have facilities for single-lead and occasionally continuous 12-lead ECG recordings of the heart rate and rhythm. The ECG is a graphic representation of the electrical events generated by the cardiac conduction system described earlier in this chapter.

Monitoring electrodes placed on the body's surface can detect these electrical events and transmit, via monitoring leads, to an oscilloscope, where the events are amplified and displayed as a series of waveforms.

The basic ECG waveforms are labelled PQRST (and U) including the PR interval, QT interval, and ST segment, and these reflect the electrical events which should trigger mechanical contraction within the heart (see Figure 3.5).

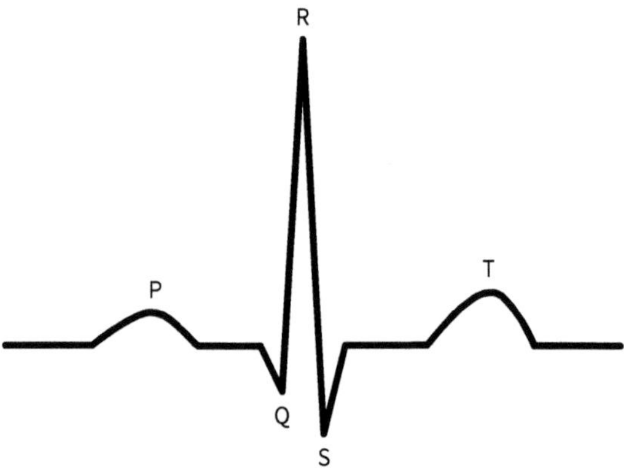

Figure 3.5 Normal ECG waveforms.

Table 3.4 ECG waveforms

Waveform	Electrical event	Mechanical event
P wave	Sino-atrial node	Atrial depolarization
P–R interval (measured from the beginning of the P wave to the beginning of the QRS complex)	Atrio-ventricular node	Ventricular filling following atrial systole
QRS complex	His–Purkinje activation	Ventricular depolarization
ST segment	Recovery	Ventricular repolarization Coronary perfusion
T wave	Recovery	Ventricular repolarization
QT interval (measured from the beginning of the Q wave to the end of the T wave)	His–Purkinje activation and recovery	Ventricular ejection

The correlation of the ECG waveforms, intervals, and segments to the electrical and mechanical events is identified in Table 3.4.

ECG paper

ECG paper is marked out in squares and the paper speed is 25 mm/s. Each small square on the horizontal axis is equivalent to 1 mm representing 40 ms. One large square (marked with a darker line on the ECG paper) is 5 mm, representing 200 ms. The vertical axis represents amplitude or voltage, thus one small square is 1 mm, equivalent to 0.1 mV. One large square (marked with a darker line on the paper) is 5 mm and two large squares represent 1.0 mV. Standardization of the ECG paper allows the accurate measurement of heart rate, regularity, and amplitude. Normal ranges of durations (in milliseconds) and amplitudes (in millimetres) of waveforms is given in Table 3.5. When there is no electrical activity present the ECG will show a flat (isoelectric) line. It is normal, for example, to see an isoelectric line between the P wave and the QRS (PR segment), between the S wave and the T wave (ST segment).

Table 3.5 Normal waveforms—duration and amplitude

Waveform/interval	Duration	Amplitude
P wave	80–120 ms	1–2.5 mm
PR interval	120–200 ms	N/A
QRS complex	60–100/120 ms	8–25 mm
ST interval	Varies with heart rate	N/A
T wave	Varies with heart rate	0.5 mV
QT interval	300–430 ms (variable with heart rate)	N/A

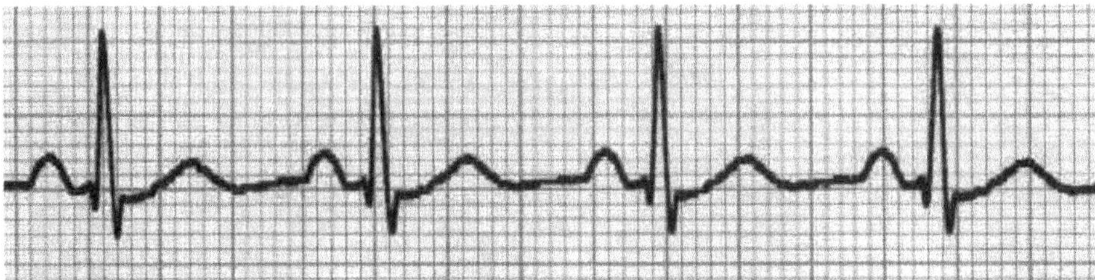

Figure 3.6 Sinus rhythm.

Sinus rhythm

Normal cardiac rhythm is identified when P waves, PR interval, QRS complexes, and T waves are present in a regular rhythm at a rate between 60 and 100/min (see Figure 3.6). Variations in cardiac rate may be precipitated in response to exercise, emotion, temperature, and exposure to stimulants such as caffeine and nicotine. Cardiac rhythm variations can occur in association with the respiratory pattern (sinus arrhythmia) generally only seen in the very young and the elderly. The heart rhythm may be either regular or irregular in both benign and malignant cardiac arrhythmias.

Rhythm interpretation

A simple approach to rhythm interpretation should be employed for all patients monitored on an acute ward. Rate, rhythm, P:QRS ratio, PR interval, QRS complex, ST segment, and T waves all require evaluation.

- Rate: bradycardia (less than 50–60 per minute), normal (50 or 60–100 per minute), tachycardia (more than 100 per minute). Rate may be measured by counting the number of small squares between two R waves and dividing the number into 1500 (the RR interval method).
- Rhythm: is it regular or irregular? Sinus rhythm may not be completely regular (heart rate may vary with inspiration as in sinus arrhythmia, for example). On the other hand, various arrhythmias may be regular; for example, ventricular tachycardia, atrial flutter, and supraventricular tachycardia (SVT) are usually regular. Atrial fibrillation usually produces an irregular rhythm.
- P:QRS ratio: There should always be a one-to-one relationship—one P wave to each QRS complex. Arrhythmias which produce more P waves to QRS complexes include heart block. In some arrhythmias such as atrial fibrillation and ventricular tachycardia there may be no evident P waves (Menzies-Gow and Spiers 2018).
- PR interval: a short PR interval may be an indication of ventricular pre-excitation, such as Wolff–Parkinson–White (WPW) syndrome (Sampson 2016). A lengthened or variable PR interval may be caused by AV node ischaemia (following acute myocardial infarction), drug-induced (β-blockers or digoxin), or age-related.
- QRS complex: the shape and duration of the QRS complex should be evaluated by closer inspection of the 12-lead ECG. However, a widened or bizarre-shaped QRS complex may indicate ventricular hypertrophy or bundle branch block (Wesley 2017). A widened QRS complex in the absence of P waves with a fast rate may indicate ventricular tachycardia.

- ST segment: this is measured at the J point and in most leads should be flat on the isoelectric line; any deviation above or below the isoelectric line of more than 1 mm is strongly indicative of myocardial infarction or ischaemia respectively (European Society of Cardiology 2017). A wandering baseline (induced by patient movement or breathing) may also cause apparent ST segment deviation.
- T waves: abnormality in either the ST segment or the T waves usually indicates coronary artery ischaemia. It is normal for the T wave to follow the same direction as the QRS complex. Hence if the QRS complex is positive (above the isoelectric line) then the T wave should also be positive. Conversely, when the QRS complex is negative (as is commonly seen in lead aVR) then it is normal for the T wave to be inverted. A negative T wave in the presence of a positive QRS complex may be indicative of myocardial ischaemia and requires further investigation. A hyperacute (tall) T wave may be indicative of early myocardial infarction or hyperkalaemia (Wesley 2017).

Many acutely ill patients may develop cardiac arrhythmias, and continuous ECG monitoring allows early identification and immediate intervention. ECG analysis should take note of the patient's clinical situation because a stressed, frightened patient may present with sinus tachycardia and a patient who is prescribed β-blockers may have a bradycardia; in the context of their clinical situation, the arrhythmia is not significant.

Arrhythmias are often classified according to the site of origin (Table 3.6). In general, atrial arrhythmias produce narrow QRS complexes, as the ventricles are depolarized normally via

Table 3.6 Origin and classification of arrhythmias

Site of origin	Arrhythmia	QRS complex
Atrial (supraventricular)	Sinus arrhythmia	Narrow
	Sinus bradycardia	
	Sinus tachycardia	
	Sinus arrest	
	Atrial ectopics	
	Atrial fibrillation	
	Atrial flutter	
Junctional (AV nodal)	Junctional ectopics	Variable
	Junctional tachycardia	
	Supraventricular tachycardia	
	Atrioventricular re-entry tachycardia (WPW syndrome)	
	AV blocks (heart blocks)	
Ventricular	Ventricular ectopics	Wide
	Ventricular tachycardia	
	Torsades des pointes	
	Ventricular fibrillation	

the AV node and bundle of His. Ventricular arrhythmias produce broad, bizarre QRS complexes because the ventricles are activated via an abnormal pathway. Junctional arrhythmias may manifest as narrow or broad morphology.

Cardiac arrhythmias may cause unpleasant symptoms such as palpitations, chest pains, syncope, or breathlessness. Serious arrhythmias may cause circulatory collapse, although occasionally patients may be asymptomatic. It is essential that an acute care nurse is able to recognize common cardiac arrhythmias, understand when to refer to senior/medical staff and be able to anticipate and understand appropriate treatment. A description of all cardiac arrhythmias is outside the range of this chapter, although the common arrhythmias will be presented. The reader is referred to a suitable textbook on cardiac arrhythmias.

Sinus arrhythmia

Sinus arrhythmia is a common (and normal) phenomenon in the very young and the elderly and rarely requires any intervention. It is characterized as an irregular sinus rhythm where the rate varies in relation to inspiration and expiration. Heart rate slows on inspiration and speeds up during expiration. The RR interval may vary in relation to the respiratory rate.

Sinus bradycardia

This is sinus rhythm with a rate less than 50–60 min. The characteristic P wave, PR interval, QRS complexes, ST segment, and T waves are present, but the RR interval is lengthened (Figure 3.7). Dependent on the cause, patients may be asymptomatic, although development of sudden bradycardia may result in circulatory collapse.

Causes

Sinus bradycardia is a normal physiological phenomenon seen during rest and in sleep and in high-performance athletes. Pathologically it may be seen in inferior myocardial infarction, hypothyroidism, raised intracranial pressure, hypothermia, and obstructive jaundice. It is induced by many commonly used drugs, including β-blockers, calcium channel blockers, and digoxin. It may be precipitated by medical procedures which cause vagal stimulation such as endotracheal suctioning or by induction of deep pain such as femoral arterial sheath removal.

Treatment

This is rarely needed unless the patient is compromised by a low blood pressure. The underlying cause should be treated if possible and in cases of circulatory collapse Atropine may be administered intravenously.

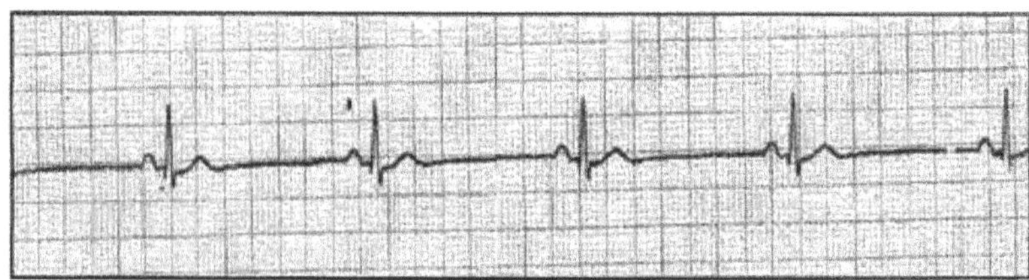

Figure 3.7 Sinus bradycardia.

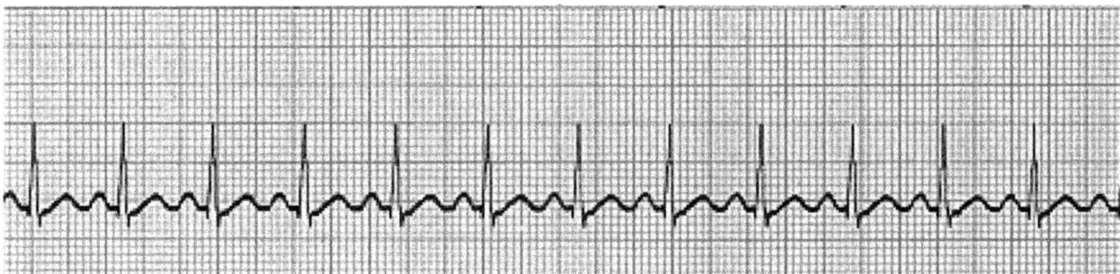

Figure 3.8 Sinus tachycardia.

Sinus tachycardia

The P wave, PR interval, QRS complexes, ST segment, and T waves are normal but occur at a rate faster than 100 per minute (Figure 3.8). Thus, the RR interval is reduced and the diastolic filling time of the heart (including the coronary arteries) is reduced.

Causes

Sinus tachycardia is a normal response to adrenergic stimuli and is a physiological response to exercise and emotional stress. It is pathological in sepsis, hyperthyroidism, cardiac disease, respiratory disease, hypovolaemia, and all shock and low cardiac output states. It may be induced by stimulants, including alcohol, nicotine, caffeine, amphetamines, and cocaine, or by prescribed drugs such as salbutamol and aminophylline.

Treatment

This is aimed at finding the cause and managing it. Hence a hypovolaemic patient may require volume replacement. Cardiac patients are particularly susceptible to sinus tachycardia as coronary artery filling time and hence coronary perfusion is reduced and sinus tachycardia may induce chest pain. Occasionally sinus tachycardia requires treatment to slow the rate and drugs such as β-blockers (atenolol) or digoxin are useful.

Extrasystoles

Extrasystoles ('ectopic beats') may arise from ectopic foci in the myocardial tissues and single isolated ectopics are not usually significant. A premature stimulus arises early and stimulates the surrounding tissue, resulting in abnormal conduction to the rest of the heart. The resulting waveform occurs early, has an abnormal shape and is followed by a 'compensatory pause'.

Causes

Ectopic beats occur in normal hearts and may be precipitated by adrenergic stimuli such as exercise, stress, caffeine, alcholol, cocaine, and β-adrenergic drugs (Figure 3.9). In cardiac disease they may result from myocardial ischaemia and, if frequent or multiform in shape, may require treatment. Hypokalaemia and acidosis are notable precipitants and maintaining the blood potassium above 4.5 mmol/L will often prevent ectopic formation (Khan *et al.* 2013).

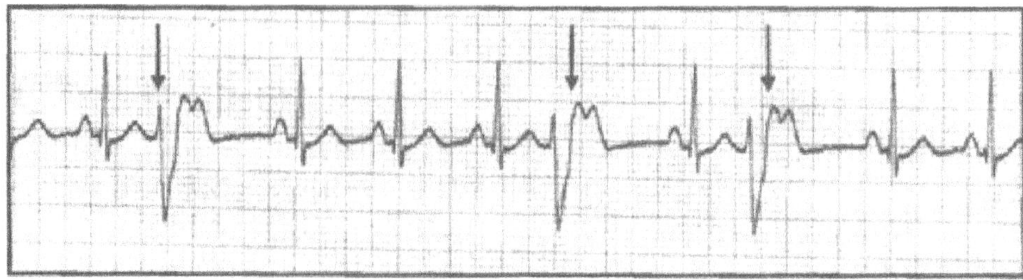

Figure 3.9 Ventricular ectopics (extrasystoles).

Treatment

Atrial ectopics are usually benign, ventricular ectopics may require treatment if they are frequent or occur every other beat. Ventricular bigeminy is defined as a ventricular extrasystole occurring every other sinus beat and is occasionally caused by digoxin toxicity. Treatment of the underlying cause (i.e. low serum potassium level or acute coronary syndrome) is essential and anti-arrhythmic drugs are occasionally used but may be arrhythmogenic and negatively inotropic (Opie and Gersch 2013).

Supraventricular tachycardia

Strictly speaking, the term 'supraventricular tachycardia' (SVT) refers to all tachycardias that originate above the level of the AV junction. In practice, however, atrial fibrillation and atrial flutter are excluded from this description.

SVT presents as a rapid, regular rhythm, with a rate between 140 and 250 beats per minute (Figure 3.10). P waves are generally absent, the QRS is narrow, and the T wave may be inverted or normal. The patient will generally be aware of the palpitations, breathlessness and dizziness. SVT may reduce the cardiac output resulting in a pale, clammy, and hypotensive patient. SVT will often start suddenly and terminate equally abruptly.

Causes

SVT may occur in normal, healthy individuals and may be precipitated by alcohol and stimulants. SVT may also occur in serious cardiac disease such as WPW syndrome (Sampson 2016) or in heart failure or acute coronary syndromes.

Treatment

Termination of the arrhythmia may be achieved in a number of ways but all require medical support. In a normally healthy person the use of carotid sinus massage or the Valsalva manoeuvre may reverse the arrhythmia. Alternatively, adenosine given as a fast intravenous bolus

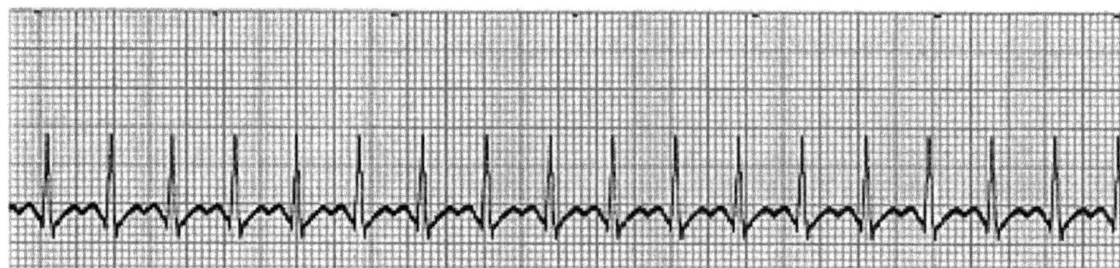

Figure 3.10 Supraventricular tachycardia.

is also very effective. Occasionally, more persistent SVT requires an amiodarone infusion or electrical cardioversion. Clinically you should be aware that adenosine can cause unpleasant symptoms for patients, including severe chest pain, flushing, and anxiety; patients should be warned prior to its administration.

Atrial fibrillation

Atrial fibrillation (AF) is a commonly encountered arrhythmia in acute care and when the onset is sudden, the rhythm is generally fast, and the patient symptomatic. It is characterized by multiple, rapid re-entry circuits within the atria which cause the atria to fibrillate, resulting in ineffective atrial contraction and the fast transmission of impulses through the AV node to the ventricles. Reduced atrial contraction (atrial 'kick') reduces preload to the ventricles and subsequently reduces cardiac output by up to 25%. The AV node protects the ventricles by reducing the number of atrial impulses transferred to the ventricles, but nevertheless at acute onset, the ventricular rate is normally fast with a variable rate between 90 and 160 beats per minute (bpm) (Figure 3.11). The patient may present with palpitations, breathlessness, and circulatory collapse if the onset is sudden. Patients with pre-existing heart disease and poor ventricular function may develop chest pain and acute left ventricular failure. Patients will be distressed and frightened by this arrhythmia especially as they will be aware of the fast, irregular heartbeat. If the arrhythmia persists there is the potential for thrombus formation due to atrial stasis and this puts the patient at risk of thromboembolic events such as embolic stroke or pulmonary embolism.

Causes

AF is the result of conditions that dilate the atria such as mitral valve disease, dilated cardiomyopathy, and hypertension. AF is the most common arrhythmia affecting individuals over the age of 65 and is often idiopathic in origin. Reversible causes of AF include excess alcohol and caffeine consumption, hypoxia, chest infections, fluid overload, and drugs that can cause tachycardia such as salbutamol (NICE 2014a).

Treatment

The management of atrial fibrillation is complex and dependent on the cause, nature, and duration of the arrhythmia. Sudden-onset AF requires urgent referral to the medical team. The urgency of treatment depends on the patient's symptoms and any underlying pre-existing heart disease that may exacerbate the physiological response. The aims of treatment include management of the patient's symptoms, ventricular rate control, restoration of sinus rhythm,

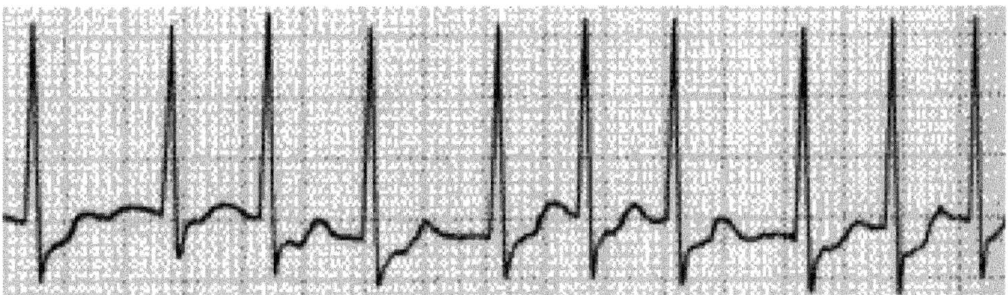

Figure 3.11 Atrial fibrillation.

Table 3.7 Treatment of acute onset atrial fibrillation

Aims of treatment	Treatment strategy
Management of patient's symptoms	Reassure patient and accompanying family to minimize distress Institute 15-min monitoring of heart rate, rhythm, blood pressure, respiratory rate, oxygen saturation If breathless sit upright and administer prescribed oxygen If hypotensive, semi-prone position to maintain blood pressure and conscious level If the patient has life-threatening haemodynamic compromise, electrical cardioversion will be carried out immediately
Ventricular rate control	This is used prior to cardioversion whilst awaiting anticoagulation therapy to achieve therapeutic levels Drugs used include β-blockers (sotalol) and calcium channel blockers (diltiazem).
Restoration of sinus rhythm	Restoration of sinus rhythm may be achieved by electrical or pharmacological cardioversion Electrical cardioversion under short-term general anaesthetic is used if the arrhythmia is less than 48 h in duration. Antiarrhythmic therapy is used following the procedure to maintain sinus rhythm Pharmacological cardioversion is also used in the first 48 h; various antiarrhythmic agents may be administered intravenously. including amiodarone or flecainide.
Prevention of thromboembolic events	The risk of thromboembolism increases after the arrhythmia has been present for 48 h Transoesophageal echocardiogram can be used to identify intracardiac thrombus in patients at risk Intravenous heparin is used acutely followed by oral anticoagulation such as warfarin or rivaroxaban

Data from Furster V et al. ACC/AHA/ESC 2006 Guidelines for the Management of Patients with Atrial Fibrillation: a report of the American College of Cardiology/American Heart Association Task Force on Practice Guidelines and the European Society of Cardiology Committee for Practice Guidelines (Writing Committee to Revise the 2001 Guidelines for the Management of Patients With Atrial Fibrillation): developed in collaboration with the European Heart Rhythm Association and the Heart Rhythm Society. *Circulation*. 2006 Aug 15; 114(7): e257–354; and NICE (2014a) Atrial fibrillation: Management Clinical Guideline 180 National Institute for Health and Clinical Excellence, London. https://www.nice.org.uk/guidance/cg180 Accessed on 12/12/2017.

and prevention of thromboembolic events (Table 3.7). Thromboembolic events are of particular concern in paroxysmal AF.

Atrioventricular (heart) block

In AV block there is a delay or absence of conduction between the atria and the ventricles. AV block is divided into first-, second-, and third-degree block with third-degree block being the most serious.

In *first-degree AV block* all sinus impulses reach the ventricles but there is a delay at the AV node resulting in a prolonged PR interval, which will measure more than 200 ms. The QRS duration and shape is normal.

First-degree AV block is a normal variant in the elderly and in athletes (Figure 3.12). It may also be induced by drugs that slow conduction through the AV node such as β-blockers and digoxin. It requires no treatment unless it occurs in association with acute myocardial infarction when it may be a precursor to second- and third-degree AV block. In this case, careful monitoring should be instituted.

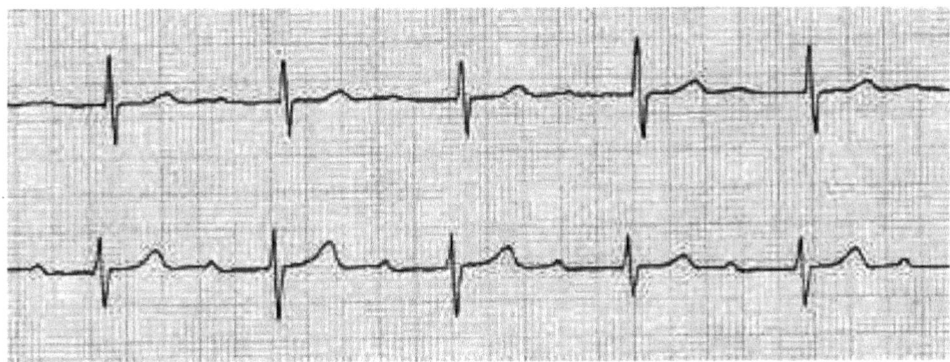

Figure 3.12 First degree AV block.

Second-degree AV block occurs when some impulses reach the ventricles and others do not. There are two types of second-degree block: Mobitz type 1 (Wenckebach) and Mobitz type 2.

Wenckebach block (Mobitz type 1) is usually relatively benign and rarely progresses to third-degree block (Figure 3.13). It is characterized by progressive prolongation of the PR interval followed by a failure of conduction to the ventricles (resulting in a 'dropped beat'). The whole process is then repeated and generally follows a pattern (i.e. fourth or fifth beat dropped). The PR interval becomes progressively lengthened, whilst the QRS complex remains normal. Treatment is not normally required, although careful monitoring should be maintained to ensure that the block does not progress further.

Mobitz type 2 block is more likely to progress to third-degree heart block. There is a varying ratio of conduction to the ventricles (i.e. two P waves to one QRS, three P waves to one QRS, etc.). The PR interval remains constant and the QRS is normal (Figure 3.14). Mobitz type 2 block indicates disease in the conduction system and is often associated with inferior myocardial infarction. If the block is 2:1 then the patient's rate may be very slow and their blood pressure significantly compromised. Temporary transvenous or transcutaneous pacing may be needed.

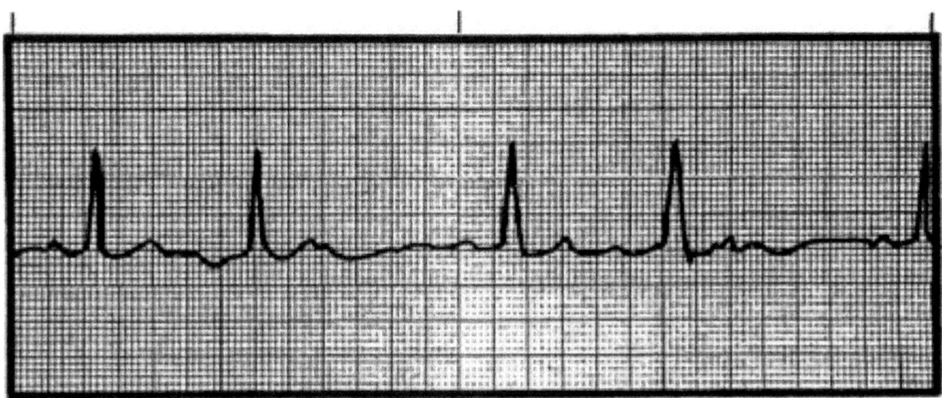

Figure 3.13 Mobitz Type 1 AV block (Wenckebach).

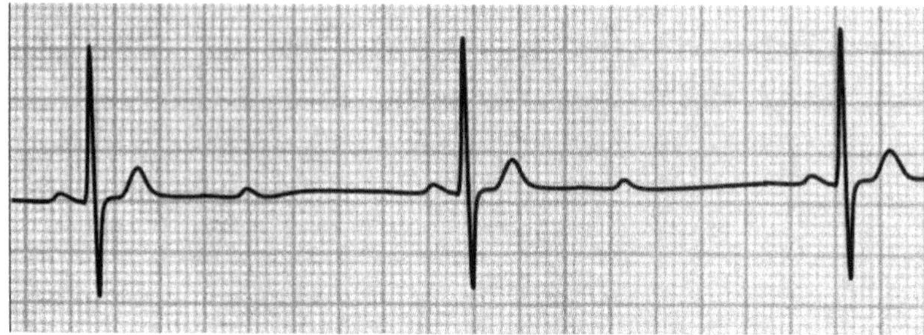

Figure 3.14 Mobitz Type 2 AV block.

Third-degree (complete) AV block occurs suddenly following acute myocardial infarction, an episode of myocarditis or cardiac surgery, or alternatively may present in a chronic form in elderly patients when the underlying pathology is progressive fibrosis of the conduction system. There is complete failure of conduction from the atria to the ventricles at the AV node. An escape pacemaker generates a ventricular rhythm and the QRS is generally wide and bizarre and at a rate between 20 and 50, dependent on where the escape pacemaker originates (AV junction, His–Purkinje system) (see Figure 3.15).

Treatment depends on the patient's haemodynamic compromise. In acute anterior myocardial infarction the presence of third-degree AV block indicates extensive infarction and urgent temporary pacing is required. Temporary pacing may be instituted either externally (transthoracic) or via the transvenous route. Permanent pacing is usually required in chronic third-degree AV block.

Ventricular tachycardia

All ventricular arrhythmias are serious and potentially life-threatening and all require urgent intervention. Further guidance on the management of patients with ventricular arrhythmias is given by the Resuscitation Council—UK (2017). Ventricular tachycardia generally occurs in patients with serious underlying heart disease. An ectopic focus in the ventricles stimulates a fast and regular rhythm that overrides the normal conduction system and results in a fast regular rate. There are no discernible P waves; the QRS complexes are wide and bizarre and the rate is between 120 and 250 beats per minute.

Causes

This commonly arises following myocardial infarction but may also result from digoxin toxicity.

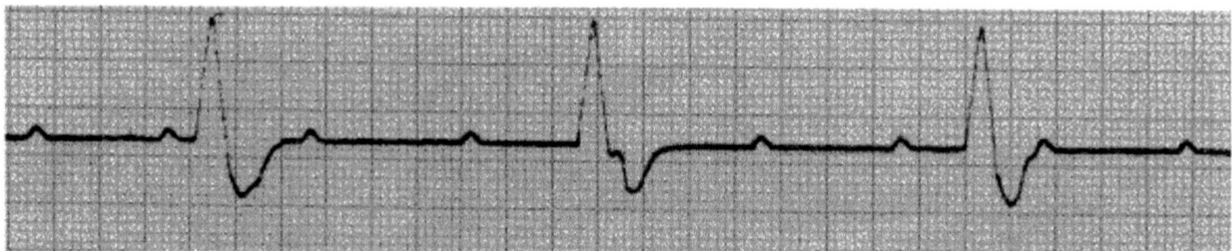

Figure 3.15 Third degree AV block.

Treatment

Treatment should be initiated urgently as the arrhythmia will result in severe haemodynamic compromise. Medical emergency teams should be summoned and emergency equipment made available at the bedside. Ventricular tachycardia is a cardiac arrest rhythm and should be treated according to current resuscitation protocols (see Chapter 11). Emergency treatment may include electrical cardioversion or anti-tachycardia therapy such as amiodarone infusion. Underlying hypokalaemia, ischaemia, or acidosis should also be treated.

Ventricular fibrillation

This is a cardiac arrest scenario and should be treated according to current resuscitation protocols (Chapter 11). It is easily identifiable on the monitor as rapid, chaotic, irregular waveforms with no discernible P waves or QRS complexes. There are no effective cardiac contractions and consequently no cardiac output; the patient will require immediate cardiopulmonary resuscitation (CPR).

Causes

Ventricular fibrillation occurs following myocardial infarction, hypoxia, metabolic disturbances, drug overdose, electrocution, and drowning.

Treatment

Immediate defibrillation is the only treatment and should be administered as early as possible in the cardiac arrest scenario (see Chapter 11).

Asystole

Sometimes referred to as ventricular standstill; this is another cardiac arrest scenario. There is effectively no electrical activity evident on the monitor and a 'flat line' will be evident. This may also occur when electrodes are detached from leads and thus is worth checking before calling arrest teams. The patient will collapse suddenly and have no cardiac or respiratory activity. Immediate CPR should be commenced, and emergency equipment organized at the bedside.

Causes

Causes are the same as for ventricular fibrillation, although the prognosis is poor.

Treatment

Treatment is as per current resuscitation protocols (see Chapter 11).

Pulseless electrical activity

Pulseless electrical activity (PEA) was previously defined as 'electromechanical dissociation'. It occurs when there is electrical activity that does not result in mechanical contraction of the heart. P waves, QRS complexes, and T waves are evident on the monitor, although the rhythm will look slightly abnormal and may be slow. There will be no discernible pulses and the patient will be collapsed. It should be treated as a cardiac arrest scenario and early CPR should be initiated (see Chapter 11).

Causes

Causes are classified under the easy to remember '4Hs and 4Ts' identified by the Resuscitation Council guidelines (2017):

- hypoxia
- hypovolaemia
- hyper/hypokalaemia (and other metabolic disorders)
- hypothermia
- tension pneumothorax
- tamponade
- toxic/therapeutic disturbances
- thromboembolism

Treatment

Treatment is directed at finding the cause, although PEA is difficult to manage and rarely successfully treated.

The clinical consequences of cardiac arrhythmias

Most cardiac arrhythmias are easily recognizable if a systematic approach is undertaken. The clinical consequences of cardiac arrhythmias are variable but are generally more pronounced in patients with pre-existing heart disease. Most cardiac arrhythmias will affect cardiac output and subsequently will affect the patient's haemodynamic state. Tachycardias are particularly serious as they lead to a reduction in ventricular filling time, with a concomitant drop in cardiac output. Tachycardias also reduce diastolic coronary artery filling time and lead to reduced myocardial perfusion. Cardiac arrhythmias thus cause many deleterious symptoms for patients, including chest pain, breathlessness, palpitations, and syncope.

Clinical link 3.1 (see Appendix for answers)

Mrs Jones, a 65-year-old lady, was admitted to the medical admissions unit for investigation of palpitations and breathlessness. In A&E her admission 12-lead ECG was 'unremarkable'. She is complaining of palpitations and says she feels dizzy. Her monitor shows the following:

Examine the arrhythmia identified above and consider:

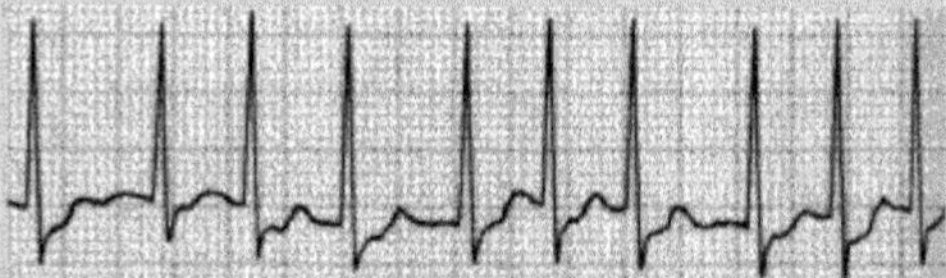

- systematic analysis of the arrhythmia, including diagnosis
- nursing actions for the next 10 m
- possible medical intervention

Common cardiovascular problems

Cardiac arrhythmias may arise in many cardiac conditions. The remainder of this chapter will focus on acute coronary syndromes, heart failure, and cardiogenic shock.

Acute coronary syndromes (ACS)

ACS describes a spectrum of cardiac conditions ranging from ST-segment elevation myocardial infarction (STEMI) and non-ST-segment elevation myocardial infarction (n-STEMI) to unstable angina (UA). ACS is a medical emergency and requires rapid treatment to reduce mortality and morbidity.

ACS can be life threatening and is the most common cause of sudden cardiac death amongst adults in the United Kingdom (British Heart Foundation 2017). Acute reduction in oxygenation to the myocardium induces chest pain and increases the likelihood of potentially fatal ventricular arrhythmias. Prompt response and early diagnosis forms the cornerstone of the management of patients with suspected ACS; treatment is time-dependent, and patients should be managed in a tertiary cardiac centre.

Pathophysiology

ACS is the clinical manifestation of rupture or erosion of the atheromatous plaque (described earlier in this chapter), followed by coronary artery occlusion with intraluminal thrombus and/or distal embolization. The exposure of the lipid-rich plaque results in the rapid accumulation and activation of platelets. The platelets induce localized vasoconstriction leading to either partial (n-STEMI/UA) or total occlusion (STEMI) of the coronary artery with thrombus. The severity of the outcome is determined by the volume of the myocardium affected and the subsequent myocardial necrosis (ESC 2017) and the management strategy depends on the occlusive nature of the thrombus. The underlying cause of ACS is similar (coronary artery disease) but the pathological process and the damage to the myocardium varies with the three types of ACS (see Table 3.8).

Table 3.8 Pathological process in different acute coronary syndromes

Type of acute coronary syndrome	Pathological processes	Myocardial damage/ cardiac marker raised
Unstable angina	Partial occlusion of coronary artery with platelet rich thrombus	Nil necrosis troponin T/I nil
N-STEMI	Partial occlusion of coronary artery with platelet-rich thrombus and vasoconstriction	Limited myocardial damage Positive troponin T/I levels
STEMI	Occlusion of coronary artery with fibrin-rich thrombus and vasconstriction	Myocardial damage. Positive troponin T/I levels

Data from European Society of Cardiology (2017) ESC Guidelines for the management of acute myocardial infarction in patients presenting with ST- segment elevation. Available at: https:// academic.oup.com/ eurheartj/ article/ 39/ 2/ 119/ 4095042; accessed 12 January 2020.

Clinical presentation

Many patients will present with acute symptoms which may result in circulatory collapse, others however may experience no symptoms at all. Classically, ACS may present with the following clinical features:

- chest pain—retrosternal, radiation to left (or less commonly right) arm, jaw, throat, back
- anxiety—some patients have a sense of 'impending death'
- increased parasympathetic (vagal) activation—nausea/vomiting
- increased sympathetic activation—sweating, pallor, tachycardia, and slightly raised blood pressure

Some patients, particularly the elderly patients and those with renal disease or diabetes, may present with more ambiguous symptoms and these patients may have atypical pain, less autonomic disturbance, a more insidious onset, or even, in the case of diabetic patients, no pain at all due to autonomic neuropathy (O'Donovan 2013). Significant gender differences have also been identified, with women who sustain ACS suffering more frequent complications and worse long-term outcome (Khamis *et al.* 2016).

High-risk patients may present with tachycardia, hypotension, or breathlessness, and these symptoms indicate a larger area of myocardial necrosis, which may form a penumbra for serious ventricular arrhythmias or acute left ventricular failure.

All patients with suspected ACS should be managed as an emergency and early medical intervention is required. Most hospitals should have fast-tracking procedures to ensure timely intervention within an acute cardiac care environment (Macdonald et al, 2016).

Clinical diagnosis

The diagnosis of ACS is made on the triad of indicators:

- clinical presentation and patient history (as above)
- 12-lead ECG
- cardiac markers.

12-lead ECG

The diagnosis of STEMI is indicated by the following criteria (in the absence of left bundle branch block or left ventricular hypertrophy):

ST-segment elevation ≥1 mm at the J point in two or more adjacent leads except for V2 and V3 where the following applies:

- Males under 40 years ST-segment elevation ≥ 2.5 mm
- Males over 40 years ST-segment elevation ≥ 2.0 mm
- Females any age ST-segment elevation ≥ 1.5 mm

(Thygesen *et al.* 2018; ESC 2017)

An example of an ST segment elevation myocardial infarction (STEMI) is shown in Figure 3.16. Note the ST segment elevation in leads II, III, aVF (inferior wall) and the reciprocal ST segment depression in leads aVL, V1–V3.

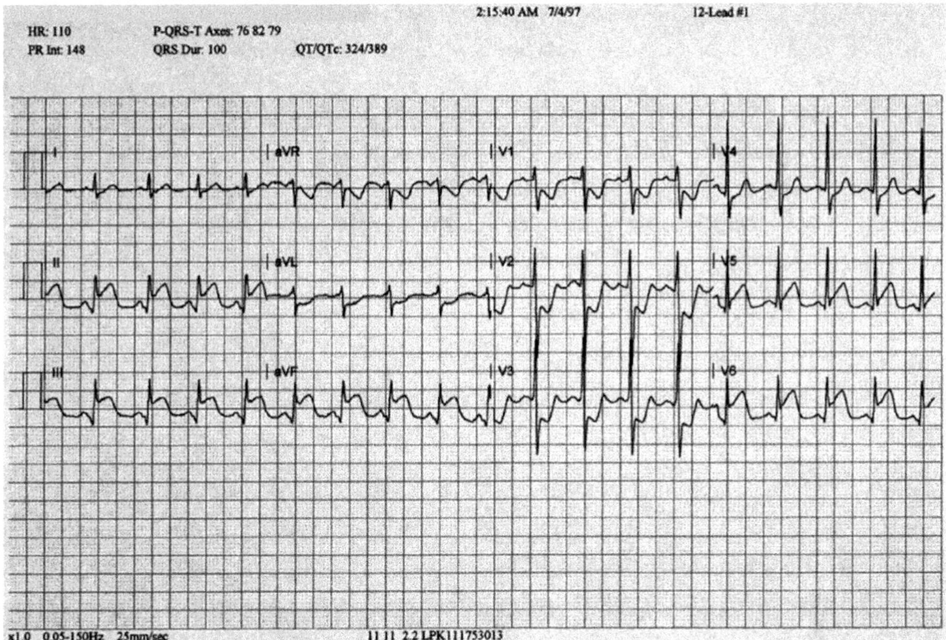

Figure 3.16 12-lead ECG showing STEMI.

12-lead ECG criteria indicative of myocardial ischaemia also include (Thygesen *et al.* 2018; ESC, 2017)

- ST-segment depression $\geq$ 0.5 mm in two adjacent leads
- T wave inversion in two adjacent leads

Cardiac markers (biochemistry)

The damaged myocardium will release enzymes or proteins into the bloodstream that can be measured within minutes/hours of presentation with chest pain. The most commonly used marker of cardiac injury is troponin T which should be measured on admission and then repeated 3–6 hours later. High sensitivity troponin can be measured at 0 hours and repeated at 3 hours (Thygesen *et al.* 2018). The troponin level will be raised in STEMI or n-STEMI but remains normal in UA.

Management of ACS

Treatment should be expedited to ensure haemodynamic stability, alleviate symptoms and establish coronary reperfusion. The main aims of treatment for the patient with a suspected ACS are to:

- relieve pain
- relieve anxiety
- use pharmacological strategies to inhibit further thrombus formation
- use mechanical strategies to achieve coronary reperfusion

Pain relief

Early relief of pain is essential, and many patients will find the pain both severe and frightening. The severity of the pain may result in a sympathetic response, which may further exacerbate the ischaemia and the potential for cardiac arrhythmias. Early intervention therefore requires the use of an opiate (morphine or diamorphine) administered intravenously with an anti-emetic. The routine use of supplemental oxygen is no longer recommended unless the oxygen saturation (SpO_2) is ≤ 90–94%. (Stub *et al.* 2015; NICE 2016b; ESC 2017). NICE (2016b) and ESC (2017) have different thresholds for the administration of oxygen and practitioners should follow their NHS Trust policy. High concentration of oxygen may increase vasoconstriction which can be deleterious to coronary artery flow. For patients with chronic obstructive pulmonary disease who may be at risk of hypercapnic respiratory failure, the aim should be to achieve a target SpO2 of 88–92% until blood gas analysis is available.

Anxiety management

Anxiety is often linked to the pain and to the patient's perception of the severity of the situation. Additionally, the sudden release of catecholamines during a stressful event, increases the risk of significant tachyarrhythmias. Some patients do describe a sense of 'impending death' and the intravenous opiates will also relieve the anxiety stimulated by catecholamine release. Constant reassurance and explanation for patients is essential and skilled nurses with enhanced communication skills are the cornerstones of good nursing care.

Most patients with ACS should be managed in a designated cardiac care unit where staff have advanced skills of clinical assessment, highly honed technological skills and are able to communicate effectively with the patient and family whilst maintaining ongoing patient monitoring (Macdonald *et al.* 2016).

The underlying pathophysiology is total or partial occlusion of a major coronary artery and this mandates early, and rapid coronary artery reperfusion preceded by pharmacological therapy. The onset of ACS results from rupture of the atheromatous plaque and exposure of the lipid core. This activates platelets which adhere to the site; platelet activation and aggregation lead to stimulation of the clotting cascade and thrombus formation.

Pharmacological therapy

Reducing platelet activity is fundamental and all patients should be prescribed aspirin which reduces production of thromboxane A_2, a powerful vasoconstrictor. Dual anti-platelet therapy (DAPT) is now the cornerstone of treatment for any patient with ACS and thienopyridines block the adenosine diphosphate receptor (P_2Y_{12}) to limit still further platelet activity. All patients will therefore be prescribed aspirin and one of the following; clopidogrel, prasugrel, or ticagrelor (ESC 2017). DAPT is potent and its use increases the risk of bleeding so the nurse should be alert to this potential complication and monitor and advise patients accordingly.

Mechanical strategies to manage ACS

The management strategy for patients with STEMI and n-STEMI differs; patients who have a confirmed STEMI will have primary percutaneous coronary intervention (p-PCI) to reopen the narrowed or occluded coronary artery to restore blood flow to the heart muscle. This involves cannulation of the radial artery, balloon angioplasty, deployment of a stent, and DAPT post-operatively to avoid the complication of in-stent thrombosis. This procedure is time-dependent and the target 'door-to-balloon time' is currently recommended as no more than 60 min and the 'call-to-balloon time' is recommended as no more than 120 min (ESC 2017).

Box 3.1 Risk criteria for early invasive strategies in n-STEMI

High risk features:

- Haemodynamic instability/cardiogenic shock
- Recurrent chest pain refractory to medical treatment
- Serious ventricular arrhythmias or cardiac arrest
- Acute heart failure
- Recurrent dynamic ST-T wave changes on ECG
- Rise in cardiac troponin consistent with MI

Patients who have n-STEMI will be stabilized with DAPT and anti-thrombin therapy such as low-molecular-weight heparin or fondaparinux. Acute risk assessment for n-STEMI guides the treatment plan, site of treatment (i.e. cardiac care unit, intermediate care unit, or in-hospital monitored bed), and the timing of angiography. Risk assessment using the Global Registry of Acute Coronary Events (GRACE) risk calculator (Fox *et al.* 2014) will enable a decision regarding the acute management plan, need for angiography, and long-term prognosis. Risk criteria requiring early invasive strategies are indicated in Box 3.1.

Nursing management of patients with ACS

Patients with ACS should preferably be nursed on an acute cardiac care unit or level 2 care area with access to continuous heart-rhythm monitoring preferably with more than a single lead; continuous 12-lead ECG monitoring is ideal. During the acute phase of ACS the patient is at risk of ventricular arrhythmias, notably ventricular ectopics which may precede ventricular tachycardia or ventricular fibrillation.

Assessment of respiratory rate, oxygen saturation, heart rate, rhythm, and blood pressure will be required at regular intervals. Assessment of any ongoing or residual chest pain or discomfort is also essential, repeat 12-lead ECG recordings to assess any dynamic ST-segment changes or arrhythmias should be carried out and analgesia offered to reduce pain levels.

The patient and their family are likely to be very anxious and it is essential to establish a good rapport at admission and to give the patient enough information to understand their diagnosis and treatment plan.

Patients who have sustained a STEMI will have a PCI procedure performed in the cardiac catheter laboratory via a radial arterial approach although in a small minority of patients a femoral approach is used. On return to the ward, assessment and management of the site is an essential skill and evaluation of peripheral pulses and the puncture site are particularly important as the patient has increased bleeding risks due to the antiplatelet and anticoagulant drugs. The contrast dye used during the procedure may affect renal function and ongoing monitoring of urinary output, urea, and electrolytes is essential, especially if the patient has pre-existing renal disease or is on other drugs which may be nephrotoxic such as metformin (Macdonald *et al.* 2016).

Patients with n-STEMI will be monitored continuously for evidence of ongoing ischaemia and for the need for an early angiogram (see Box 3.1). Regular assessment for haemodynamic instability, chest pain/other discomfort, arrhythmias, and heart failure is a vital part of the nursing role. All patients with n-STEMI will undergo a coronary angiogram and/or angioplasty within 72 hours of admission but earlier if any of the risk criteria in Box 3.1 arise (ESC 2015).

Complications of acute coronary syndrome

The patient with acute coronary syndromes may develop complications during the in-hospital stay. The main complications are arrhythmias; atrial fibrillation and ventricular arrhythmias (previously discussed), acute heart failure, and cardiogenic shock.

Heart failure—diagnosis

Heart failure can be defined as the inability of the heart to maintain sufficient output to meet the metabolic demands of the peripheral tissues. It is a clinical syndrome with typical clinical symptoms such as breathlessness, tachycardia, hypotension, and anxiety, accompanied by signs such as elevated jugular venous pressure (JVP), pulmonary and peripheral oedema. Heart failure is diagnosed by identification of these clinical symptoms and evidence of cardiac dysfunction on an echocardiogram (Ponikowski *et al.* 2016). Echocardiography evaluates the ejection fraction, which is the percentage of blood ejected by the ventricles per beat and it is normally ≥ 50%. Heart failure may occur with reduced ejection fraction < 40% (HFrEF), this is also known as left ventricular systolic dysfunction (LVSD). Heart failure with preserved ejection fraction (HFpEF) is termed diastolic dysfunction and is due to elevated filling pressures in the heart caused by conditions such as hypertension and hypertrophic cardiomyopathy. Acute decompensated heart failure (ADHF) is defined as the rapid onset of symptoms or a change to existing symptoms of heart failure (Riley 2013). It may be the patient's first presentation of the condition or it may represent an acute deterioration of an existing problem. This chapter will focus upon the management of ADHF which is usually due to sudden onset of an arrhythmia or following an acute myocardial infarction. It is essential that acute care nurses can recognize an episode of ADHF, assess the patient appropriately, and initiate rapid treatment to relieve the patient's symptoms and stabilize their condition.

Acute decompensated heart failure

Pathophysiology

ADHF occurs as a response to factors that increase the workload of the heart reducing its ability to maintain stroke volume. Initially compensatory measures designed to maintain cardiac output evolve which, whilst helpful in normal physiological circumstances, play a role in the development of acute heart failure (Young 2017).

Compensatory measures

When left ventricular function is impaired there is a fall in cardiac output and the following neuro-hormonal compensatory mechanisms develop:

- The sympathetic nervous system is stimulated and this adrenergic stimulation increases heart rate and myocardial contractility. The elevated catecholamine activity results in

increased peripheral vasoconstriction. This results in increased heart rate and blood pressure, reduced peripheral perfusion to the skin and vital organs, and increases in venous return.
- The heart dilates in response to the pressure and volume load. This increases the degree of myocardial fibre stretch to maintain stroke volume (Starling's Law). However, in the presence of cardiac injury, the cardiac reserve does not permit an increase in cardiac output and there is increased myocardial energy consumption.
- The renin–angiotensin–aldosterone system (RAAS) is activated due to stimulation of the β_1-adrenergic receptors on the juxta-glomerular apparatus in the kidney. Additionally, reduced renal perfusion activates baroreceptors in the renal arterioles stimulating renin production. Stimulation of the RAAS increases concentrations of renin, plasma angiotensin II, and aldosterone. This leads to marked vasoconstriction, an increase in sodium and water retention, and increased potassium excretion (Young 2017).

Thus, a vicious spiral of events results in the symptoms observed in the patient and constitutes a clinical emergency. Movement of fluid into the pulmonary alveoli causes oedema of the pulmonary membranes and airway narrowing. This reduction in lung compliance makes breathing difficult and reduces gaseous exchange in the alveoli. This leads to extreme breathlessness, arterial hypoxaemia, increased mucus production, and cough.

Clinical presentation

The patient presents with the following signs and symptoms:

- acute breathlessness
- extreme anxiety
- tachycardia
- hypotension
- cough, wheeze
- pink, frothy sputum (pulmonary oedema)

The priorities of management include reassuring the patient, reducing volume and pressure overload, and enhancing fluid excretion.

Management of acute decompensated heart failure

This is an acute medical emergency and successful management requires physicians and nurses to work together to relieve the patient's symptoms rapidly.

The patient should be sat upright as this reduces venous return to the heart, thus reducing the formation of pulmonary oedema. *Oxygen* should not be used routinely in the non-hypoxaemic patient as it causes vasoconstriction and further reduction in cardiac output. It should be given if the patient's oxygen saturation ($Sp0_2$) is < 94% and continuous positive airway pressure (CPAP), non-invasive positive pressure ventilation (NIPPV), or non-invasive ventilation (NIV) may be useful for those with respiratory distress (Ponikowski *et al.* 2016). NICE (2014) only recommend the use of NIPPV for cardiogenic pulmonary oedema with severe dyspnoea and acidaemia when the patient has failed to respond to other medical therapy. CPAP/NIPPV or NIV with high flow oxygen via nasal specs provide respiratory support during inspiration and expiration. CPAP and NIPPV have beneficial effects on both the respiratory and cardiac function of a patient with heart failure. During continuous positive airway pressure, the pressure splints open the alveoli, preventing the small airways from collapsing under the high pressure of pulmonary vascular congestion. NIV also prevents further fluid from moving into the alveoli, improving hypoxaemia. However, CPAP can also be deleterious to cardiac function and should be used with caution in patients who are hypotensive or who have cardiac arrhythmias. For a further discussion of NIV methods, see Chapter 2.

An *intravenous loop diuretic*, such as furosemide, should be administered. This is a powerful diuretic and venodilator and will help the failing heart by reducing circulating blood volume and reducing preload. It will have an immediate effect on the patient's breathlessness by reducing pulmonary pressures, the patient's fluid balance, renal function and electrolyte levels should be closely monitored. An indwelling urinary catheter will facilitate careful monitoring of the urine output.

Intravenous *nitrates* reduce preload by venodilation and help to reduce pulmonary congestion rapidly. IV nitrates are useful for symptomatic relief when the blood pressure is > 90 mmHg. Continuous blood pressure monitoring is essential.

Inotropes may be required if the patient is severely compromised with reduced organ perfusion. Intravenous inotropes such as dobutamine or dopamine increase cardiac output and peripheral perfusion, but complications include tachycardia and myocardial ischaemia and they should be used with caution and only administered in an acute cardiac care or level 2 care facility (Ponikowski *et al.* 2016).

Routine use of *opiates* is not recommended but they are occasionally used cautiously in patients with severe dyspnoea and pulmonary oedema. The side effects include hypotension, bradycardia, and respiratory depression which may potentially increase the need for invasive ventilation (Ponikowski *et al.* 2016).

For the management of chronic heart failure in adults, see NICE (2018) guidelines for a comprehensive discussion of the diagnosis and management plans for these patients.

Cardiogenic shock

Cardiogenic shock is the final result of failure of the compensatory mechanisms described above. Cardiogenic shock is defined as decreased cardiac output with critical end-organ hypoperfusion in the presence of adequate intravascular volume (Tharmaratnam *et al.* 2013; Thiele *et al.* 2015). It is caused by myocardial damage most commonly following an acute myocardial infarction.

Clinical diagnosis

Established criteria (Thiele *et al.* 2015) are

- systolic blood pressure < 90 mmHg for > 30 mins or inotropes required to achieve a blood pressure of ≥ 90 mmHg.
- pulmonary congestion
- impaired organ perfusion with at least one of the following
  - altered mental status
  - cold, clammy skin
  - oliguria
  - increased serum lactate

Management of cardiogenic shock

Early comprehensive assessment with 12-lead ECG, echocardiography, and angiography is indicated and invasive monitoring with an arterial line is advocated; the patient should be transferred to a level 2 care facility such as an Acute Cardiac Care Unit or Intensive Care Unit (Ponikowski *et al.* 2016).

Intravenous pharmacological therapy aims to increase blood pressure, increase cardiac output, and improve organ dysfunction. Various inotropic drugs are used; noradrenaline is used to maintain the mean arterial pressure, dobutamine, milrinone, or levosimendan are used alone or in combination. Finally, intra-aortic balloon pump (IABP) may be used for intractable patients although recently the IABP-SHOCK II trial did not demonstrate improved outcomes in patients with acute myocardial infarction and cardiogenic shock (Thiele *et al.* 2013).

Clinical link 3.2 (see Appendix for answers)

You are caring for a 60-year-old female patient who sustained STEMI two days ago. She is due for discharge tomorrow. She has seen the cardiac rehabilitation team and has also discussed her discharge medications with the pharmacist.

It is 18:00 and you record a routine set of vital signs:

Temperature: 36.4°C.
Radial pulse: 95 bpm irregular (recording at 14:00 was 65 bpm regular).
Blood pressure: 110/50 mmHg (recording at 06:00 was 126/70 mmHg).
Respiratory rate: 26 breaths/min (recording at 06:00 was 14/min).
O_2 saturations: 88% on air.

You note that she is breathless on minimal exertion and you also note that she appears slightly cyanosed peripherally. Capillary refill is 3 s. She denies any chest pain.

- What would your next immediate actions be and why?
- What other investigations is the doctor likely to perform and why?
- What are the potential problems evolving in this situation?

End of chapter test

The following assessment will enable you to evaluate your theoretical knowledge of cardiovascular assessment and management as well as your ability to apply this theory to clinical practice. You should undertake the following assessment with an appropriately trained member of staff in clinical practice. If you are unable to answer any questions it may be helpful to revisit the section in this chapter.

Knowledge assessment

With the support of your mentor/supervisor from practice, work through the following prompts to explore your knowledge level about cardiovascular assessment, care, and management.

- Describe the anatomy and blood flow through the heart.
- Describe the normal compensatory mechanisms that help regulate blood pressure.
- Discuss the coronary artery circulation and the anatomical regions supplied by each coronary artery.
- Describe the normal waveforms on the ECG and discuss the normal amplitude and duration parameters.
- Explain the important aspects of taking a cardiac history and discuss commonly presenting symptoms of cardiac disease.
- Differentiate the various causes of chest pain.
- Critically analyse factors which contribute to the formation of atherosclerosis.
- Recognize commonly encountered arrhythmias (supraventricular tachycardia, atrial fibrillation, and third-degree AV block) and discuss nursing and medical interventions.
- Define acute coronary syndromes and differentiate between the presentation of different types of acute coronary syndromes.
- Discuss the underlying pathophysiology for acute decompensated heart failure and explain how management strategies are used to treat patients with this condition.
- Discuss signs of impending cardiogenic shock and appropriate management.
- Differentiate types of shock, including; hypovolaemic, cardiogenic, anaphylactic, neurogenic, and septic shock.

Skills assessment

Under the guidance of your mentor/supervisor, undertake a cardiovascular assessment followed by appropriate interventions for any significant abnormality. Your mentor/supervisor will assess your ability and provide feedback based on the following skills:

- Takes a cardiac history, including key points in relation to assessment of cardiac symptoms.
- Conducts a comprehensive cardiovascular assessment and explains normal/abnormal findings related to the patient's symptoms and presentation.
- Demonstrates an ability to perform 12-lead ECG, continuous cardiac monitoring, oxygen saturation monitoring, and other vital signs.
- Identifies the need for and frequency of vital signs observation.
- Facilitates the completion of relevant clinical investigations such as blood, urine, X-ray, and ECG tests, and evaluates results.
- Liaises with other members of the healthcare team as necessary, including nurse in charge, doctor, pharmacist, and healthcare assistant.

- Recognizes the need for fast and appropriate response if cardiovascular function is deteriorating.
- Reports any new or worsening chest pain and records appropriate assessments.
- Reviews need for cardiovascular assessment and frequency of vital signs monitoring.
- Informs patient/relative of any changes.
- Demonstrates clinical reasoning and provides justification for all interventions for a patient with acute decompensated heart failure.

References

Bhatnagar, P., Wickramasinghe, K.E. Wilkins, E., *et al.* (2016) Trends in epidemiology of cardiovascular disease in the UK. *Heart*, 102(24):1945–52.

Bridges, E. (2017) Assessing patients during septic shock resuscitation. *Am J Nursing*, 117(10):34–40.

British Heart Foundation (2017) Cardiovascular Disease Statistics 2017. London: BHF. Available at: https://www.bhf.org.uk/research/heart-statistics; accessed 8 December 2019.

Bunce, N.H., Ray, R. (2017) Cardiovascular disease, in: P. Kumar and M. Clark (eds), *Clinical Medicine* 9th edn. Edinburgh: Elsevier, 931–1056.

Chaterjee, K., Topol, E.L. (2015) *Cardiac Drugs* 2nd edn. New Delhi: Jaypee Brothers Medical Publishers.

European Society of Cardiology (2015) ESC Guidelines for the management of acute coronary syndromes in patients presenting without persistent ST-segment elevation. Available at: https://doi.org/10.1093/eurheartj/ehv320; accessed 6 January 2020.

European Society of Cardiology (2017) ESC Guidelines for the management of acute myocardial infarction in patients presenting with ST-segment elevation. Available at: https://academic.oup.com/eurheartj/article/39/2/119/4095042; accessed 12 January 2020.

Fox, K.A.A., FitzGerald, G., Puymirat, E., *et al.* (2014) Should patients with acute coronary disease be stratified for management according to their risk? Derivation, external validation and outcomes using the updated GRACE risk score. *BMJ Open* 4(2): e004425. Available at: https://bmjopen.bmj.com/content/bmjopen/4/2/e004425.full.pdf; accessed 20 January 2020.

Kato, K., Lyon, A.R., Ghadri, J-R., *et al.* (2017) Takotsubo syndrome: Aetiology, presentation and treatment. *Heart*, 103(18):1461–69.

Khamis, R.Y., Ammari, T., Mikhail, G.W. (2016) Gender differences in coronary heart disease. *Heart*, 102:1142–49.

Khan, E., Spiers, C., Khan, M. (2013) The heart and potassium: A banana republic. *Acute Cardiac Care*, 15:17–24.

Menzies-Gow, E., Spiers, C. (2018) *Rapid Cardiac Care*. Chichester: Wiley Blackwell.

Macdonald, N.J., Jones, I., Leslie, S.J. (2016) Acute coronary syndromes—the role of the CCU nurse. Part 1: initial management. *Br J Cardiac Nurs*, 11:453–8.

Mok, W., Wang, W., Cooper, S., *et al.* (2015) Attitudes towards vital signs monitoring in the detection of clinical deterioration: A Scale development and survey of ward nurses. *Int J Qual Health Care*, 27:207–13.

NICE (2014a) *Atrial Fibrillation: Management Clinical Guideline* 180. London: National Institute for Health and Care Excellence. Available at: https://www.nice.org.uk/guidance/cg180; accessed 8 December 2019.

NICE (2014b) *Acute Heart Failure: Diagnosis and Management* 184. London: National Institute for Health and Care Excellence. Available at: https://www.nice.org.uk/guidance/cg187; accessed 20 January 2020.

NICE (2016b) *Chest Pain of Recent Onset: Assessment and Diagnosis*. London: National Institute for Health and Care Excellence, London. Available at: https://www.nice.org.uk/guidance/cg95/chapter/Recommendations#people-presenting-with-acute-chest-pain; accessed 8 December 2019.

NICE (2018) *Chronic Heart Failure in Adults: Diagnosis and Management.* London: National Institute of Health and Care Excellence. Available at: https://www.nice.org.uk/guidance/ng106; accessed 8 December 2019.

O'Donovan, K. (2013) Nursing assessment of the causes of chest pain. *Br J Cardiac Nurs*, 8:483–8.

Opie, L.H., Gersh, B.J. (2013) *Drugs for the Heart* 8th edn. Philadelphia, PA: WB Saunders.

Public Health England (2016) *Action on Cardiovascular Disease: Getting Serious About Prevention.* London: Public Health England.

Ponikowski, P., Voors, A., Anker S., *et al.* (2016) ESC Guidelines for the diagnosis and treatment of acute and chronic heart failure of the European Society of Cardiology (ESC). *Eur Heart J*, 37(27):2129–200.

RCP (2017) *National Early Warning Scores: Standardizing the assessment of acute illness severity in the NHS.* London: Royal College of Physicians.

Resuscitation Council (UK) (2017) *Adult Advanced Life Support Guidelines.* London: Resuscitation Council UK. Available at: https://www.resus.org.uk/resuscitation-guidelines/adult-advanced-life-support/; accessed 8 December 2019.

Riley, J. (2013) Acute decompensated heart failure: Diagnosis and management. *Br J Nurs*, 22(22):1290–95.

Sampson, M. (2016) Understanding the ECG. Part 5: Pre-excitation. *Br J Cardiac Nur*,. 11(3):123–30.

Stub, D., Smith, K., Bernard, S., *et al* (2012) A randomised controlled trial of oxygen therapy in acute myocardial infarction. Air Verses Oxygen In myocardial infarction study (AVOID Study). *Am Heart Journal*, 163(3): 339–45.

Tharmaratnam, D., Nolan, J., Jain, A. (2013) Acute coronary syndromes: Management of cardiogenic shock complicating acute coronary syndromes. *Heart*, 99:1614–23.

Thiele, H., Zeymer, U., Neumann, F-J., *et al.* (2013) Intra-aortic balloon counterpulsation in acute myocardial infarction complicated by cardiogenic shock (IABP_SHOCK II): Final 12 month results of a randomized open-label trial. *Lancet*, 382:1638–45.

Thiele, H., Ohman, E.M., Desch, S., *et al.* (2015) Management of cardiogenic shock. *European Heart Journal*, 36:1223–30.

Thygesen, K., Alpert, J.S., Jaffe, A.S., *et al.* (2018) Fourth universal definition of myocardial infarction. *Eur Heart J.* Available at: https://doi.org/10.1093/eurheartj/ehy462; accessed 8 December 2019.

Wesley, K. (2017) *Huszar's ECG and 12-Lead Interpretation* 5th edn. St Louis, MO: Elsevier.

Young, S. (2017) An overview of current treatments in heart failure *Br J Cardiac Nurs*, 12(3):120–7.

4
Neurological care

Fiona Creed

Chapter contents

In order to understand how to assess and manage the patient with neurological conditions it is essential to have an understanding of the structure and function of the brain and how injury/illness can affect this. This chapter will examine:

- normal anatomy and physiology
- physiological changes following illness and injury
- the physiology of raised intracranial pressure and cerebral oedema
- immediate assessment of neurological function
- formal neurological assessment (to include Glasgow Coma Scale (GCS))
- nursing care of the patient with neurological injury, to include:
    - stroke
    - mild brain injury
    - seizures

Learning outcomes

This chapter will enable you to:

- develop understanding of the normal structure and function of the nervous system
- develop an understanding of changes during illness/injury
- understand the significance of neurological assessment
- examine the practice of neurological assessment
- discuss the management of common neurological problems
- understand common treatments for neurological illness
- understand when the patient with deteriorating neurological function requires urgent medical attention
- understand the impact of neurological problems on the patient and their carers
- use a skills assessment tool to assess your clinical practice

Introduction

The human brain is composed of billions of specialized cells (neurons). All the neurons a person has are present at birth. These specialist cells do not have mitotic capacity and are not replaceable. In cases of illness and injury it is therefore essential that care is delivered to prevent cell death and to preserve nervous system functioning. An adequate understanding of the nervous system's structures and functions is essential to ensure adequate assessment of this complex system, and timely and appropriate care delivery.

Normal anatomy and physiology

The nervous system is divided into two main anatomically different parts:

- the central nervous system, which includes structures and nerves within the cranium and spinal cord
- the peripheral nervous system, consisting of nerves outside the brain and spinal cord and which is further subdivided into somatic and autonomic nervous systems

The main focus of this chapter will be role of the central nervous system and the function of the brain. Reference will be made to the autonomic system in Chapters 2, 3, and 7. It may be beneficial to refer to a specific neurophysiology text if more detail is required.

The brain

The brain constitutes about 2% of total body weight. Simplistically, the brain is divided into three main areas: the cerebrum, the brain stem, and the cerebellum. Other subdivisions are explained in specialist literature. The brain is protected by the skull, the meninges, and the cerebrospinal fluid (CSF).

The skull

The purpose of the skull is to protect the most vulnerable parts of the brain. The skull provides a bony framework and consists of 8 bones of the cranium and 14 bones of the face. At around the age of 14 the bones become fused and the brain is encapsulated in a closed box. This means there is little space for swelling or bleeding within the cranial cavity.

The meninges

Immediately below the skull are the three layers of the meninges (see Figure 4.1). These cover both the brain and the spinal cord and are detailed below.

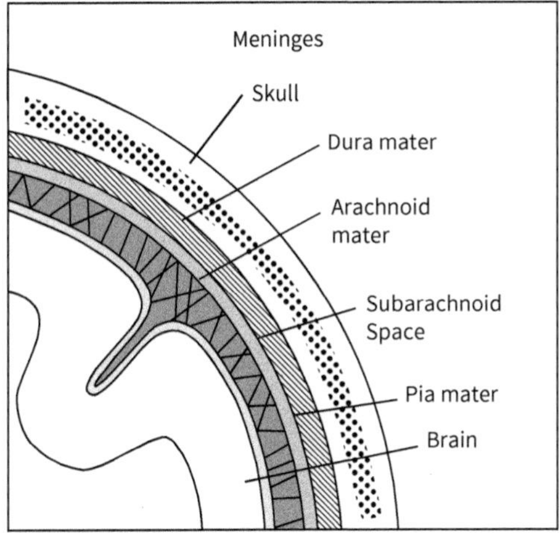

Figure 4.1 The meninges.

Dura mater

The dura mater is a double-layered, white, inelastic membrane that lies beneath the bone. Folds of dura are also situated within the skull cavity to support and protect the brain. These folds of dura mater further divide areas of the brain. The most important of these is the tentorium cerebri. The area above the tentorium is supratentorial, the area below infratentorial.

Arachnoid membrane

The arachnoid membrane is an extremely thin and delicate layer. It is separated from the dura by the subdural space. CSF flows around the subarachnoid space. It contains a large number of blood vessels. The arachnoid membrane also contains pressure sensitive 'valves', or arachnoid villi, that allow reabsorption of CSF. Blockage of these villi can cause communicating hydrocephalus.

Pia mater

The pia mater is a mesh-like vascular membrane that covers the entire surface of the brain.

Spaces of the meninges

The meninges are not fused together, and three important potential spaces occur:

- the extradural (epidural) space, between the periosteum and outer layer of dura;
- the subdural space, between the inner layer of dura and the arachnoid membrane;
- the subarachnoid space, between the arachnoid membrane and pia mater.

These potential spaces are of significance in clinical practice as they may become the focus of bleeding/haematoma formation following traumatic brain injury.

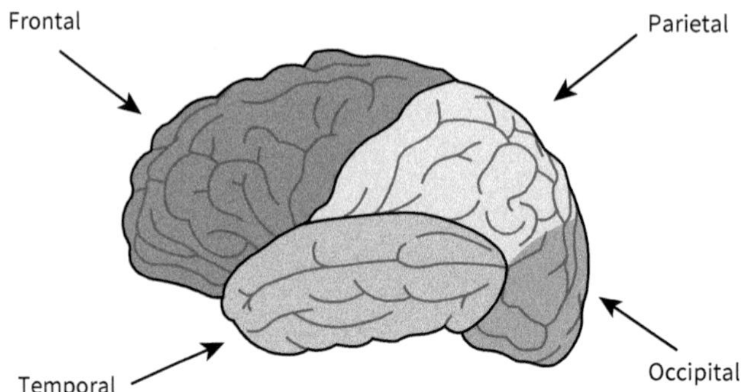

Figure 4.2 The cerebrum.

The cerebrum

The first major subdivision within the brain is the cerebrum. The cerebral cortex is often linked to higher functioning of the nervous system. The cerebrum is made up of two cerebral hemispheres, separated by the sulcus. The surface of the cerebral hemispheres consists of gyri that substantially increases the surface area of the brain. Each hemisphere is covered by a cerebral cortex of grey matter that contains billions of neurons. Under the cerebral cortex is white matter that contains nerve fibres. The cerebrum is further divided into pairs of lobes. Historically, attempts have been made to match the functions of these lobes and therefore predict expected damage following injury and illness. The advent of functional magnetic resonance imaging (MRI) scans has allowed for further classifications, but this work is not complete and more research is required. The following section highlights some of the functions of the cerebrum and discusses some symptoms of lobe damage that may occur in the patient with neurological damage. The cerebrum is divided into frontal, parietal, occipital, and temporal lobes (see Figure 4.2).

The frontal lobe

Major functions of the frontal lobe include:

- higher-level cognitive functioning such as reasoning and concentration
- memory
- emotional states
- control of voluntary eye movement
- speech production (Broca's area)
- motor function

Frontal damage can lead to some of the following:

- inability to solve problems
- personality changes
- disordered eye movement
- speech problems (expressive dysphasia)
- decreased memory

The parietal lobe

Major functions of the parietal lobe include:

- analysis of gross aspects of sensation (touch, position, pressure, etc.)
- awareness of body
- orientation in space
- perception of body positioning

Parietal damage can lead to:

- lack of conscious sensation on half of the body
- neglect of half of the body
- disorders of spatial awareness
- agnosia (difficulty in perceiving objects normally)

It should be noted that the frontal and parietal lobes work closely together to control motor/sensory function, since the sensory and motor cortex is located between these two lobes.

The temporal lobe

Major functions of the temporal lobe include:

- primary auditory receptive area
- comprehension of speech (Wernicke's area)
- memory
- learning
- intellect

Temporal lobe damage can lead to:

- disorders in learning verbal information
- memory loss
- speech problems (receptive dysphasia)

The occipital lobe

Major functions of the occipital lobe include:

- visual perception
- visual reflexes
- involuntary smooth eye movements

Occipital lobe damage can lead to:

- visual disturbances
- alterations in visual reflexes

Cerebral dominance

At birth, both cerebral hemispheres have an equal capacity for development. In adulthood most adults will have one dominant hemisphere. Left cerebral dominance is found in approximately 90% of the population. It is generally held that the patient's speech centres are located in the dominant region of the brain, hence for the majority of the population the speech centre is in the left cerebral hemisphere. This can cause significant problems with the perception and production of speech if the dominant side of the brain is affected by injury.

Corpus callosum

Although studies suggest that the right and left cerebral hemispheres function independently, it is important to acknowledge that the areas are linked. The cerebral hemispheres are connected by the corpus callosum, a thick area of nerve fibres connecting one part of the hemisphere with its corresponding part on the other side. Because of this connection the two hemispheres are intricately linked. Studies in children with damage suggest that if one hemisphere is damaged the other can take over its role. In adults neurological damage may be more debilitating as the capacity for compensation is limited.

Other structures within the cerebrum

Basal ganglia: control movement that involves both cognitive and motor processing.
Dicephalon: a major division of the cerebrum, divided into four regions, including:

- the thalamus
- the epithalamus
- the hypothalamus
- the subthalamus

The brain stem

The brain stem is the second major subdivision of the brain. The brain stem has specific functions and contains the nuclei of several of the cranial nerves. It is made up of:

- the midbrain
- the pons
- the medulla

Damage to the brain stem can be confirmed by a specific examination of cranial nerve function.

The midbrain

The midbrain's function is to act as a pathway for the cerebral hemispheres and lower brain. It is the centre for auditory and visual reflexes and contains the nuclei of the occulomotor and trochlear cranial nerves.

The pons

The pons acts as a bridge between the midbrain and the medulla. A large number of tracts (nerve pathways) go through the pons, connecting higher cerebral regions with the lower levels of the nervous system. The pons also has some control over respiratory function, including the apneustic centre and the pneumotaxic centre.

The medulla oblongata

This part of the brain stem joins the spinal cord. It is level with the foramen magnum. The decussation of pyramids occurs here (this means that the motor fibres from the left side of the brain cross over to the right side of the body, enabling the left brain to control right body movement and vice versa). The medulla also contains the cardiac, respiratory, and vasomotor centres.

Special systems within the brain

The reticular activating system

The reticular activating system (RAS) is a diffuse system that extends from lower brain to cerebral cortex. The RAS controls sleep/wake cycles, consciousness, and focused attention. Stimulation of the brain stem portion of the RAS results in wakefulness throughout the entire brain. The RAS is the physical basis of consciousness. Certain drugs can affect RAS. It is suppressed by alcohol and tranquillizers, and enhanced by some mood-altering drugs, for example LSD.

The reticular formation

The reticular formation is a group of neurons originating within the brain stem that project towards the higher parts of the nervous system. It is involved in:

- sleep/waking cycles
- control of sensory information (either inhibit or allow sensory messages to pass)
- control of responsiveness

The cerebellum

The cerebellum is the last major subdivision within the brain. It is located at the posterior fossa and is attached to the brain stem. The cerebellum has a large number of functions. These include control of fine motor movement, coordination of muscle groups, and maintenance of balance (through feedback loops). It is quickly affected by alcohol consumption and is often damaged in patients with a history of alcohol abuse.

Blood supply to the brain

About 20% of oxygen consumption in the body occurs in the brain and this is used for metabolism. A lack of oxygen, and hence glucose metabolism, for more than 5 m can cause irreversible brain damage.

The blood supply to the brain is via two pairs of arteries (the internal carotid and vertebral basilar arteries). These vessels join together to form the circle of Willis. In favorable instances

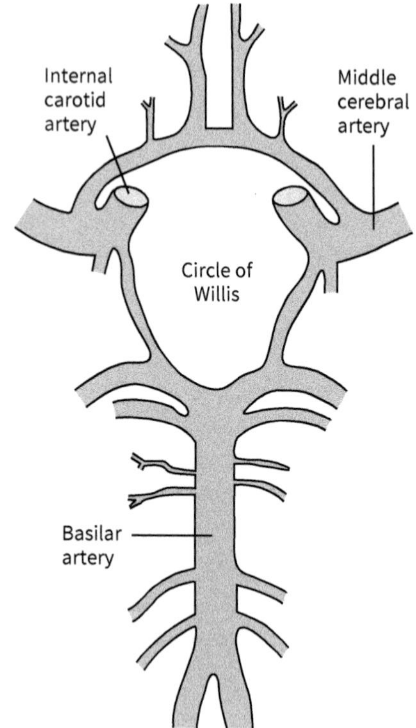

Figure 4.3 The circle of Willis.

the circle of Willis may allow an adequate blood supply to circulate in the event of damage such as occlusion (see Figure 4.3).

The venous drainage is largely managed by two vascular channels, the dural sinuses. The dural sinuses empty into the jugular veins and then back to the heart.

The blood–brain barrier

In order for the brain to function normally, it must maintain its own stable environment. The blood–brain barrier is a term used to describe the tight network of cells and capillaries that prevent anything not required by the brain from entering. Substances that cross the blood–brain barrier easily include lipids, oxygen, carbon dioxide, water, and glucose. In clinical practice it is important to note that drugs, unless bound in lipids (e.g. propofol), do not cross the blood–brain barrier easily. This is of particular significance when considering antibiotics for cerebral infection.

Cerebral spinal fluid

It was highlighted earlier that CSF has a role in the protection of the brain by acting as a 'shock absorber'. It also has a significant role in the carriage of nutrients to the brain and is sometimes referred to as a 'third circulation'. CSF is composed of water, a small amount of protein, oxygen, and carbon dioxide. It also carries electrolytes and glucose. CSF is produced in the choroid plexus, this produces about 25 mL of CSF per hour. This flows through the ventricular system and around the brain and spinal cord, where it is reabsorbed by pressure-sensitive arachnoid villi. Sometimes in neurological damage there can be problems with obstruction to flow or problems with reabsorption and this can lead to communicating hydrocephalus.

The spinal cord

The spinal cord is continuous with the medulla oblongata; it runs from the upper borders of the atlas (first cervical vertebra C1) to the lower border of the first lumbar vertebra (L1). The spinal cord is protected from injury by the spinal column and the meninges. The spinal cord allows messages to travel from the peripheral nervous system to the brain and messages from the brain to get to the peripheral nervous system. It can on occasion act as an activating centre in its own right by receiving incoming sensory impulses and initiating outgoing motor signals. This is seen in reflex arcs and is an important consideration in neurological assessment (where spinal reflex may mimic movement; this will be discussed under neurological assessment).

Damage to the central nervous system

The nursing management of patients with any neurological condition requires an understanding of the pathophysiology of the disease process and complications that can arise as a result of these changes.

Cerebral metabolism

The brain is very dependent on blood flow to provide oxygen and nutrients to the neurons and remove the end products of metabolism. Damage will quickly occur to the neuron if it is deprived of oxygen or blood for a short period or if excessive carbon dioxide accumulates. Following damage, because of their inability to replicate, neurons die and are not replaced. If sufficient numbers of neurons are damaged the patient will exhibit significant loss of neurological function. A number of factors have been shown to influence the amount of blood the brain receives (cerebral blood flow). These are often described as extracerebral (outside the brain) or intracerebral (within the brain).

Extracerebral factors

These are primarily related to the cardiovascular system and include changes in blood pressure, cardiac function, and viscosity of blood. Usually in adults, cerebral blood flow is held constant unless the mean arterial pressure (MAP) falls below 50–60 mmHg. Factors that may reduce cardiac function, for example atherosclerosis, advancing age, and cardiac dysfunction, will again only impact on cerebral blood flow if pressure is low. Cerebral blood flow is

Table 4.1 Factors affecting cerebral blood flow

Chemical change	Net effect
Increased CO_2	Cerebral vasodilatation
Decreased CO_2	Cerebral vasoconstriction
Decreased oxygen	Vasodilatation
Increased H^+ concentration	Vasodilatation

generally held constant by the ability of the brain to autoregulate its own blood flow all the time systemic pressure is sufficient. Blood viscosity changes may have an impact on flow and it is acknowledged that if the patient is anaemic, flow is increased (less resistance to flow) whereas polycythaemia may decrease flow (increased resistance to flow).

Intracerebral factors

The primary intracerebral factors are cerebral vascular artery disease and increased intracranial pressure (ICP). Widespread cerebral vascular disease can cause increased cerebral vascular resistance and hence decrease flow. Raised intracranial pressure increases the pressure within the brain that the blood has to flow against, deceasing overall perfusion. Additional changes to blood flow will occur in relation to chemical changes within the brain (see Table 4.1).

In terms of blood flow to the brain, it is usually considered more appropriate to consider cerebral perfusion pressure (CPP). Normal CPP is 60–70 mmHg. It is not directly possible to measure this in a ward/high dependency unit environment, since the equation for CPP necessitates the measurement of ICP. It is useful to monitor systemic blood pressure whilst considering any impact potential neurological damage may have on ICP.

Compensation

The brain is able, to an extent, to compensate for slight changes in ICP. According to the Monro–Kelly hypothesis, the skull is a rigid box filled to capacity with non-compressible contents: 80% brain, 10% CSF, and 10% blood. The volume of each of these should remain constant. If there is an increase in any of these then ICP will rise unless compensation occurs. Compensation within the skull is limited and is dependent on altering one of the contents, usually blood or CSF (since it is not possible to decrease amount of brain tissue). This can be done by:

- increasing CSF absorption
- decreasing CSF production
- shunting of CSF to the spinal column
- alterations in cerebral blood flow (vasoconstriction)

The ability to compensate is small and if not treated quickly the patient's ICP will rise and cause further problems with cerebral blood flow.

Pathophysiology of cerebral ischaemia

Patients with neurological damage are usually affected by secondary injury that worsens the effect of their original condition/injury. The secondary injury is usually related to problems where metabolism of neurons exceeds blood flow, resulting in ischaemia. When the brain is deprived of oxygen (for whatever reason) a chain of events occurs called the ischaemic cascade. The end point of this cascade is neuronal dysfunction and then death. In the centre of the ischaemic area (referred to as the penumbra) are a number of minimally surviving cells. The lack of O_2 causes these cells to switch to anaerobic metabolism, with a resultant decrease in adenosine triphosphate (ATP) production. ATP is required to power neurotransmission. The process of anaerobic metabolism causes the release of an excitatory neurotransmitter glutamate, which has a neurotoxic effect and ultimately causes cell lysis and eventual neuronal death. The survival of the penumbra of neurons is dependent on the re-establishment of effective cerebral circulation. If the cells of the penumbra die, the core of dead tissue increases and ultimately causes cerebral oedema and eventual death if not treated quickly. Nursing management needs to be effective to prevent further deterioration.

Nursing management of neurological conditions

Nursing management of this group of patients has some common features. Specific management will be detailed under specific subheadings. The main aim of treating patients with neurological injury is to prevent secondary damage and the cascade of problems that may lead to cerebral ischaemia and further neuronal death. It is vital that neuronal function is optimized to facilitate patient recovery and prevent further neurological deterioration. Care should be aimed at:

- accurate and timely neurological assessment
- management of symptoms to prevent secondary damage
- timely nursing/medical intervention

Of these management tools, the most important is neurological assessment and this will be discussed in detail as it is a fundamental part of neurological care. Early diagnosis of problems will lead to timely treatment that may reduce the impact of damage. It is essential that all staff should understand how to perform neurological assessment correctly so that early changes can be identified and treated promptly. Timely escalation of the patient with neurological problems is vital.

Nursing assessment of consciousness

Simplistically, consciousness is defined as state of general awareness of oneself and the environment (Hickey 2013). Consciousness is a dynamic state and levels of consciousness can change very rapidly. Consciousness may be affected by neurological or non-neurological changes (see Table 4.2).

Table 4.2 Factors affecting consciousness

Neurological causes	Systemic/metabolic causes
Acquired brain injury	Altered gaseous exchange
Tumours	Hypoglycaemia
Cerebral oedema	Hypotension
Cerebral abscesses	Hepatic failure
Brain stem infarction	Drug induced
Convulsions	Alcohol induced

Assessment of consciousness is an integral part of patient assessment. It may be simplistic or more in-depth and professional judgment and clinical care bundles will indicate the most appropriate tool.

ACVPU

The AVPU (Alert, Verbal, Pain, Unresponsive) tool has been superseded by the ACVPU following publication of the NEWS2 assessment format (RCP 2017). ACVPU is a very simplistic assessment that allows quick evaluation of conscious levels. It is not and should not replace a full neurological examination if the patient's condition requires this. It is a tool designed to be used in emergency situations to enable a very quick assessment of consciousness. It is ideal in the initial rapid ABCDE assessment of the acutely ill patient.

The ACVPU scale is:

- Alert
- Confusion (new)
- responds to Voice
- responds to Pain
- Unconscious (Resuscitation Council 2015).

The ACVPU scale is usually linked to a track-and-trigger scoring system and is used as part of the scoring system to detect acute deterioration (see Chapter 11). It may be necessary to conduct an in-depth neurological assessment following initial scoring.

There are a number of reasons to conduct an in-depth neurological assessment. These include:

- to establish a baseline of the patient's neurological function
- to determine whether the patient has a neurological condition
- to determine if the neurological condition is deteriorating
- to detect life-threatening situations and those that require immediate intervention
- to establish the impact of neurological illness on a patient

The Glasgow Coma Scale

The Glasgow Coma Scale (GCS) was introduced initially in 1974 (Teasdale and Jennett 1974) and updated recently to provide greater clarity and structure (Teasdale *et al.* 2014).

The key categories remain and these are:

- eye opening
- verbal response
- motor response

However, the descriptions of these categories have changed in an attempt to standardize assessment and enhance understanding of the process still further. A useful website explaining the assessment is found at http://www.glasgowcomascale.org/.

Teasdale and colleagues (2014) advocate the use of a structured process that will enable standardization of neurological assessment. Four steps are suggested:

- **Check**: look for factors that may interfere with assessment within the three domains of verbal eye opening and motor function; for example inability to move due to substantial fracture. Treatment regimens that may affect responses; for example tracheostomy *in situ*, trauma to eyes which may prohibit eye opening.
- **Observe**: the patient should be observed and the nurse should note whether there is spontaneous eye opening, 'normal' speech patterns, and content and bilateral movement.
- **Stimulate**: if needed, additional stimulation should be used to generate a response. This can be speech (at varying intensities) or graded pressure (note that this has replaced painful stimuli).
- **Rate**: the patient should be rated against specific criteria (see Table 4.3) and the *best* response noted (Teasdale *et al.* 2014)

When testing eye opening it is acceptable to use peripheral pressure such as pressure on side of finger. However, motor function *always* requires the use of central pressure. This should initially be a trapezius squeeze and if no response to a graded increase in pressure then supraorbital pressure should be applied (N.B. this is only acceptable in the absence of facial injury in the supraorbital area).

Following recording of GCS pupillary responses, haemodynamic observations and limbs also require assessment.

Pupil responses

Normal pupil size ranges from 2 to 6 mm, and this can be influenced by a number of factors in clinical practice (see Box 4.1) Pupil assessment is important and is the only cranial nerve assessment to be performed by ward staff.

In health, the activation of a reflex arc will cause pupil constriction if a bright light is shone into the pupil. Additionally, the other pupil should produce a consensual reaction (i.e. constrict when a light is shone into the other pupil). Pupil abnormality is a late but important indicator of neurological deterioration and, taken in association with other neurological changes, is an indication of increasing ICP (De Sousa and Woodward 2016). Cerebral oedema causes a partial herniation of the temporal lobe through the tentorium and places pressure on the oculomotor nerve, causing pupillary changes. Initially, pupil changes will be on the same side as the cerebral damage (ipsilateral changes), but as cerebral oedema worsens the other side will

Table 4.3 Criteria for response

Eye-opening		
Criterion	**Rating**	**score**
Eyes already open and require no stimulus	Spontaneous	4
Eyes open after normal speech or raised voice	To sound	3
Requires pressure to promote eye opening	To pressure	2
No eye opening and checks for interfering factor	None	1
Eyes closed due to another factor	Not testable	NT
Verbal response		
Criterion	**Rating**	**Score**
Correctly able to provide details relating to name, place, and date	Orientated	5
Not orientated but able to communicate/speaks in sentences	Confused	4
Intelligible single words	Words	3
Moans and groans	Sounds	2
No response and interfering factors checked	None	1
Factors interfering with communication, e.g. tracheostomy	Not testable	NT
Motor response		
Criterion	**Rating**	**Score**
Obeys two-part command, e.g. squeeze my fingers and let go	Obeys command	6
Pressure applied to shoulder and patient brings hand over clavicle	Localize	5
Pressure applied to shoulder* and patient bends elbow	Normal flexion	4
Pressure applied to shoulder and patient bends elbow. Movement noted to be abnormal	Abnormal flexion	3
Pressure applied to shoulder and patient extends arm at elbow	Extension	2
No movement in any limbs despite stimulation	None	1
Patient paralysed or another factor prohibiting movement	Not Testable	NT

data from Teasdale G, Allen D, Brennan P, McElhinney E, Mackinnon L. The Glasgow Coma Scale: an update after 40 years. *Nursing Times* 2014; 110: 12–16.

Box 4.1 Factors affecting pupil response

Amount of light in the clinical area
Use of medication, e.g. atropine/opiates
Use of recreational drugs
Accommodation reflex (patient focusing on an object)
Physical attraction
Aging processes
Ophthalmic damage

be affected and the patient will have contralateral changes. As the pressure increases on the cranial nerve the patient may present with the following progression of changes:

- pupil shape becomes ovoid
- pupil begins to dilate on affected side (ipsilateral changes)
- pupil fixes on affected side
- pupil fixes on the unaffected side (contralateral changes)

The speed of these changes is dependent on the speed of the swelling and may happen very quickly in some patients. Pupils should be examined for size, shape, and equality. The size documented on the chart should be the size of the pupil prior to direct light testing. It is worth noting that about 12–17% of the population have unequal pupils, with no underlying pathophysiology (Hickey 2013). However, in clinical practice abnormalities should be considered abnormal until proven otherwise.

Any changes to pupil shape and size should be quickly reported as urgent action/treatment may be required.

Assessment of motor function

The GCS is only required to assess best motor function and any differentiation in sides is not noted in a GCS assessment. The motor function assessment provides additional information about the overall function of the nervous system. It is here where weaknesses and hemiparesis are recorded. An increasing weakness on one side may indicate further damage/swelling and is often a good indicator of further deterioration in patients with traumatic brain injury. It is important to note that motor weakness is seen on the opposite side of the body to the damage. This is because the motor fibre tracts or pyramids swap sides at the medulla oblongata (decussation of pyramids), hence the right side of the brain controls the left side of the body below this level.

Motor function is assessed through the patient's ability to overcome weakness. There is a tendency for this to be a little subjective and it is recommended that Medical Research Council tool criteria is used (see Table 4.4) to enable a structured, objective approach.

It is acceptable practice to note whether there is a difference between limbs and to plot this accordingly using L (left) or R (right) symbols. If motor response is the same there is no need to differentiate between sides and a single dot will suffice.

Table 4.4 Objective classification of motor function

Classification	Criteria
Normal power	Patient is able to match resistance applied by the observer; i.e. they are able to hold up the limb and resist moderate efforts to push limb down
Mild weakness	Patient is able to hold up limb against mild resistance but this may be overcome if resistance is increased slightly
Severe weakness	Patient is able to move limb but not against resistance
Flexion	This is in response to central pain stimulus
Extension	Pain should only be used if there is no spontaneous movement from the patient
No response	No response to stimuli

Assessment of physiological status

It is important to record the patient's physiological status once the other parts of the neurological assessment are complete. There is a pattern of recognized changes in physiological measurements that may indicate that the patient's condition is deteriorating. These comprise quite a late sign and it is probable that changes in levels of consciousness will have been noticed first.

As the patient's neurological condition deteriorates as a result of increasing ICP (see section on damage to the nervous system), changes in physiological measurements occur. These are referred to as the Cushing's triad and include the following.

Increased blood pressure

There is an increase in blood pressure with a widening of the pulse pressure. The increasing blood pressure is the body's attempt to maintain cerebral perfusion as the ICP increases.

Bradycardia

Bradycardia is caused by midbrain compression. As ICP increases, pressure is increased on the vagus nerve, which in turn causes a slowing of the heart rate.

Alterations to respiratory rate

As the respiratory centres within the brain are compressed, the patient may show signs of respiratory alteration. In the initial stages there may be a decrease in respiration, but as ICP increases there is sometimes an increased respiratory rate. Abnormal patterns of respiration may be seen.

Temperature

Temperature is not part of the Cushing's triad but damage to the hypothalamus due to oedema may result in pyrexia. Pyrexia can be of other origins and it is important to exclude infection as cause of pyrexia.

Any indications that the patient is presenting with Cushing's triad signs (hypertension, bradycardia, decreased respirations) should be reported promptly as they may indicate a potentially lethal rise in ICP.

Frequency of neurological observations

There is no real consensus about the frequency of neurological observations and professional judgement is needed in this process. It is important that the practitioner uses the assessment tool with care. It is vital to note that no single change is more important than another and changes must be reported to enable timely and appropriate intervention. NICE head injury guidance CG176 (NICE 2014) has issued some guidelines relating to changes that may require review. Although these are explicitly written for head-injured patients they are also applicable to other patients and urgent attention should be sought if:

- there is development of agitation or abnormal behaviour;
- there is a sustained drop of 1 point in GCS (greater weight if this is related to motor function);
- there is any drop in the GCS of greater than 2 points, regardless of the time or GCS subscale;
- there is development of new or increasing headache;
- there are new or evolving neurological symptoms, for example pupil, limb movement, or facial asymmetry.

Rapid escalation of the deteriorating patient is vital and any cause for concern in relation to neurological deterioration should be reported to the medical staff immediately.

Common neurological disorders

Stroke

Care of the acute stroke patient

In England and Wales, 80,000 patients are hospitalized with stroke every year (Intercollegiate Stroke Working Party 2016). Cerebral vascular disease is the third leading cause of disability in the United Kingdom (RCP 2016). The most recent guidance (RCP 2016) identifies that:

- 85% of strokes are ischaemic in origin;
- 10% are due to intracerebral bleed;
- 5% are due to subarachnoid haemorrhage.

The need for urgent access to treatment is acknowledged by the RCP (2016) and it highlights that the initial aim of treatment is to minimize the consequence of stroke at the cellular and organ level. Later interventions are aimed at modifying the impact of the stroke on patients to enable the best level of functional recovery. Initial care will be considered in this chapter as stroke rehabilitation is beyond the scope of this book.

It is important to acknowledge that over the last four years stroke treatment has rapidly expanded, and new techniques aimed at modifying the impact of the stroke continue to be developed. At the time of writing the most current guidance (RCP 2016) will be referred to but the practitioner is reminded to remain vigilant to changes in guidance recommendations and treatment modalities as the pace of change in stroke intervention and management is rapid.

Delivery of acute stroke care is being modified to ensure that where available, patients are admitted to regional specialist services offering hyper acute management (RCP 2016). Hyper acute management is recommended for the first 72 hours of care. Thereafter patients should be transferred to acute stroke services and rehabilitation services.

It is important for staff to acknowledge that 1 in 20 strokes occur in patients already hospitalized for another condition. The Intercollegiate Working Party (2016) has identified that strokes typically occur in cardiology, renal, and cardiothoracic areas, and it is vital that staff in these areas are alert to the possibility of stroke and can recognize and quickly escalate these patients to specialist stroke servicers. Arguably it is vital for *all* staff to understand the presentation of stroke and need for urgent attention as stroke could occur in any acute hospital area. The guidance emphasizes that patients admitted with stroke should have access to:

- specialist medical staff trained in the acute management of people with stroke;
- specialist nursing staff trained in the acute management of people with stroke, covering neurological, general medical, and rehabilitation aspects;
- stroke specialist rehabilitation staff;
- access to diagnostic, imaging, and cardiology services;
- access to tertiary services for neurosurgery and vascular surgery.

Pathophysiology of stroke

Ischaemic stroke

Ischaemic stroke accounts for 85% of all strokes. This is further broken down into:

- atherosclerotic cerebral vascular stroke: extra- and intracranial arteries are narrowed by arteriosclerotic changes; this is worsened by associated atheroma which can be the site for thrombus development. Around 40% of these patients will experience transient ischaemic attack (TIA) before the stroke occurs (Hickey 2013).
- small artery penetrating stroke (lucunar stroke): a lucune describes a small cavity that develops after the necrotic tissue from a deep infarct is removed. Although often small in size, the consequences can be devastating and are dependent on the area of injury.
- cardiogenic embolic stroke: often caused by emboli from atrial fibrillation, valve disease, and other cardiac problems. Microemboli from the left side of the heart move, commonly through the carotid arteries. This often blocks the left middle cerebral artery as it is a relatively straight vessel and offers little resistance.
- cryptogenic stroke: cause unknown.
- other causes: these include coagulopathies, vasospasm, and substance misuse.

Haemorrhagic stroke

Haemorrhagic stroke accounts for 15% of strokes. This is further subdivided into:

- intracerebral stroke (10%): bleeding into the brain caused by rupture of a small artery, often related to prolonged periods of poorly controlled hypertension.
- subarachnoid haemorrhage (5%): bleeding into the subarachnoid space usually related to aneurysm (refer to section on subarachnoid haemorrhage (SAH)).

Haemorrhagic stroke leads to an immediate rise in ICP because blood from the bleeding artery causes an intracerebral haematoma that displaces brain tissue. Some degree of compensation may occur, but if the bleed is large enough then the associated ischaemic cascade discussed earlier will be triggered.

Subarachnoid haemorrhage

SAH is a bleed into the subarachnoid space (space between the arachnoid layer and the pia mater). It may be caused by bleeds from cerebral vessels, aneurysms, venous malformations, and sometimes trauma.

Patient presentation for SAH is very different to stroke. Whilst there may be some sign of neurological deficit the patient's first symptoms are normally a thunderclap headache accompanied by signs of severe meningeal irritation (neck stiffness, photophobia and vomiting) and therefore subarachnoid haemorrhage must be considered as a potential diagnosis if these symptoms are exhibited

Patient presentation for ischaemic and haemorrhagic stroke

This will vary according to the area of the brain involved and the severity of stroke. Signs and symptoms include:

- reduced levels of consciousness
- hemiparesis or hemiplegia
- right or left hemianopia (loss of visual fields unilaterally)
- deviation of head/eyes to one side (same side as stroke)
- dysphasia
- inattention to one side of the body (opposite side to stroke)

An advertising campaign has been developed that aims to encourage people to recognize and respond to signs and symptoms of acute stroke. The campaign uses the FAST acronym to help identify changes:

Facial weakness
Arm weakness
Speech disturbance
Time to seek help

It is important for nursing and medical staff to appreciate that the FAST tool will not identify forms of stroke that affect vision and cerebellar function and clinicians should be aware that changes to vision and balance may represent stroke and require urgent escalation.

Treatment

As highlighted earlier, the interventions for stroke management are rapidly progressing. Current recommendations continue to emphasize the need for rapid assessment of the suspected stroke patient. RCP (2016) identifies the need for:

- admission into a hyper acute stroke unit
- access to imaging within one hour of onset of symptoms
- access to angiography if an endovascular approach is indicated

Treatment is dependent on the cause of the stroke and immediate computerized tomography (CT) to establish whether the stroke is ischaemic or haemorrhagic is essential, as the treatment is different and misdiagnosis could have disastrous consequences.

Ischaemic stroke

The driving principle behind rapid intervention for acute stroke is the fact that 'time equals brain' (Papanagiotou and White 2016). Treatment options have altered significantly since the publication of the previous guidance (RCP 2012). The latest guidance (RCP 2016) identifies the continued use of thrombolysis, the additional use of an endovascular approach, and consideration of neurosurgical intervention.

Thrombolysis

Intravenous thrombolysis (IVT) continues to be an effective treatment and a recent review of safety into thrombolysis by the Medicines and Healthcare Products Regulatory Agency (MHRA 2015) reaffirmed the potential benefit of this therapy. A recent Stroke Thrombolysis Trialists Collaboration (2015) identified that IVT remains an important treatment and that treatment should not be age restricted, especially in the first three hours following stroke symptoms. The risk of cerebral bleeding remains problematic but a recent meta-analysis (Whitely *et al.* 2012) identified that risks were increased in patients with certain comorbidities such as atrial fibrillation, congestive cardiac failure, renal impairment, and previous use of antiplatelet treatment.

Current recommendation for IVT is that it can be administered to:

- All suitable patients within the first three hours of onset of symptoms.
- For patients under the age of 80 the treatment window may be extended to 3–4.5 hours.
- For patients over the age of 80 treatment window may be extended to 3–4.5 hours following a case-by-case risk assessment.
- Patients must be nursed in an acute stroke/hyper acute stroke area where the use, monitoring, and interventions for complications is fully understood by the multidisciplinary team.

Endovascular treatment

A relatively recent innovation in stroke management is the introduction of endovascular approaches. These are usually used in conjunction with IVT but may be used alone in patients for whom IVT is contraindicated. A meta-analysis of the randomized control trials into endovascular approaches identified a significant improvement in functional outcomes 90 days post stroke (Goyal *et al.* 2015). Endovascular approaches utilize mechanical means of embolectomy to revascularize the affected vessel and restore blood supply to the brain. Endovascular treatment is most effective when undertaken in the first 2 hours of stroke, however Saver and colleagues (2016) identified benefits for up to 7.5 hours following onset of symptoms

Current recommendations for mechanical embolectomy are:

- Patients should be considered for this treatment alongside IVT if they have a large vessel proximal occlusion, alongside a National Institute for Health Stroke Score (NIHSS) of 6 or more.

- Patients should be considered for this treatment if they have contraindications to IVT and a large vessel proximal occlusion: alongside a NIHSS score of 6 or more within 5 hours of onset of treatment.

Patients may be considered for a mechanical embolectomy if they continue to have significant neurological deficit (NIHSS score of 6 or more) beyond the five-hour window if they have:

- A large artery occlusion in the posterior circulation (up to 24 hours may be indicated)
- A favorable indication that salvageable brain tissue remains (up to 12 hours may be indicated)

Neurosurgical intervention

Neurosurgical intervention of a decompressive hemi-craniectomy is recommended for patients with significant middle cerebral artery (MCA) stroke (RCP 2016). Selection for this intervention is based upon:

- Pre-stroke Modified Rankin Score of less than 2; (2 = slight disability; unable to carry out all previous activities, but able to look after own affairs without assistance).
- Clinical deficits indicating MCA regional territory of stroke.
- NIHHS of 15 or more.
- Signs of an infarct covering at least 50% of MCA territory.

Management of haemorrhagic stroke

The RCP (2016) highlights the need to admit patients with haemorrhagic stroke to a hyper acute stroke unit as these patients have potential for rapid deterioration in neurological condition. There has been much debate about the need to lower blood pressure and the use of surgical intervention in this group of patients. Recent guidance from the RCP (2016) following reviews of randomized controlled trials has made several important recommendations.

It is obvious that these patients need to be identified as they are *not* appropriate candidates for IVT. Previous management has been conservative in nature with little suggested intervention into management of hypertension unless blood pressure was excessively high and referral to neurosurgeons for review was recommended. The current guidance recommends:

- Management of hypertension to reduce blood pressure to 140 mmHg systolic unless:
  - The GCS is 5 or less
  - Death is the expected outcome
  - Immediate surgery is indicated
- Referral to neurosurgeons may not normally be indicated for patients with primary intracerebral supratentorial bleeds unless there are signs of hydrocephalus. Patients with post fossa bleeds should be referred.
- Patients who develop hydrocephalus should be referred for potential insertion of external ventricular drains.
- Coagulation abnormalities caused by medications should be treated with an appropriate reversal agent.

Subarachnoid haemorrhage management

It is encouraging to see that the overall survival rate for patients admitted with subarachnoid haemorrhage has increased to approximately 70% over the last decade (RCP 2016). Subarachnoid haemorrhages are classified depending on their severity using the World Federation of Neurosurgeons Scale. Grade 1 is the lowest score with a grade 4 normally indicating severe neurological deficit and potentially poorer prognosis.

The emphasis on this group of patients remains to transfer them to specialist neuroscience centres for urgent investigation and treatment.

First-line management in acute hospitals includes:

- Immediate brain scan and angiography if agreed by neurosurgeons.
- Instigation of frequent neurological observations to detect early signs of deterioration or re-bleed.
- Current recommendations are for treatment with 60 mg of nimodopine six hourly unless contraindicated.
- Pain control and appropriate hydration and management of nausea and vomiting may be significant issues for this group of patients.
- Once at a neurological centre the aneurysm will be secured (normally either via an endovascular route but surgical intervention may be required in some patients).
- Complications of subarachnoid haemorrhage include hydrocephalus and cerebral ischaemia.

Nursing care

The immediate focus of nursing care of the patient following stroke involves many different factors (see Table 4.5). Long-term stroke care and rehabilitation is significant but beyond the focus of this book.

Traumatic brain injury

Each year 1.4 million people attend the emergency departments with traumatic brain injury (TBI); of these 200,000 are admitted to hospital (NICE 2014). The incidence of death in patients with head injury is relatively low (0.2% of all emergency department attendees) and the majority of patients (95%) have a minor head injury (defined as a GCS between 12 and 15). Patients with moderate and severe injury are normally transferred to a trauma centre which provides specialist neurosurgical care.

Pathophysiology of head injury

Several classification systems exist for traumatic injury. Significant classifications are:

- Mechanism of injury
- Primary or secondary injury
- Gross pathology

Table 4.5 Nursing care of the patient following stroke

Potential problem	Nursing care
Ineffective airway due to deteriorating consciousness levels	• Careful positioning to maintain airway • Elevation of head of bed to 30° • Use of airway adjuncts; consider anaesthetic referral if Glasgow Coma Scale below 8 • Suctioning and oxygen as required
Potential deterioration of respiratory function	• Monitor respiratory rate • Provide supplemental oxygen if saturations below 95% (RCP 2016) • Appropriate respiratory assessment (see Chapter 2) • Physiotherapy
Risk of aspiration (see Chapter 6)	• A swallow screen should be carried out before anything is given orally. • This should occur in first 24 h. Patients should remain nil by mouth until this time. • Patients with swallow difficulties should have a swallow assessment by an appropriately trained specialist • Elevation of head of bed to 30°
Potential neurological deterioration	• Neurological assessment is paramount • Maintain venous return from brain by elevation of head of bed to 30° • Maintain patient's head in neutral alignment • Avoid activities that may increase ICP • Ensure analgesia is administered if required
Hypertension	• Monitor blood pressure/pulse • Report significant changes immediately • Hypertension may only be treated if evidence of a hypertensive emergency (RCP 2016) • Blood pressure reduction to 185/110 mmHg should be considered if thombolysis indicated (RCP 2016)
Pyrexia	• Monitor temperature • Temperature may increase post stroke but important to eliminate infection as cause • Conservative management of pyrexia
Blood glucose instability	• High glucose levels will increase intracranial pressure • Maintenance of blood glucose within range of 5–15 mmol (RCP 2016)
Risk of dehydration	• Regular review of hydration status using multiple methods • Aim to achieve normal hydration status as soon as possible but at least in initial 4 hours • Observe for signs of dehydration/fluid overload (see Chapter 7)
Nutrition	• Patients should have nutritional assessment and assessed regularly for risk of malnutrition
Communication difficulties	• Assess type of deficit • Develop appropriate communication methods • Speech and language therapist assessment

Data from Hickey JV. Clinical Practice of Neurological and Neurosurgical Nursing (Clinical Practice of Neurological & Neurosurgical Nursing). Lippincott Williams and Wilkins. 2013 Dec 1; and Royal College of Physicians. (2016). National Clinical Guideline for the Management of Stroke, Fifth edition. Royal College of Physicians 2016. Prepared by the Intercollegiate Stroke Working Party.

Mechanism of injury

In the United Kingdom: blunt head injury is the commonest form of injury seen (motor vehicle accidents, falls, and assault). However, in the United States, penetrating injuries (gunshot or blast wounds) are the most common (Baxter and Wilson 2012).

Primary/Secondary injury

A primary injury is damage that occurs at the scene of the accident and is irreversible damage. A secondary injury occurs after the initial injury and is therefore potentially treatable. Examples of secondary injury include:

- Hypoxia secondary to airway obstruction
- Poor cerebral perfusion
- Prolonged raised intracranial pressure

Baxter and Wilson (2012) highlight that secondary injury often causes the most impact to the patient with TBI who survive their primary injury.

Gross pathology

Head injuries are also classified according to their effect on brain pathology. These include:

- Extradural haematoma (EDH)
- Subdural haematoma (SDH)
- Contusions
- Concussion/diffuse injury
- Penetrating injury

Some injuries (EDH and acute SDH) may require immediate surgery. Irrespective of injury, it is important that care is aimed at minimizing the consequence of secondary injury.

Nursing management

Nursing management of the patient with minor head injury largely revolves around initial assessment, admission, accurate neurological assessment, and immediate reporting, and action on deteriorating neurological function.

Initial assessment

Bethal (2012) suggests that immediate assessment for minor TBI should include:

- Assessment of mechanism of injury
- Assessment for red-flag criteria: fall from height, direct blow/fall, high-speed injuries)
- Associated signs and symptoms (loss of consciousness, amnesia, vomiting, or pain).
- Other likely injuries (dependent upon mechanism of injury)
- Factors that may worsen TBI (e.g. anticoagulation)

Admission

Criteria for admission are clearly identified by NICE (2014) and include:

- Patients with abnormal imaging findings
- Patients with a GCS < 15
- Patients who have continuing worrying signs (e.g. vomiting, headache)
- Patients presenting with alcohol or recreational drug intoxication

NICE (2014) stresses the importance of accurate and timely neurological assessment conducted by professionals who are competent in the assessment of patients with head injury and care should be aimed at assessment and prevention of secondary injury (see Table 4.6).

Neurological assessment and alcohol consumption

Alcohol plays a significant contributory factor in TBI. Whilst definitive statistics are unavailable, Shahin and Robertson (2012) identify that alcohol plays a contributory factor in approximately 35–40% of all admissions with TBI. Alcohol can cause problems in assessment and management of the TBI patient. Intoxicated patients may not be able to provide an accurate history and the signs and symptoms of intoxication (slurred speech, confusion, amnesia, vomiting) can be interpreted as symptoms of TBI.

Shahin and Robertson (2012) highlight that alcohol intoxication can cause either over diagnosis (misinterpretation of signs of alcohol intoxication for TBI) or under diagnosis (ignore signs of TBI and attribute to alcohol). Research into the impact of alcohol on TBI is ongoing. It is suggested that caution is used in this vulnerable group and that assessment concerns are escalated immediately.

Head injury and vulnerable adults

The need to consider potential safeguarding issues is stressed by Trout (2014) and is a recent addition to the NICE (2014) guidance. If safeguarding issues are suspected patients should be assessed by a specialist trained in safeguarding and age-appropriate procedures should be put in place if safeguarding concerns are evident.

Managing discharge

Once fit for discharge, the need for appropriate written instructions and appropriate advice regarding potential further deterioration/long-term consequences of mild head injury is emphasized by NICE (2014).

Seizure

Care of the patient following seizure

Seizures may be defined as episodes of paroxysmal neurological dysfunction which occur as a result of abnormal neuronal firing. This may manifest as changes in behavior, sensory

Table 4.6 Nursing care of the patient following head injury

Potential problem	Nursing care
Neurological deterioration 1	Neurological assessment to include GCS, pupil size and reactivity, limb movement, respiratory rate, heart rate, blood pressure, temperature, oxygen saturation The NICE guidelines (2014) suggest the frequency should be half hourly for 2 h, hourly for 4 h, 2 hourly thereafter until discharge Care should be taken to report any deterioration immediately. Doctors should be prepared to liaise with neurosurgical team if patient's condition deteriorates
Neurological deterioration 2	The following criteria should be used as a guide for reporting any deterioration (NICE 2014): • there is development of agitation or abnormal behaviour • there is a sustained drop of 1 point in GCS (greater weight if this is related to motor function) • any drop in the GCS of greater than 3 points in eye and verbal response score or 2 points in motor score. • development of new or increasing headache • new or evolving neurological symptoms, e.g. pupil, limb, or facial movement asymmetry
Potential dehydration	Dehydration is damaging to the neurological patient, so it is important to ensure adequate fluid intake. This may be oral fluids if tolerated or intravenous infusion. This is of particular importance if the patient appears to have been drinking alcohol because of the diuretic effects. Fluid balance should be recorded.
Headache	Patients may experience pain due to injury. It is important to offer adequate analgesia, but at the same time important to ensure that analgesia will not affect neurological assessment. Paracetamol and codeine are useful analgesia in the management of headache. Small doses of intravenous opiates may be required, however opiate-based analgesia may make the patient drowsy and compound the difficulties with adequate assessment.
Maintaining a safe environment	It is important to ensure a safe environment is maintained at all times. Consideration should be given to: • location of patient's bed to enable close supervision • use of pillows and other protective equipment to protect patient from injury • close supervision at all times
Patient positioning	A quiet environment is useful especially if the patient has severe headache/photophobia Patient should not be nursed flat and kept at 30° to facilitate venous return
Treatment of other injuries	Other injuries should have been assessed and documented in the emergency department Observe for any other injuries and take appropriate action

perception or motor activity. Seizures, depending upon their type, may or may not impact upon consciousness (Spray 2015).

The World Health Organization (2015) highlights that seizures can occur as a 'one off' occurrence and that careful investigation should be undertaken before a patient is diagnosed with a seizure disorder (epilepsy) as this can impact on the individual's lifestyle and still may cause stigmatization in many countries in the world. Statistically recurrent seizure activity is quite common in the United Kingdom, with estimated figures of occurrence affecting 362,000–415,000 adults (NICE 2012). Given the occurrence of 'one-off' seizures and relatively high incidence of epilepsy, it is particularly significant that the Registered Nurse should understand the pathophysiology, presentation, and management of seizures in acute care settings (Spray 2015).

Pathophysiology

Seizures can be triggered by a variety of causes including drug and alcohol intoxication, metabolic disturbance, acute neurological injury, hypoglycaemia, pregnancy, and electrolyte imbalances. Classifications of epilepsy have recently been updated (Smith *et al.* 2015a) and describe the cause of epilepsy as either:

- Resulting from genetic predisposition; or
- Resulting from a structural or metabolic problem; or
- Resulting from an unknown cause (idiopathic).

In health there are two different types of neuron that control neurological activity. Simplistically, excitatory neurons send messages and inhibitory neurons stop messages. In seizure activity, an imbalance occurs between these neurons leading to simultaneous hyper excitation and hyper synchronization of a neuronal network. Therefore, the cells begin to fire repeatedly, producing sustained neural activity that results in seizure activity as the inhibitory neurons fail to stop the neuronal activity. During the period of the seizure there is a dramatic increase in cellular metabolism, increasing the neurons' need for glucose, oxygen, and ATP. Cerebral blood flow will increase to meet the demands of the overactive neural cells. If the seizure continues for a long period, this excessive increase in metabolic requirements can lead to cellular exhaustion and cellular destruction. The goal of nursing intervention is to prevent cellular damage caused by excessive seizure activity.

It is argued that seizure activity is often underestimated in clinical practice as the majority of non-neurological nurses tend to define seizure activity when it impacts upon motor function and other seizure types may be overlooked. In terms of classification seizures may be grouped as focal or generalized.

Focal seizures

In focal seizures (previously known as partial seizures), seizure activity is limited to one part of the cerebral hemisphere. They may be subdivided further into simple or complex focal seizures depending on whether consciousness is lost.

- Simple focal seizures: consciousness is not lost, and the effects of seizure activity will be dependent upon area of brain affected. The patient may have abnormal movement or jerking of limbs/twitching of facial muscles. In some patients, sensation is changed and they may complain of feelings of numbness/tingling in an area. The patient will often be quite frightened and can often explain the effects of their seizure on them. Simple seizures may evolve into complex seizure activity.
- Complex focal seizures: consciousness is impaired /lost and the patient will not be aware of their surroundings. Patients may present with bizarre behaviour (automatisms) or absences, or may experience hallucinations and motor disturbances such as fumbling, repeated rubbing, and semi-purposeful movement. They are not aware of their behaviour (Marshall and Crawford 2013).

Both types of partial seizures may terminate on their own or develop into a generalized seizure.

Generalized seizures

Generalized seizures reflect involvement of both cerebral hemispheres and there is always a loss of consciousness but not necessarily convulsive activity. Presentation of generalized seizure will depend on type and can range from:

- a tonic/clonic seizure (see below);
- generalized absence that may be brief and can be mistaken for 'daydreaming';
- atonic seizure, where the patient abruptly loses muscle tone (often mistaken for fall or faint);
- myoclonic seizure activity (sudden jerking movements affecting most of the body);
- clonic seizure activity (sudden stiffening of all limbs causing the patient to collapse);
- tonic seizure activity (sudden brief stiffening of limbs).

Recovery from seizure depends on the type. Most seizure activity will have spontaneous recovery. However, a post ictal phase, characterized by drowsiness, confusion, weakness, and a need to sleep normally is normally seen following tonic-clonic seizures and tonic seizures and it is important to document patient presentation post seizure. Note that a seizure is not deemed to have completed until full recovery returns (Smith *et al.* 2015b).

Tonic-clonic seizure

The patient may or may not experience an aura (a warning that a seizure is starting). In the tonic phase the voluntary muscles contract, the body, legs, and arms stiffen, and the patient falls to the ground if standing. The muscles of the jaw cause the mouth to close tightly (this may cause the patient to bite their tongue). The bladder and (rarely) bowel will empty, the pupils dilate and are unresponsive to light. The patient will stop breathing and may become pale/cyanosed. This period usually lasts 1 m (Hickey 2013). In the clonic phase the patient will begin to develop violent, rhythmic muscular contractions accompanied by strenuous breathing (hyperventilation). The eyes may roll and there is excessive salivation/frothing at the mouth. The clonic phase usually lasts for 30 s but may be longer. After the clonic phase the patient is usually unconscious for a period of time, their extremities may be limp, they will breathe quietly, and pupils may be unequal but should respond to light. After awakening there is usually a period of confusion and amnesia and the patient may be very drowsy and sleepy.

A more worrying form of seizure is status epilepticus.

- *Status epilepticus* is defined as either a prolonged seizure (more than 5 m) or serial seizures without recovery of consciousness between seizures (Smith *et al.* 2015b). Status epilepticus usually presents as tonic-clonic seizures but it must be remembered that partial seizures can also cause continuous seizure activity and should be suspected if the patient with partial seizures have sustained significant alterations in consciousness. Status epilepticus is a medical emergency as neuronal death will quickly ensue if seizure activity is not halted.

Nursing care

Nursing care of the patient having a focal seizure largely involves observation, protecting the patient from harm, and documentation of seizure on the seizure chart. Documentation of seizure activity should include detail about:

- levels/alteration of consciousness;
- presentation of seizure;
- length of seizure; and
- patient's condition post seizure.

Care of the patient having a tonic-clonic seizure evolves around seizure first aid, protecting the patient from injury during the seizure, monitoring seizure activity, and calling for help if required (see Table 4.7).

Table 4.7 Nursing management of a seizure

Potential problem	Nursing care
Prevention of injury	If patient falls to ground, ensure area is free from hazards or remove hazards, e.g. hospital furniture
	Remove any glasses or objects that may cause injury
	Loosen constricting clothing
	Do not attempt to force anything into mouth
	Do not restrain the patient
	Stay with the patient
	Maintain patient dignity
Observation of seizure	You will need to note and document the following: • any aura or warning • part of body where seizure activity began • spread of movement • type of movement • duration of time (tonic and clonic) • pupils • continence/incontinence • post-ictal state
Aftercare following seizure	ABC assessment (crash call if respiration does not return)
	Ensure patient placed in comfortable position/recovery position because of risk of post-ictal vomiting
	Move the patient to bed from floor when able
	Psychological support and clear communication
	Allow rest
	Observe for repeated seizure activity
	Check compliance with medication/medication levels

Note: Seizure activity can be a side effect of under/over dose of phenytoin—levels should be monitored.

Management of status epilepticus

This is considered a medical emergency and immediate medical attention is vital this may be using a medical emergency call or follow hospital policy, NICE (2012) guidance identifies differing stages of management (see Box 4.2).

Medication is generally the remit of the doctor in status epilepticus (SE) and the following medications are currently recommended by NICE and some are weight related (see https://www.nice.org.uk/guidance/cg137/resources/epilepsies-diagnosis-and-management-35109515407813)

- Initial treatment: short-acting diazepam
- Consider lorazepam and normal dose of anti-epileptic drugs (AED) (N.B. patients receiving phenytoin may require drug-level testing)

Box 4.2 Management of status epilepticus

1st stage (0–10 minutes)

Secure airway and resuscitate
Administer oxygen
Assess cardiorespiratory function
Establish intravenous access

2nd stage (0–30 minutes)

Begin regular monitoring
Consider the other causes of seizure
Emergency anti-epileptic drug therapy
Treat acidosis if severe
Consider risk of seizure related to alcohol abuse and follow protocol (Pabrinex and 50% glucose)

3rd stage (0–60 minutes)

Establish aetiology
Alert anesthetist and ITU

4th Stage

Transfer to intensive care
Establish intensive care and EEG monitoring
Initiate intracranial pressure monitoring where appropriate
Initiate long-term, maintenance anti-epileptic drug therapy

- Consider phenytoin infusion
- Critical care treatment may include administration of propofol, midazolam, thiopental sodium, and anaesthesia (with electroencephalogram (EEG) monitoring)

The patient may require additional assessment/tests post scan especially if they have not experienced a seizure before. This may include CT scan, EEG tests, and referral to a neurologist. Long-term management of epilepsy revolves around patient education to increase compliance with treatment and prevent the risk of sudden unexpected death in epilepsy. Most treatment revolves around new-generation medications but surgery and neuro-stimulation are also long-term options (Smith *et al.* 2015).

Clinical link 4.1 (see Appendix for answers)

Part 1

You are caring for a 24-year-old patient admitted with mild concussion after a fight in a nightclub. He has a severe headache and is feeling very nauseated; his breath smells strongly of alcohol. On admission his GCS is 13. He is quite sleepy, awakes to verbal command, but is aggressive and agitated when awake. He is speaking in sentences and is able to respond to command. Physiological observations are normal and pupils a size 3 and reacting to light consensually. Consider how you will:

- manage this patient's aggression.
- ensure neurological assessment is appropriate.

Part 2

One hour after admission you note that he is sleepier and is requiring painful stimuli to awaken him; he is less agitated and once awake is able to obey commands. His pupils are a size 3 but they are ovoid and a little sluggish in reacting to light. Consider the following:

- What is his GCS now?
- What other assessments will you do?
- When will you report these changes?
- What other actions may be required?

Clinical link 4.2 (see Appendix for answers)

You are called to see a patient in a side room. The patient has been in hospital for several weeks following a stroke and his room is quite cluttered. On your arrival the student nurse reports that the patient has just collapsed on the floor and is now beginning to shake violently. He is blue in the face and is foaming at the mouth.

- What are your immediate actions?
- What will you need to observe in relation to his seizure?
- How can you protect this patient from injury?

After about 1 min the seizure appears to stop and then the patient starts shaking again. This is still continuing after 3 min.

- Discuss your initial actions.
- What help will you summon?
- What equipment/treatment may you need?
- How will you organize this patient's transfer to ITU?
- What will you need to consider prior to transfer?

End of chapter test

It is important that you understand both the theory related to neurological care and the practice of specific neurological skills in order to care safely for patients with neurological problems. In order to test your knowledge and apply this knowledge to clinical practice you should undertake the following assessment with an appropriately trained member of staff in clinical practice. If you are unable to answer any questions it may be helpful to revisit the section in this chapter.

Knowledge assessment

Work with your mentor/supervisor in practice and ask them to test your knowledge in relation to the following. Incorrect answers/lack of knowledge will require further revision/re-reading of this chapter.

- Discuss the normal divisions within the central nervous system.
- Discuss why it is important to prevent damage to the neurons.
- Discuss the ischaemic cascade that occurs as a result of neuronal damage.
- Discuss the factors that can influence consciousness.
- Analyse common causes of decreasing levels of consciousness.
- Discuss the use of quick assessment of neurological function (ACVPU).
- Discuss the need for formal objective neurological examination.
- Discuss how accurately to perform each stage of assessment.
- Describe responses to each assessment.
- Describe the difference between central and peripheral painful stimuli.
- Discuss the significance of pupil response.
- Analyse the reliability and validity of neurological assessment tools.
- Discuss indicators for further nursing/medical intervention.
- Analyse treatment options for patients with deteriorating conscious levels.
- Identify causes of seizure and discusses management.
- Discuss risk issues related to transfer of patients with decreasing levels of consciousness to CT and other areas.
- Discuss signs of swallowing difficulty and appropriate management.

Skills assessment

Work with your mentor/supervisor in practice and ask them to assess your ability to care for patients with neurological injury using the following criteria, where appropriate. Note that you may not be able to demonstrate all these skills. Ask your mentor/supervisor to give you feedback on areas that you did well and areas that may require improving.

- Identifies need and frequency of observation.
- ACVPU: systematically makes quick neurological assessment and determines need for GCS testing.
- Tests blood glucose if suspected cause of loss of consciousness.
- GCS: systematically tests eye-opening, verbal response, and motor function using appropriate assessment.
- Tests pupils, noting for reaction and consensual reactions.
- Highlights any treatment/cause of change in pupil size.
- Reports any new or worsening confusion.
- Reports changes in consciousness.
- Ensures patient safety and appropriate positioning if required.
- Summarizes neurological findings and initiates appropriate management as required.
- Liaises with multidisciplinary team.
- Informs patient/relative of any changes.
- Recognizes need for fast and appropriate response if conscious levels deteriorating.
- Demonstrates neurological assessment technique at handover if appropriate.
- Reviews need for neurological assessment and frequency of neurological assessment.

References

Baxter, D., Wilson, M. (2012) The fundamentals of head injury. *Neurosurg*, 30(3):116–21.

Bethal, J. (2012) Emergency care of children and adults with head injury. *Nurs Stand*, 26(43):49–56.

De Sousa, I., Woodward, S. (2016) The Glasgow Coma Scale in adults: Doing it right. *Emerg Nurse*, 24(8):33–8.

Goyal, M., Demchuk, A.M., Menon, B.K., *et al.* (2015) Randomized assessment of rapid endovascular treatment of ischemic stroke. *N Engl J Med*, 372:1019–30.

Hickey, J.V. (2013) *The Clinical Practice of Neurological and Neuroscience Nursing* 7th edn. Philadelphia, PA: Lippincott.

Intercollegiate Stroke Working Party (2016) *National Clinical Guideline for Stroke* 5th edn. London: Royal College of Physicians.

Jennett, G., Bennett, B. (1974) Assessment of coma and impaired consciousness: A practical scale. *Lancet*, 2:81–4.

Marshall, F., Crawford, P. (2013) *Coping with Epilepsy.* London: Sheldon Press.

MHRA (2015). Alteplase for treatment of acute ischaemic stroke: Independent review. London: Medicines and Healthcare products Regulatory Agency.

NICE (2012) CG137. *Epilepsies: Diagnosis and Management.* London: National Institute for Health and Care Excellence.

NICE (2014) CG176. *Head Injury: Assessment and Early Management.* London: National Institute for Health and Care Excellence.

Papanagiotou, P., White, C. (2016) Endovascular reperfusion strategies for acute stroke. *Cardiovascular Interventions*, 9(4):307–16.

Resuscitation Council (2015) *Resuscitation Guidelines*. London: Resuscitation Council.

RCP (2012) *National Clinical Guideline for the Management of Stroke* 4th edn. London: Royal College of Physicians.

RCP (2016) *National Clinical Guideline for the Management of Stroke*, 5th edn. London: Royal College of Physicians.

RCP (2017) National Early Warning Scores 2: Standardising the Assessment of Acute Illness Severity in the NHS. London: RCP.

Saver, J., Goyal, M., der Lugt, A., *et al.* (2016) Time to treatment with endovascular thrombectomy and outcomes from ischemic stroke: A meta-analysis. *JAMA*, 316(12):1279–88.

Shahin, H., Robertson, C. (2012) Alcohol and the head injured patient. *Trauma*, 14(3):233–42.

Smith, G., Wagner, J.L., Edwards, J.C. (2015a) Epilepsy update, Part 1: Nursing care and evidence-based treatment. *J Adv Neurosci*, 115(5):40–7.

Smith, G., Wagner, J.L., Edwards, J.C. (2015b) Epilepsy update, Part 2: Nursing care and evidence-based treatment. *J Adv Neurosci*, 115(6):34–44.

Spray, J. (2015) Seizures: Awareness and observation in the ward environment *Br J Nurs*, 24(19):946–55.

Stroke Thrombolysis Trialists Collaboration (2015) STT: Stroke thrombolysis trialists' collaboration. Available at: https://www.ctsu.ox.ac.uk/research/st; accessed 9 December 2019.

Teasdale, G., Jennett, B. (1974) Assessment of coma and impaired consciousness: A practical scale. *Lancet*, 2:81–4.

Teasdale, G., Allan, D., Brennan, P., *et al.* (2014) Forty years on: Updating the Glasgow Coma Scale. *Nurs Times*, 110(42):12–16.

Trout, R. (2014) Updated NICE head injury guidelines. *Brit J Neurosci Nurs*, 10(2):97.

Whiteley, W.N., Slot, K.B., Fernandes, P., *et al.* (2012) Risk factors for intracranial hemorrhage in acute ischemic stroke patients treated with recombinant tissue plasminogen activator: A systematic review and meta-analysis of 55 studies. *Stroke*, 43:2904–09.

World Health Organization (2015) Epilepsy factsheet. Geneva: WHO. Available at: http://www.who.int/mediacentre/factsheets/fs999/en/; accessed 9 December 2019.

5

Acute kidney injury

Cristina Osorio and Theofanis Fotis

Chapter contents

Assessing and supporting kidney function is an integral aspect of acute care. The purpose of this chapter is to examine:

- the anatomy and physiology of the kidney
- the pathophysiological changes in acute kidney injury
- the assessment of kidney function
- the conservative management of the patient with reduced kidney function
- renal replacement therapies

Learning outcomes

This chapter will enable you to:

- apply knowledge of the normal anatomy of the kidney to greater understand the pathological mechanisms which cause acute kidney injury (AKI)
- identify tools for the assessment of kidney function and understand the relevance of findings to define the extent of kidney failure
- select appropriate interventions to alleviate symptoms, control severity, and halt AKI
- demonstrate knowledge of renal replacement therapies and when to start them, as well as a working knowledge of which choices are best for solute clearance, restoration of fluid and electrolyte homeostasis, or physiological stability
- discuss with insight the importance of multidisciplinary work towards proactive and effective resolution of AKI
- appreciate patient participation in their recovery and vested interest for long-term kidney health

Introduction

Acute kidney injury (AKI) is a serious and rapid-onset condition that complicates other pathologies and threatens human life. AKI also increases the long-term risk of chronic kidney failure.

Acute care nurses will make good use of an understanding of their patients' kidney function because protective measures and early detection of anomalies greatly reduces the risk of AKI. Technology has improved patient outcome in many areas of healthcare, yet the increase in invasive actions such as contrast and angiographic procedures, and the use of artificial devices have also increased the risk of kidney injury (NICE 2013). This chapter will review kidney anatomy and physiology followed by the nursing care involved in assessing and managing abnormal kidney function. The focus is on relevance and applicability to clinical practice and this will be aided by reference to clinical link activities.

The UK-based 'Think Kidneys AKI Programme' outlines that up to 100,000 deaths in hospital each year are associated with AKI, 65% of AKI starts in the community, and as many as 1 in 5 emergency patients admitted to hospital has AKI on presentation (Bassett *et al.* 2017). Surgery remains a leading cause of AKI in hospitalized patients with the incidence ranging from 18% to 47% depending on the definition used (Calvert and Shaw 2012). The risk of AKI is widespread, making prevention of kidney injury, early intervention, and suitable follow-up important aspects of patient care to improve survival and reduce length of hospital stay. For the patient, an equally important outcome is life without dialysis or significant kidney disability.

Applied anatomy and physiology of the kidney

People will normally have two functioning kidneys. Figure 5.1 indicates their location and anatomic size.

The primary functions of the kidney are:

- to filter and excrete metabolic waste products; and
- to sustain homeostasis of blood pH, electrolytes, and body water.

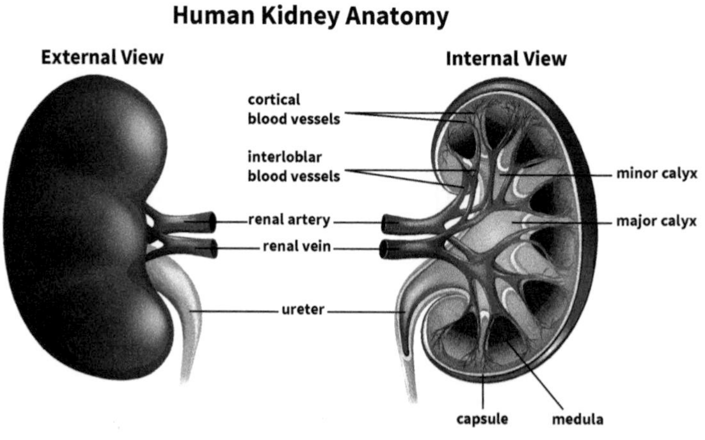

Figure 5.1 Location and macroscopic view of uro-kidney body system.
BlueRingMedia / Shutterstock.com.

Additional functions of the kidney are:

- regulation of blood pressure;
- production of erythropoietin; and
- regulation of parathyroid activity.

It is generally helpful to distinguish between the macroscopic and microscopic structures of kidney.

Macroscopic overview

The kidneys receive 20–25% of the cardiac output from the heart. This is equivalent to approximately 180 L/day, circulated via the renal arteries. An extensive vascular system delivers blood supply to every cell of the kidney, enabling quick and responsive filtration and homeostatic regulation.

The anatomic size and shape of each kidney is important in clinical investigations. The simplest and quickest way to identify deviation from normal size and shape is to undertake a kidney ultrasound. A reduction in kidney size indicates chronic damage, often too advanced to enable diagnosis of underlying cause. Damage to kidney tissue would have progressed silently and by the time the patient reports signs or symptoms, there is not enough tissue to investigate cause on biopsy or angiogram. This is described as 'small kidneys', first detected on ultrasound for size, shape, and presence of the two kidneys. Significant atrophy of the kidneys rules out AKI, deprives the patient of a cause of kidney failure, and, most of all signals, the need to commence life-saving dialysis treatment.

The large proportion of patients presenting with 'small kidneys' illustrates the silent nature of chronic kidney failure and also the possibility that patients admitted into hospital may already have kidney failure, unbeknownst to them. The Renal Registry (2015) monitors reasons for starting dialysis and over 20% of patients in England and Wales do not know why they have kidney failure.

Those who present clinically with symptoms of AKI and are found to have small kidneys on ultrasound visualization are considered to have had silent chronic kidney failure and are not likely to recover function. The therapeutic aim changes from recovery to halting progression. NICE (2013) recommends 24-hour access to kidney ultrasound facilities in all hospitals to improve early and proactive identification of small kidneys in all UK hospitals.

The signs and symptoms of chronic kidney failure are non-specific and numerous, making it easily confused with other possible differential diagnosis. Box 5.1 outlines signs and symptoms although very rarely would they present simultaneously. The presence of two to three parameters, followed with a blood test for creatinine and urea, would confirm kidney damage.

Microscopic overview

The vascular network of arteries and arterioles of the kidney ends near the cortex, where just over 1.1 million nephrons are located. The nephron is a microscopic structure and the functional unit where the filtration and secretion functions of the kidney take place, culminating

Box 5.1 Signs and symptoms of chronic kidney failure

Sodium and fluid retention:
- pitting oedema
- shortness of breath
- weight gain

Uraemia:
- sallow colour and uraemic breath
- nausea and vomiting, loss of appetite
- tiredness, lethargy, and jerkiness
- lack of concentration, poor cognitive functioning
- disseminated itching

Endocrine alterations, causing:
- hypertension
- anaemia
- abnormal bone turnover

in the formation of urine, drained into the collecting duct. Figure 5.2 shows the anatomical structure in some detail.

Blood entering the glomerular capsule is filtered at a rate of 120–150 mL/min/1.73 m^2 body surface, known as the glomerular filtration rate (GFR). Few substances or solutes remain unfiltered; for example, protein and red blood cells do not normally filter through the

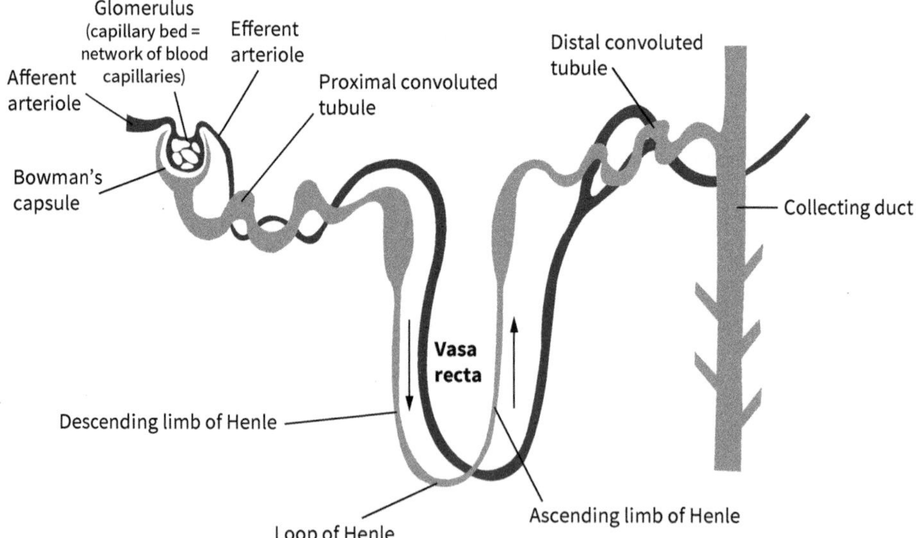

Figure 5.2 Anatomic structure of the nephron.

basement membrane. As the filtrate moves through the tubule, 99% of the water and glucose are reabsorbed into body circulation and several electrolytes are secreted, excreted, or actively transported through the tubular cells. Damage to the glomerular membrane or the tubular cells leads to the presence of protein and blood in urine. In acute care, urinalysis is a simple, quick tool to detect early signs of kidney injury, both chronic and acute (Bassett *et al.* 2017). It is good nursing assessment to undertake urinalysis on admission and repeat at intervals according to changes in patient condition.

Kidney function, assessment, and investigations

Pathology laboratories in the United Kingdom now report routinely on the estimated GFR (e-GFR). This tool for the assessment of kidney function is most useful if the patient does not have acute sepsis, recent amputation, and is an adult. It is used to monitor chronic kidney failure or suspected acute-on-chronic kidney failure. It has no use in monitoring AKI, which causes more immediate physiological changes and needs to be investigated through other means, explored later in this chapter.

Estimation of e-GFR is currently based on the Modified Diet Renal Disease (MDRD) calculation formula as follows:

$$\mathrm{e-GFR} = 186 \times (\text{serum creatinine})^{-1.154} \times (\text{age})^{-0.203} \times 0.742 \text{ (if female)}$$

The formula considers the person's measured serum creatinine and mathematically corrects for predictable variations associated with gender and age, making the result more accurate than serum creatinine alone. It is an approximate estimation and more complex formulae will make further corrections for other variables also known to influence GFR, for example body weight and ethnicity. However, more complex calculations are not practical for acute setting laboratories because it is unlikely that doctors and nurses will routinely enter the patient's weight and ethnicity on blood forms, whereas gender and age are easier to elicit from hospital computer records.

The e-GFR is helpful when chronic kidney failure is suspected, but serological changes are not noticeable until the e-GFR drops below 60 mL/min/1.73 m^2. This represents loss of 50% kidney function before the e-GFR result causes concern. People can tolerate up to 70% loss of function without detriment to daily functioning and this helps explain silent progression. However, high blood pressure and urinalysis alterations with positive blood and protein are non-specific early signs of reduced kidney function.

Estimated GFR is an unreliable calculation in AKI, including instances of sepsis, when the patient is catabolic and has disturbed muscle physiology affecting creatinine levels.

Whether chronic over a long period or the result of acute onset, various investigations and detailed patient history assist differential diagnosis of kidney failure. Patient history in particular is of great value when diagnosing AKI, especially for those admitted from the community with signs and symptoms. There may be environmental and patient-specific factors that only history taking and good communication among health professionals will bring to the fore.

However, nurses who work in hospital-based acute settings are more likely to come across AKI as a complication rather than a reason for patient hospitalization. This makes it especially relevant for nurses to undertake regular patient assessment and use early warning scores as a means for early recognition of AKI (NICE 2007; RCP 2017).

Whilst glomerular damage affects the content of urine and is a feature of chronic kidney injury, damage to the tubular structure affects *urinary output* more directly and is a feature of AKI. Tubular cells have the ability to regenerate and recover with therapeutic support, further highlighting the central role of the acute care nurse in assisting in the early detection and intervention on kidney injury.

To assess AKI, the preferred markers continue to be serum creatinine levels together with serum urea levels and urinary output. In acute care the first sign may be reduced urinary output. This is known as oliguria, which is further defined as urinary output lower than 0.5 mL/kg body weight/hour (NICE 2013).

Physiological measurements of urinary output and serum electrolytes are already supported by early warning scores and outreach care (NICE 2007; RCP 2017). A National Confidential Enquiry into Patient Outcome and Death (NCEPOD) found that 29% of the AKI cases reviewed had inadequacies in the management of their kidney injury, with lack of physiological monitoring a common feature (Stewart *et al.* 2009). Worryingly for nurses, they found a proportion of patients with AKI whose urine had not been tested with a urinalysis reagent strip. This is a simple, inexpensive test that should be part of all hospital admissions, offering the opportunity to identify abnormalities immediately.

Table 5.1 summarizes clinical investigations to determine kidney function and move towards a diagnosis.

Vital signs

As a regulatory organ, the kidney has mechanisms to compensate physiologically for imbalance and it may take a while for abnormalities to be noted in the routine vital signs observations done by nurses and healthcare assistants.

The first abnormality to be noted is an increase in respiratory rate to compensate for metabolic acidosis. Respirations rise when kidney cells cannot recycle and create new molecules of bicarbonate and therefore respiratory excretion of CO_2 increases in accordance with the Hasselbach formula for acid–base balance. Regular monitoring of respiratory rate will be an early indicator of deterioration, more so when a trend can be identified over time. It is a key vital sign routinely monitored in NEWS2 (National Early Warning Score 2).

Blood pressure is not likely to change until there are marked compensatory physiological changes. Hypovolaemia will usually translate into hypotension, and hypervolaemia into hypertension. However, by these extremes stages other physical signs are present on examination.

Chronic kidney failure

Health professionals in acute hospital settings need to remain alert to the possibility that patients may have kidney failure unknown to them; that is, silent progression of chronic damage. This means patients initially suspected to have AKI in fact have acute aggravation of underlying chronic kidney failure.

Table 5.1 Renal investigations

Diagnostic investigation	How it is done	Utility
Kidney ultrasound	Sound waves are used to obtain visualization on screen of organs and surfaces of varying densities Gel is applied to the patient's skin and the probe moved round as images are observed on screen in real time This is a painless procedure that can be done anywhere: the machine can be taken to where the patient and an available technician are	Confirms size and presence of two kidneys It will give indication of cysts, if any accumulations of fluid can be indicated but are less clearly defined
Urinalysis	A fresh urine sample is dipped with a suitable reagent strip and readings taken in the given time, which will be up to 2 min	Leucocytes will indicate urinary infection, which can also be suspected from the presence of blood, protein, and nitrates. Where it is known the patient has acute renal failure, specific gravity can indicate acute tubular necrosis due to poor kidney perfusion
Urine creatinine:protein ratio	Urine is collected any time of the day, but not the first void after waking up	Determine urinary loss of protein If more than 3 g/24 h, the patient has nephrotic syndrome
Urine pheresis and cytology	A fresh urine sample is spun and examined under the microscope.	Presence of Bence–Jones protein suggests chronic renal failure from amyloid disease
Kidney angiogram	Contrast substance is injected into the bloodstream and timed X-ray films taken of the kidneys	Stenosis and aneurysms will show up on the X-ray films, indicating problems in the blood circulating to the kidneys
Kidney biopsy	Under local anaesthesia and ultrasound guidance, a biopsy needle is pushed into the kidney to obtain a small number of nephrons for microscopic study	Damaged nephrons are inspected to determine causes Many glomerular and tubular pathologies can be diagnosed immediately

Routine reporting of e-GFR helps long-term monitoring of people who have reduced kidney function and assists care management plans, as outlined in Table 5.2.

Acute kidney injury in hospital settings

AKI is characterized by rapid reduction in kidney excretory function. It is classically divided into pre-renal, renal, and post-renal, depending on where the cause of the insult originated. Table 5.3 shows a selection of common causes.

Table 5.2 Stages of chronic kidney disease, internationally recognised and sanctioned by the UK Renal Association (2014)

Stage	Glomerular filtration rate*	Description	Treatment stage
1	90+	Normal kidney function but urine findings or structural abnormalities or genetic trait point to kidney disease	Observation, control of blood pressure
2	60–89	Mildly reduced kidney function and other findings (as for stage 1) point to kidney disease	Observation, control of blood pressure and risk factors
3A	45–59	Moderately reduced kidney function	Observation, control of blood pressure and risk factors
3B	30–44		
4	15–29	Severely reduced kidney function	Planning for end-stage renal failure
5	< 15 or on dialysis	Very severe, or end-stage kidney failure (sometimes called established renal failure)	Planning for renal replacement therapies, based on lifestyle

* All glomerular filtration rate values are normalised to an average surface area (size) of 1.73 m^2.

Reprinted from *American Journal of Kidney Diseases*, 39, 2, National Kidney Foundation, K/DOQI Clinical Practice Guidelines for Chronic Kidney Disease: Evaluation, Classification and Stratification, pp. S1-S266, Copyright 2002, with permission from Elsevier and the National Kidney Foundation.

In addition to physiological causes of AKI, kidney damage can arise from treatments and investigations offered to patients whilst in hospital. Table 5.4 below outlines common risk factors for kidney injury during hospital admission.

Pathophysiology of acute kidney injury

AKI in the acute setting is most likely to affect the tubules in the nephron. There are two primary mechanisms of injury: acute tubular necrosis, which accounts for approximately 75% of acute renal failure, and interstitial nephritis (Renal Association 2014). Both pathological processes cause oliguria and anuria defined as urinary output less than 0.5 mL/kg/h. A third

Table 5.3 Pre-renal, renal, and post-renal causes of acute kidney injury

Pre-renal	Renal	Post-renal
Hypovolaemia: • vomiting and diarrhoea • haemorrhage	Glomerular damage: • glomerulonephritis • vasculitis	Obstruction: • calculi • tumours
Reduced effective circulating volume: • heart failure • septic shock	Tubular damage: • acute tubular necrosis • interstitial nephritis	

Reproduced from Lopes, J.A. The RIFLE and AKIN classifications for acute kidney injury: A critical and comprehensive review. *Clinical Kidney Journal*. 2013 Feb; 6(1):8–14.

Table 5.4 Risk factors for kidney injury during inpatient episodes

Risk factor	Risk enhancer	Risk reduction measure
Use of intravenous contrast for diagnostic tests, such as angiogram, magnetic resonance	Dehydration Metformin Type and dose of contrast	Rehydration prior to procedure Withhold metformin Adjust choice of contrast, according to e-GFR
Sepsis	Dehydration Hypotension Influx on septic debris for kidney clearance	Intravenous rehydration Prompt antibiotic treatment
Prolonged periods of hypotension	Surgery Continued use of hypotension-inducing drugs such as diuretics and drugs for blood pressure control and heart function	Use of the Enhanced Recovery After Surgery (ERAS) programme Daily medication reviews alongside vital signs—reduce dose or withhold
Use of nephrotoxic drugs	Over-medication Lack of adjustment in dose and need in established prescriptions	Medication review and Medication holiday as needed

mechanism is the nephrotic syndrome, which may be acute or chronic and is characterized by lack of protein reabsorption and consequent low serum levels.

Acute tubular necrosis

Acute tubular necrosis (ATN) accounts for approximately 75% of the AKI episodes that occur in hospital. In ATN, the injury may occur within the tubule, caused by nephrotoxic solutes suspended in the glomerular filtrate, or it may stem from reduced perfusion, as is the case in hypovolaemia and prolonged hypotension. It is known that a sustained drop in mean arterial pressure (MAP) below 60 mmHg increases the risk of acute tubular necrosis.

Tubular cells receive nourishment and excrete some waste products directly on to the glomerular filtrate. Poor perfusion can starve them and lead to acute tubular ischaemia or acute tubular necrosis and AKI.

Interstitial nephritis

In interstitial nephritis the injury occurs in the interstitial space that surrounds tubules, compromising normal tubular flow. The mechanism is different than in acute tubular necrosis. Damage is caused by swelling of the space between the tubules and this may be caused by certain drugs, such as non-steroidal anti-inflammatory drugs. General causes of interstitial nephritis are:

- drug reactions, for example to vancomycin, especially if given too fast.
- allergic processes, for example peanut allergy and wasp stings.

The result is AKI through interstitial nephritis.

Acute kidney injury (AKI) and the nephrotic syndrome

Nephrotic syndrome refers to patient presentation with protein loss in urine. Physiologically the glomerular basement membrane becomes excessively permeable and vast amounts of serum albumin and protein are constantly lost in urine. The nephrotic syndrome is associated with inflammation of the glomerulus, known as glomerulonephritis. There may be an underlying condition or the result of a skin or throat streptococcal infection, generating too much bacterial debris for the glomerular filter of the nephron.

Kidney injury with nephrotic syndrome is identified by measuring extensive loss of protein in urine greater than 3 g/24 h. This will be first suspected when performing urinalysis with a reagent strip that will react intensely to protein. It is then confirmed by 24-hour urine sample or a protein/creatinine ratio in a single void (see Table 5.1 for details of the test).

Patient presentation

The patient with nephrotic syndrome develops low levels of serum protein: creatinine and urea often remain in acceptable range; albumin is less than 25 mmol/L, despite efforts to replace it by breaking down muscle protein. Blood proteins and especially albumin are needed to create oncotic pressure which is a type of osmotic pressure that normally draws water from the body tissues into blood circulation. Loss of oncotic pressure changes the fluid distribution across body compartments, as explained in Chapter 7. The patient becomes fluid-depleted in the vascular space but fluid-overloaded in the interstitial space. The elements of the nephrotic syndrome are:

- hypotension;
- pitting oedema and large amounts of fluid retention, to the point that mobility is difficult and weight rises sharply every day;
- muscle breakdown and malnutrition;
- clotting disturbances, with high risk of embolism.

Nursing management

To protect patient well-being, nursing care is directed to manage symptoms, monitor progress, and prevent clotting complications, such as deep-vein thrombosis and embolisms. Table 5.5 outlines a nursing care plan.

Once the cause of the nephrotic syndrome is known, the medical team will be able to formulate a treatment plan to address the underlying cause. As the glomeruli recover, so the protein loss in urine improves and the signs and symptoms recede.

In extreme cases where protein loss does not improve despite individualized treatment, kidney embolization may be required under angiographic guidance. This means a section of kidney will be lost but it is a justifiable step to prevent long-term complications of unstoppable urinary excretion of protein and hypoalbuminaemia.

Table 5.5 Nursing plan of care for nephrotic syndrome

Potential problem	Nursing care
Rapid malnutrition and oedema due to protein loss and low serum albumin	• Encourage food intake • Explain to patient that appetite is impaired due to internal oedema to the stomach and bowel and advise to eat little and often • Check weight daily • Monitor blood pressure, which may be low; postural hypotension will indicate hypovolaemia due to lack of oncotic pressure from low serum protein levels, particularly albumin • Monitor and document level of pitting oedema • Take regular blood tests to monitor trend in serum albumin level • Encourage light exercise to prevent rapid tissue deterioration and type 2 pressure ulcers
Emboli caused by serum accumulation of lipoprotein as a by-product of muscle breakdown	• Measure, supply and help the patient wear anti-thromboembolism stockings • Ask doctor to prescribe thrombus prevention sub-cutaneous heparin • Observe for respiratory distress/chest tightness or deep leg pain—all possible sites for thrombotic obstruction

Clinical link 5.1 (see Appendix for answers)

Consider this case. Mr T, 72-year-old man, living alone and managing independently, had a fall on the street, landing on his coccyx. Next day he presented to hospital with back pain, which had started with his fall and gradually became worse. There were no detectable abnormalities on X-ray and the pain was thought to be musculoskeletal. The plan was to discharge once the analgesics were sufficiently effective. Mr T was not thriving in hospital, appeared unexpectedly bed-bound despite physiotherapy collaboration, and in day 2 of admission appeared disorientated, had a temperature of 37.5°C, and was complaining of urinary urgency. At the same time his abdomen appeared distended and he reported diarrhoea.

Urine

Leucocytes Present ++
Protein Present +++
Blood Present ++
Ketones Negative
Glucose Negative

Blood results

K^+ 2.9 mmol/L
Na^+ 139 mmol/L

Urea 45 mmol/L
Creatinine 400 µmmol/L
White blood cells 18.0×10^9/L
Haemoglobin 12.3 g/dL
Blood pressure 124/86 mmHg
Pulse 130 bpm
Respirations 24 rpm
Past medical history: bowel cancer in remission for five years, hypertension, awaiting urology appointment for suspected prostate enlargement.

- What would your priorities be for this patient? Justify your actions.
- What interventions from the doctors would you anticipate?
- What types of assessment and monitoring will you continually undertake?
- Why would serum potassium be low and how can this be resolved?
- What type of acute kidney failure may be occurring here? Identify how it can be compensated.

Notes

- Hypokalaemia is a rare presentation and hyperkalaemia is much more likely in AKI, but Mr T reports diarrhoea.
- Refer to Table 5.7 for conservative nursing plan of care.

Conservative management of acute kidney injury

International interest and collaboration to define stages of AKI has led to two main classification systems: RIFLE and AKIN. Published in 2001, RIFLE (Risk, Injury, Failure, Loss, End-stage) has proved useful in clinical practice and popular in research. Clinicians however reported overlap between failure, loss, and end-stage in terms of the optimal timing for intervention. As a result, in 2004, the Acute Kidney Injury Network (AKIN) adapted RIFLE by advocating that invasive treatment should be introduced earlier, at the stage of F for failure (Bassett *et al.* 2017; Bellomo *et al.* 2004; Stevens *et al.* 2001) (Table 5.6).

Whatever the gravity of AKI experienced by the patient, there are two priorities for the healthcare team:

- to help the patient survive—mortality varies between 20% and 80% depending on comorbidity and speed of diagnosis and treatment.
- to rehabilitate kidney function for the long term—although survival is an immediate priority, avoidance of dialysis and filtration therapies is an important outcome. This is because survival with irretrievable and disabling loss of kidney function offers patients poor long-term prognosis and worsening quality of life.

Initially, AKI can be managed conservatively in all clinical settings. Once doctors have diagnosed AKI, conservative management is standardized. It revolves around measurement of

Table 5.6 RIFLE classification of acute kidney failure, including later revision by Acute Kidney Injury Network

	Non-oliguria	Oliguria	Intervention
Risk	Abrupt—1–7 days, decrease (> 25%) in GFR Or serum creatinine × 1.5. Sustained for more than 24 h	Decreased urine output relative to the fluid input. Urine output less than 0.5 mL/kg/h for longer than 6 hours	
Injury	Adjusted creatinine or GFR decrease more than 50%, or serum creatinine × 2	Urine output less than 0.5 mL/kg/h for longer than 12 hours	
Failure	Adjusted creatinine or GFR decrease > 75%, serum creatinine × 3 or serum creatinine > 4mg% or 5 mg/% when acute	Urine output less than 0.5 mL/kg/h for longer than 24 hours and/or anuria for longer than 12 hours	Earliest point for provision of RRT
Loss	Irreversible AKI or persistent AKI for more than 4 weeks	Irreversible AKI or persistent AKI for more than 4 weeks	
ESRF	ESRF for longer than 3 months	ESRF for longer than 3 months	

GFR, glomerular filtration rate; AKI, acute kidney injury; ESRF, end-stage renal failure; RRT, renal replacement therapy.

Reproduced from Lopes, J.A. The RIFLE and AKIN classifications for acute kidney injury: A critical and comprehensive review. *Clinical Kidney Journal.* 2013 Feb; 6(1):8–14, by permission of European Renal Association - European Dialysis and Transplant Association and Oxford University Press.

urine output and clinical judgement to instruct fluid challenge in the presence of oliguria and fluid replacement in the presence of polyuria.

Nursing management

In contemporary nursing care, management of AKI starts with prevention. Patients admitted for elective procedures and surgery need routine assessment with simple tools such as urinalysis and blood pressure measurement, lying and standing. Certain patient groups are at greater risk of silent chronic kidney failure, for example those with diabetes, history of hypertension, or heart failure. Medication reviews are important to protect kidney health with measures such as withholding medications known to be nephrotoxic.

A simple and effective preventative measure for all patients is to avoid pre- and post-operative hypovolaemia with proactive management of patient fasting. Enhanced recovery after surgery (ERAS) guidelines recommend the use of balanced crystalloids as the fluid of choice (Hahn 2016). The Royal Society of Anaesthetists collaborated with nurses and other health professionals to publish much-needed guidance on fasting for surgery in the UK (Hamid 2014; RCN 2005). They recommend clear fluids to be drunk up to two hours pre-surgery. In reality, effective hydration by hospital inpatients continues to be a daily challenge aggravated by lack of clarity on times for procedures. Routine measurement of blood pressure lying and standing on admission is a rough indicator of hydration status; a drop greater than 20 mmHg is often found in dehydrated patients, unaware that they need to drink more fluids.

Nurses are optimally placed to ensure effective hydration and educate their patients accordingly. Good hydration is a positive step to protect kidney function that can be improved greatly with patient involvement.

The effect of low water intake could be further aggravated by the administration of diuretic medication. The same follows for medications known to have a nephrotoxic effect, such as metformin and angiotensin-converting enzyme inhibitors. Whilst the patient may continue to have a clinical need to take these medications, sustained hydration with intravenous fluids during operative procedures that use contrast substances is a simple intervention to help preserve good kidney perfusion. Once discharged and in the community regular medication reviews that include patient symptom and hydration history follow the same proactive thinking to protect kidney health.

In conclusion, the role of acute care nurses in identifying patients at risk and implementing simple but highly effective measures cannot be underestimated. Good communication with patients and other health professionals is essential, for example reviewing the need for diuretic and nephrotoxic medication, clarifying fasting times, and evaluating and discussing response to fluid challenges (Bassett *et al.* 2017). Table 5.7 summarizes the nursing plan of care for conservative management.

Fluid challenge and replacement

Fluid challenge is the practice of administering a large volume of intravenous fluids, possibly combined with diuretics. There is a long tradition of using this approach in an attempt to stimulate return to improved levels of kidney function. Its success is not guaranteed where the kidney function does not respond to the drugs. More recent randomized controlled trials are adding evidence that popular drugs used in acute renal failure such as furosemide and dopamine are ineffective or have benefits neutralized by side effects and complications (NICE 2013). In the majority of cases, AKI can be resolved by adequate fluid challenge or replacement and the treatment of underlying medical conditions, such as sepsis and haemorrhage, as well as avoidance of nephrotoxic drugs.

Clinical link 5.2 (see Appendix for answers)

You are caring for Lydia, a patient 48 h post appendicectomy. Yesterday she had a pyrexia of 39.4°C and a peripheral blood culture sample was taken. The results yields MRSA septicaemia, and Lydia commenced intravenous vancomycin. Lydia is aged 57 and known to have congestive heart disease and takes ramipril and furosemide regularly. However, today her breathing is laboured, bubbly, and distressed. Lydia reports a sense that something terrible is about to happen. Her oxygen saturation is 85% on air, so you start her on oxygen therapy.

- What other immediate actions would you undertake and why?
- What other signs and symptoms would indicate pulmonary oedema?
- If pulmonary oedema was confirmed, how would you coordinate care of the patient including interaction with the nurse in charge and medical team?

Table 5.7 Nursing plan of care for conservative management of acute kidney injury

Potential problem	Nursing care
AKI evidenced by oliguria. One of the first signs of AKI is reduced urinary output, less than 0.5 mL/kg body weight/h.	• Advocate and implement urinary catheterization for the purpose of accurate, hourly measurement of urinary output • Maintain fluid balance chart • Work closely with doctor to implement fluid challenge as soon as possible • Take vital signs observations four times a day and look for changes in breathing and blood pressure • Listen to chest sounds for crackles and observe for dyspnoea • Observe for cyanosis and take oxygen saturation readings; if below 94% (BTS 2017) review oxygen therapy
Infection risk indicated by the presence of invasive devices such as urinary catheter and central line	• Review need for urinary catheter daily and aim to remove on day 5 (NICE 2012) if possible • Observe intravenous cannula daily for signs of infection, give it a phlebitis score once daily, shift, and re-site after 72 h in-situ • Use aseptic non-touch technique when opening the central line • If central line is used for renal replacement therapies, do not use it for anything else—to remain a dedicated line • Support good hygiene practice around the patient environment and with their person, including catheter cleansing • Assess temperature fluctuations four times a day • Encourage nutrition and hydration
Fluid imbalance aggravating AKI	• Encourage patient to keep up fluid intake and keep hydrated. Observe progress and investigate obstacles • If there is a central line in place, take regular readings for central venous pressure • If the patient appears dry, take lying and standing blood pressure; differential greater than 20 mmHg is indicative of dehydration, unless he/she takes medications likely to cause it • If patient is hypotensive review diuretic and anti-hypertensive medication with medical staff
Lack of recovery from AKI	• Notify doctor urgently and contact outreach team if available in hospital (RCP 2017) • Review nephrotoxicity of all medications and discuss with medical team • Take urgent blood sample for urea and electrolytes • Take ECG looking for hyperkalaemic changes—inverted T wave and longer PR interval
Polyuria during recovery phase from AKI	• Polyuria is likely to take 2–3 days to normalize; in the meantime polyuria has to be managed • Monitor hourly urine output and give variable fluid replacement therapy • Educate the patient and reassure that polyuria is transitional, a sign that tubular cells are recovering and it is important to continue drinking and avoid dehydration

AKI, acute kidney injury.

Invasive management of acute kidney injury

A case is made for invasive management of AKI in the presence of the following problems:

- *Metabolic acidosis*, identifiable in elevated respiration rate and hyperkalaemia. Hyperkalaemia is the result of potassium migrating from normal high intra-cellular concentration in an acidotic state.
- *Oliguria* or *anuria*, expressed as urinary output less than 0.5 mL/kg/hour. Reduced fluid output may combine with nausea and vomiting as physiological ways to compensate fluid overload. Anuria can result in pulmonary oedema.
- *Uraemia*—products from normal metabolism are not excreted in urine, resulting in the uraemic syndrome. Amidst its most serious consequences is interference in the clotting cascade, causing extension of bleeding times, and gastrointestinal irritation. The risk of severe and uncontrolled bleeding is life-threatening.

Each problem, on its own and with sufficient gravity in presentation, is enough reason to commence renal replacement therapies (RRT), a decision made after specialist review by a nephrologist or intensivist. Patients with a degree of heart or respiratory failure suffer quicker escalation of the above problems.

When the clinical problems listed above are present and serious, AKI becomes life-threatening. Survival rate is reported in the region of 20–80% depending on comorbidity. RRTs improve both survival and prognosis, but are resource-intensive, not readily available outside intensive care or renal units, and carry new risks associated with their invasive requirements.

All forms of RRT share the following new risks to the patient:

- embolism, accidental puncture of a central vein, and septicaemia due to the need for a double-lumen central vascular catheter
- loss of blood due to clotting in the RRT circuitry or excessive bleeding from use of anticoagulation during treatment

When a patient needs RRT, failure to act worsens prognosis rapidly. Once a decision is made to instigate RRT, the physician has to choose the best option available at the time. That decision should be primarily guided by the clinical priority around one of these life-threatening parameters:

- correction of metabolic acidosis to reduce the cardiac threat of *hyperkalaemia*
- fluid removal across body compartments to correct *pulmonary oedema*
- solute removal to improve *uraemic syndrome*

Clinical link 5.3 (see Appendix for answers)

Following on from Clinical link 5.2, 12 h have passed. Her condition has deteriorated further but she is still able to sustain her own breathing. The chest X-ray shows upper lobe blood diversion, urinary output is a total of 200 mL in the last 12 h.

Vital signs

Blood pressure 92/58 mmHg
Pulse 136 bpm
Respirations 32 rpm
Oxygen saturations 82%
Temperature 37.4°C

Recent blood results

K^+ 6.9 mmol/L
Na^+ 139 mmol/L
Urea 45 mmol/L
Creatinine 450 μmmol/L
Bicarbonate 13 mEq/L

- What may be causing Lydia's problems?
- Why is potassium high?
- What will the medical team do next?

Renal replacement therapies (RRT)

RRTs aim to replace the homeostatic function of the kidney normally regulated by the production of urine. They offer safe, effective means to support kidney function and maintain acceptable levels of fluid and electrolyte balance.

Despite a wide range of small studies comparing RRTs in the treatment of AKI, small samples often make the evidence base inconclusive. What is known with certainty is that recurrent hypotensive episodes will cause further kidney injury and increase the likelihood of long-term dialysis as a patient outcome. Hence the choice most likely to preserve haemodynamic stability for the individual patient is the optimal RRT.

There are several choices to compare in Table 5.8

Clinical link 5.4 (see Appendix for answers)

Following on from Clinical link 5.3, Lydia was prescribed 50 mL of 50% glucose mixed with 10 units of human insulin administered over 30 m. She was also given intravenous calcium gluconate 10%.

A double lumen central line was inserted into the femoral vein and arrangements were made for Lydia to receive 6 h of haemodiafiltration.

- Why was Lydia prescribed the above drugs?

The physician opted for haemodiafiltration as RRT. This decision was based on the need to remove both fluid and solutes.

- Why was haemodialysis not given instead, when the same outcome can be delivered?

Table 5.8 Choices of RRT, all of which require extra-corporeal blood circulation and anticoagulation

Therapy	Overview of therapy	Best suited to these patients	Advantages and shortfalls
Haemofiltration	Blood is pushed through a filter in a closed circuit. Plasmatic fluid is drained, depending on the flow pressure through the filter Treatment will continue for more than 8 h, and up to 24 h	Patients whose clinical priority is fluid removal Patients who need up to 15 L removed from their blood circulation in 24 h	Gradual fluid removal helps sustain blood pressure levels Equipment easier to set-up and cheaper than the other options Requires sustained anticoagulation for a long period
Haemodialysis	Same as above but therapy takes 2–4 h only Blood is exposed to purified water across a semi-permeable membrane, allowing for diffusion	Patients whose clinical priority is solute removal and correction of acidosis, with fluid removal no more than 3 L per session	Physiological shifts of solutes and fluid are rapid and effective Water treatment facilities and sophisticated dialysis machines are required Anticoagulation is needed but can be dispensed with if necessary
Haemodiafiltration	Same as above but therapy takes 6–8 h. In this option sterile water is used. Blood is exposed to it across a membrane as in haemodialysis, however water is also mixed with blood, usually in a pre-filter dilution regimen but can also be post-dilution.	Patients whose clinical priority is solute removal and large fluid removal Patients who need to achieve this and are severely hypotensive.	Good diffusion of larger molecules than any of the above, good for removal of body toxins produced in septicaemia Good fluid and solute removal with least hypotension risk Requires sterile water, which can be provided in large bags Sterile water requirement added to the limited availability of machines makes this is the most expensive therapy Anticoagulation is needed during therapy

RRT is linked to approximately 4.9% of admissions to intensive care units. Patients with single-system failure or recovering well from other complications may, however, be able to transfer to level 2, high-dependency areas, of which there is a recognized lack in the United Kingdom (NICE 2013; RCP 2017). Level 2 patients are those needing high dependency care, usually due to one organ failure. Managed in clinical areas with the right nursing skills and ratio, level 2 patients do not require an intensive care bed. Level 3 patients also require highly dependent care, but have multi-organ failure and need intensive care accommodation and one-to-one specialist nursing. Lydia could have been managed in a level 2 facility if one was available, provided her heart and respiratory systems remained stable.

The ideal model of care offers fluidity and collaborative critical care networks that are responsive to patient need in a timely fashion. If care remains patient-centred, professional boundaries and systems are less likely to drive their clinical outcome. More level 2 high-dependency areas increase the flexibility to offer the patient RRT without having to take an intensive or renal unit bed.

Acute care nursing

Nurses help protect patients from kidney injury by understanding that every individual with a health problem is at risk. Hospital admission, and all that comes with it, enhances that risk. National early warning scores widely introduced across the NHS include respiration rate. A rising early warning score based on faster respiration and observation of lower urinary output in the previous 6 h should be escalated for medical attention. In the meantime, seeking further information from the patient and obtaining additional clinical data would help a timely, differential diagnosis of AKI, for example:

- fluid intake
- urinalysis
- medication review
- urgent urea and electrolytes blood test
- postural blood pressure readings to assist fluid assessment
- 12-lead ECG looking for rhythm changes related to accumulated serum potassium or calcium

Finally, life without dialysis is an important outcome for any patient recovering from kidney injury. Effective intervention to avoid permanent kidney injury requires sound clinical judgment but also equipment and expertise that are not available in every hospital. It is important to build networks of care and support across NHS Trust organizations, knowing how to access specialist advice at tertiary level. Renal services in the United Kingdom are organized centrally for each county. Through networks of care and local contacts, acute care nurses can be made aware of the location and services offered at their tertiary renal unit, for example access to renal pharmacy, dieticians, and advice from nursing colleagues with expertise in renal care.

The patient experience of acute kidney injury

AKI has sudden onset and the patient may be too ill to comprehend the full extent of their progress, risk, and prognosis. This will be different for loved ones, observing rapid changes to more invasive devices such as urinary catheterization, intravenous infusions, filtration, or dialysis, and stepping up of nursing and medical monitoring. They require much reassurance and especially to be kept informed.

A frequent concern expressed by visitors is weight loss, poor appetite, and fatigue. Taking into account existing evidence, aggressive nutritional supplementation is generally discouraged and viewed as detrimental to kidney recovery. Nurses can reassure relatives and visitors that a short period of fasting is not damaging and equally that a change in clinical condition is expected within days, therefore malnutrition is not likely to become a problem. Nevertheless, early dietetic referral is an essential multidisciplinary plan for patient recovery from AKI. Dietitians will assess patients individually and promote oral intake, followed by sips and supplements, enteral feeds, and, in extreme cases, parental nutrition. The emphasis is on the less invasive options supported by frequent review and adjustments (Mafrici and Williams 2015).

During the recovery phase of AKI, an excessive amount of urine, known as polyuria, is passed in the first two to three days. This reassures patients and their loved ones because it indicates a return to normal kidney function. It is still a critical period when the kidney cells are readjusting; it carries risk of dehydration before aldosterone reabsorption returns to normal. It is a timely opportunity for nursing staff to educate patients on the need to keep up fluid intake and to quantify this effectively, based on continued measurement of urine output.

Patient engagement

Information and understanding are necessary for patients to consent and adhere to treatment. In recent years use of digital resources has increased to understand health problems and help make decisions. A reliable and informative example is managed by NHS Choices at http://www.nhs.uk. The acute care nurse can recommend it to patients as a resource to find comprehensive information on AKI (NHS Choices 2016a) in everyday language. It has the added advantage of inclusiveness for patients with sensory deficit or those who require translation (NHS Choices 2016b).

End of chapter test

The following assessment will enable you to evaluate your theoretical knowledge of acute kidney injury and its management as well as your ability to apply this theory to clinical practice.

Knowledge assessment

With the support of your mentor/supervisor from practice, work through the following prompts to explore your knowledge level about assessment of kidney function and management of acute kidney injury.

- Describe the functions of the kidney and relate common signs and symptoms to kidney failure.
- Differentiate between acute, chronic, and acute-on-chronic kidney failure.
- Recognize risk factors for kidney failure.
- Explain what makes AKI life-threatening.
- Explain your role and responsibilities as a nurse to protect kidney health.
- Explain how blood tests, investigations, and observations are needed to assess kidney function.
- Choose a case from personal practice where the patient experienced AKI and explore what happened, what worked well, and what could have been different.

Skills assessment

Under the guidance of your mentor/supervisor, plan care for an individual in acute renal failure, followed by appropriate interventions and evaluation. Your mentor/supervisor will be able to assess your ability and provide feedback based on the following skills:

- Conducts a patient history and physical assessment to support a clinical judgment on their likelihood of developing AKI.
- Monitors and interprets patient's urinary output, fluid intake, vital signs, and blood test results to comment on kidney function.
- Undertakes urinalysis, postural blood pressure, and study of fluid balance to comment on kidney health and risk of injury.
- Undertakes appropriate medication review to protect kidney health.

References

Bassett, S. *et al.* (2017) *Think Kidneys National AKI Programme- Review and Evaluation Report.* London: NHS England. Available at: https://www.thinkkidneys.nhs.uk/aki/wp-content/uploads/sites/2/2017/02/NHS-Think-Kidneys-AKI-Programme-Review-and-Evaluation.pdf, accessed 13 January 2020.

Bellomo, R., Ronco, C., Kellum, J.A., and the ADQI workgroup (2004) Acute renal failure—definition, outcome measures, animal models, fluid therapy and information technology needs. The second international consensus conference of Acute Dialysis Quality Initiative (ADQI) Group. *Crit Care,* **8**:R204–R212.

British Thoracic Society (BTS) (2017) BTS Guideline for oxygen use in healthcare and emergency settings. Available at: https://www.brit-thoracic.org.uk/standards-of-care/guidelines/bts-guideline-for-emergency-oxygen-use-in-adult-patients/; accessed 9 December 2019.

Calvert, S., Shaw, A. (2012) Perioperative acute kidney injury. Available at: https://perioperativemedicinejournal.biomedcentral.com/track/pdf/10.1186/2047-0525-1-6; accessed 13 January 2020.

Hahn, R. (ed.) (2016) *Clinical Fluid Therapy in the Perioperative Setting* 3rd edn. London: Cambridge University Press.

Hamid, S. (2014) Pre-operative fasting—a patient-centered approach. Available at: http://qir.bmj.com/content/2/2/u605.w1252.full.pdf+html; accessed 9 December 2019.

Mafrici, B., Williams, H. (2015) *Overview of Nutritional Considerations in the Treatment of Adult Patients with Acute Kidney Injury in Hospital.* London: NHS England.

NHS Choices (2016a) Acute Kidney Injury. Available at: http://www.nhs.uk/conditions/acute-kidney-injury/Pages/Introduction.aspx; accessed 9 December 2019.

NHS Choices (2016b) Accessibility Statement. Available at: http://www.nhs.uk/aboutNHSChoices/aboutnhschoices/accessibility/Pages/Accessibilitystatement.aspx; accessed 9 December 2019.

NICE (2012) *Healthcare-Associated Infections: Prevention and Control in Primary and Community Care* CGD 139. London: National Institute for Health and Care Excellence.

NICE (2007) *Acutely Ill Patients in Hospital: Recognition of and Response to Acute Illness in Adults in Hospital.* London: National Institute for Health and Care Excellence.

NICE (2013) *Acute Kidney Injury: Prevention, Detection and Management*

Clinical Guideline CG169. London: National Institute for Health and Care Excellence.

Renal Association (2014) *Treatment of Adults and Children with Renal Failure: Recommended Standards And Audit Measures,* 6th edn. London: Royal College of Physicians.

Renal Registry (2015) *The Eighteenth Annual Report*. London: The Renal Association.

RCN (2005) *Perioperative Fasting in Adults and Children*. London: Royal College of Nursing.

RCP 2017 *National Early Warning Scores (NEWS) 2: Standardising the Assessment of Acute Illness Severity in the NHS*. London: Royal College of Physicians.

Stewart, J., Findlay, G., Smith, N. *et al.* (2009) *Adding Insult to Injury—A Report by the National Confidential Enquiry into Patient Outcome and Death*. London: National Confidential Enquiry into Patient Outcome and Death.

6
The care of patients with gastrointestinal disease and nutritional support for the acutely ill patient

Katharine Martyn and Fiona Creed

Chapter contents

This chapter will explore the:

- care and management of patients presenting with symptoms of the gastrointestinal (GI) tract and associated organs with related anatomy and physiology
- management of raised blood glucose in the acutely ill patient including patients with diabetes
- nutritional support of the patient in the acute care setting, including enteral and parenteral nutrition

Learning outcomes

This chapter will enable you to:

- explain common symptoms associated with GI disorders and dysfunction using the relevant anatomy and physiology
- explain the significance of a raised blood glucose and the importance of its management for patients with and without type 1 or type 2 diabetes
- understand the importance of nutritional support in the acutely ill patient

Patients with acute gastrointestinal disease

In 2014–15, 5.7% of attendances to an Accident and Emergency (A&E) department in England were due to gastrointestinal conditions with the highest number of admissions related to pelvic and abdominal pain (HSCIC 2017). An understanding of the normal physiology of the gut is therefore essential to facilitate delivery of appropriate care to this group of patients.

Physiology of the gastrointestinal tract

Mouth and swallowing

Swallowing is controlled by a swallowing centre in the brain and is in three distinct stages. The first stage is the formation of a bolus.

At the mouth, mastication or chewing of food forms a bolus, which can then be swallowed into the oesophagus. The teeth break the food into small segments and movement of the tongue and cheek mixes the food with saliva, salivary amylase, and lingual lipase. During the chewing process the food is gradually moved to the back of the throat, the oropharynx, where the swallowing reflex is initiated. The second stage, the pharyngeal phase, is triggered as soon as the bolus reaches the tonsils and is automatic.

During this phase the soft palate closes against the back wall of the throat, separating the oral cavity from the nasal cavity to prevent food or liquid from coming up through the nose. The vocal cords close, shutting access to the trachea to prevent food or liquid from being aspirated into the lungs. Next the throat muscles contract in a rhythmic, coordinated fashion to propel the bolus downwards towards the oesophagus. There is movement of the larynx and epiglottis to both protect the vocal cords and to ensure the bolus goes in the correct direction. Finally, the oesophageal sphincter relaxes and the bolus enters the oesophagus.

The third and final phase occurs once the bolus is in the oesophagus, the oesophageal phase, describes the active movement of the bolus through peristalsis into the stomach.

The stomach and small intestine

The stomach allows food to be consumed in large amounts, mixing the food with mucus, hydrochloric acid (HCl), and gastric enzymes (pepsin and lipase). Food often contains many microbes and during swallowing a large number of microbes will be swallowed. Parietal cells secrete HCl into the lumen of the stomach, which reduces the bacterial load as the contents of the stomach fall to a pH of 1–3. This acid environment denatures proteins, making them more accessible to enzyme activity, and activates the enzyme pepsinogen.

Parietal (also known as oxyntic) cells are stimulated by:

- acetylcholine, released by parasympathetic neurons;
- gastrin, secreted by G cells;
- histamine, secreted by mast cells.

The movement of food along the GI tract is due to rhythmic contractions, known as peristalsis, which are controlled by the vagus nerve through the parasympathetic divisions of the autonomic nervous system. The type of movement will reflect the function of that component. In the body of the stomach, peristalsis takes the form of waves of vigorous muscle contraction that mix the food with HCl, mucus, gastric lipase, and pepsin, until a thick paste called chyme is formed. The rate at which chyme leaves the stomach through the pyloric sphincter, gastric emptying, depends on the composition and volume of food or liquid consumed. Water leaves the stomach quickly, whilst

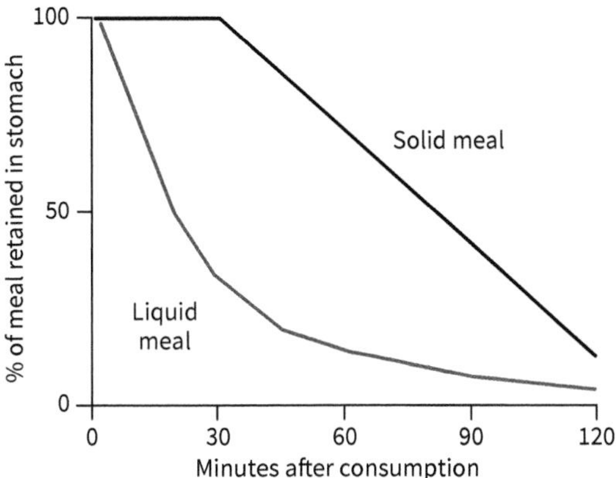

Figure 6.1 Estimated gastric emptying time.

Adapted from Degen, L.P., and Phillips, S.F. Variability of gastrointestinal transit in healthy women and men. *Gut*, 39(2): 299–305. Copyright © 1996, BMJ Publishing Group Ltd and the British Society of Gastroenterology. With permission from BMJ Publishing Group Ltd. http://dx.doi.org/10.1136/gut.39.2.299.

complex meals begin to leave after a lag time of between 20 min and 30 min, 2–4 h after consumption. For an estimation of the time taken for gastric emptying see Figure 6.1.

The stomach joins with the small intestine by the pyloric sphincter, regulating gastric emptying. The small intestine comprises the duodenum (25 cm), the jejunum (1 m), and ileum (2 m), and joins with the large intestine at the ileocaecal sphincter. The movement of chyme begins as a slow wave at the lower portion of the stomach, reaching the end of the ileum in 90–120 min, before another wave begins. In this way chyme remains in the small intestine for three to five hours. A second type of peristalsis, segmentation, is a localized contraction that mixes the chyme with the digestive juices and brings the digested food into contact with the mucosa for absorption.

As the chyme enters the duodenum, the presence of lipids (fatty acids) and peptides trigger the release of the hormone cholecystokinin that stimulates secretion of pancreatic juice and contraction of the wall of the gall bladder. In addition, it:

- slows gastric emptying by promoting the pyloric sphincter to contract;
- enhances satiety by acting on the hypothalamus;
- maintains the normal growth of the pancreas and enhances the effect of secretin.

The presence of chyme also triggers the release of the hormone secretin from S cells in the duodenum to increase the flow of pancreatic juices containing bicarbonate ions, buffering the acidic chyme and inhibiting the secretion of gastric juices.

The structure of the small intestine is modified by the presence of circular folds, villi and micro villi (the brush border), which enhance its absorptive function. The circular folds also ensure that the chyme spirals as it is moved through the small intestine by muscle contractions, known as the migratory motility complex.

The villi are finger-like projections that have a central lymphatic capillary (lacteal), arteriole, venule, and capillary network which is essential for nutrient absorption. These vessels

Table 6.1 Brush border enzymes

Substrate	Enzyme	End product
Sucrose	Sucrase	Glucose and fructose
Lactose	Lactase	Glucose and galactose
Maltose	Maltase	Glucose
Dipeptides	Dipeptidases	Amino acids

are embedded in the lamina propria, which also contains mucosa-associated lymphoid tissue. The outer layer of a villus is composed of several different cells:

- absorptive cells that have microvilli (the brush border) on their surface, which increases the surface area, and have brush border enzymes (see Table 6.1);
- goblet cells that secrete mucus;
- enteroendocrine cells that secrete secretin, cholecystokinin, or glucose-dependent insulinotropic peptide;
- paneth cells, which secrete lysozyme and are capable of phagocytosis.

Functions of the small intestine

The main function of the small intestine is the absorption of nutrients, water, and drugs through the mucosal membrane and into the hepatic portal vein or lymphatic system. Absorption of nutrients, amino acids, glucose, fructose and galactose, fatty acids, vitamins, minerals, and trace elements is through several distinct mechanisms. Some areas of the small intestine have precise roles in absorbing micronutrients. Vitamin B12 is only absorbed in the ileum because of the presence of intrinsic factor and carrier proteins (Table 6.2).

Absorption of nutrients and fluids may be compromised during periods of ill-health or due to specific disease processes that alter the length and surface area of the small intestine.

Common symptoms associated with malabsorption include:

- osmotic diarrhoea (carbohydrate malabsorption);
- steatorrhoea (fat malabsorption);
- pernicious anaemia (vitamin B12 malabsorption);
- iron deficiency anaemia (iron malabsorption).

Protection

In addition, the GI tract is an integral part of the first line of defence immune mechanism, by limiting entry of ingested pathogens or toxins to the body. The acid environment of the stomach created by the release of HCl reduces the bacterial load of any food ingested. The lymphoid tissue along with lymphatic nodules throughout the small intestine form Peyer's patches making the GI tract the largest immune organ in the body.

Table 6.2 The absorption of macronutrients

Food	Enzymes	Absorption
Carbohydrates found in foods such as bread, pasta, rice, fruit, and vegetables	Salivary amylase Pancreatic amylase Sucrase Maltase Lactase Galactase	Fructose is absorbed by facilitated diffusion, so there is no need for metabolic energy, but a specific carrier is required. Once inside the cell, fructose is phosphorylated and converted to glucose prior to entering the portal blood. Galactose and glucose are actively transported into the mucosal cell by a common transport protein. The energy for this active transport is provided by the electrochemical Na + gradient. The glucose carrier has binding sites for Na + and glucose. When both are bound, the protein translocates across the membrane.
Protein found in meat, fish, dairy products, fruit, vegetables, pulses, and grains	Pepsin Pancreatic peptidases	Dipeptides and tripeptides are transported across the brush border membrane. Amino acids are transported across the brush border plasma membrane into the intestinal mucosal cell by way of certain specific amino acid transport systems. There are three main sodium-dependent active transport systems for amino acids that occur in brush border membranes. The neutral brush border system transports most of the neutral amino acids, both hydrophobic and hydrophilic.
Fat found in all food groups, with most dietary fats coming from animal and dairy products	Gastric lipase Pancreatic lipase The absorption of fat requires bile salts to emulsify fat and aid formation of micelles	The fat digestion products, i.e. monoglycerides, fatty acids, cholesterol, and phospholipids, are present in the intestinal lumen in the form of micelles (aggregates). Micelle formation is aided by the presence of bile acids. These products are absorbed into the intestinal mucosal cell from these micelles. They enter the lacteals in the villi in the form of chylomicrons entering the blood stream at the vena cava. As the micelles travel down the small intestine they become more concentrated with cholesterol. Although the duodenum and jejunum are active in absorbing fatty components, most of the ingested fat is absorbed at the mid jejunum. Free fatty acids diffuse across the brush border membrane.

The structures of the lining of the small intestine do not normally come into direct contact with nutrients, potential pathogens, or allergens, and as such the immune tissues are not stimulated. However, it is possible for individuals to develop intolerance to a nutrient if the functions of the GI tract are altered, or an allergy to a specific nutrient if the lining of the small intestines is compromised and the immune system is activated.

The large intestine

At the end of the ileum, the ileocaecal sphincter or valve allows the remnants of food to enter the large intestine. This valve has an important regulatory function as it slows the flow from

Table 6.3 Infections caused by bacteria found in the colon

Infection	Bacterium
Urinary tract infections	*E coli*, enterococci and Proteus species
Intra-abdominal infections	Bacteriodes fragilis
Diarrhoea and vomiting	*E. coli*

the ileum into the caecum. Distension and irritation to the caecum results in a reflex increase in the tone of the ileocaecal valve and inhibits ileal peristalsis. The large intestine is 1.5 m in length and is divided into the caecum, colon, rectum, and anus. The food remnants from digestion and absorption are slowly moved along its length by peristalsis. As the contents move towards the transverse colon a strong peristaltic wave begins (mass propulsion), quickly driving the contents of the colon into the rectum. Once in the rectum, stretching of the rectal wall stimulates stretch receptors, initiating a defaecation reflex. After consuming food, a gastrocolic reflex is initiated in the colon, triggering mass peristalsis three to four times per day during or shortly after a meal.

Functions of the large intestine

The functions of the large intestine include chemical digestion, absorption of water and the end products of fermentation, and faeces formation. The colon contains 10^{12} per cubic millilitre (mL^3) of commensal bacteria. These bacteria are essential for maintaining the health of the colon but can easily be transmitted to other tissues and organs, causing infection (Table 6.3). In the colon, bacterial fermentation breaks down remaining carbohydrates, proteins, and fats. In the fermentation process, methane is produced causing flatulence, which can cause distress to patients. In addition, short chain fatty acids (butyric acid and propionic acid) are produced, maintaining colonic health, with the excess entering the bloodstream for use by other body tissues.

The remaining faecal matter contains a mixture of inorganic salts, sloughed off epithelial cells, products of bacterial fermentation, unabsorbed digested materials, and the indigestible parts of food.

Fluids and fluid balance

Approximately 2000 mL of fluid are consumed each day, with a further 7000 mL of water made up from saliva, gastric secretions, bile, pancreatic juice, and intestinal secretions entering the lumen of the GI tract.

Food will have been in the GI tract for as long as 10 h and during this time 90% of the water will have been reabsorbed along with nutrients in the small intestine. Of the remaining 0.5–1 L of water that enters the large intestine, up to 800 mL will be reabsorbed, making the large intestine an important organ for maintaining fluid balance.

Inflammation of the mucosal membranes due to infection or disease will compromise this function, leading to diarrhoea (see section on altered bowel function). Excessive water and electrolytes loss can be seen in:

- ulcerative colitis;
- Crohn's disease; and
- gastroenteritis.

The liver and gall bladder

The liver is the major metabolic organ and, weighs almost 1.4 kg in adults, it occupies most of the right hypochondriac region. It is divided into two principal lobes: a large right lobe and smaller left lobe, made up of functional units called lobules; each containing hepatocytes, a central vein, highly permeable capillaries called sinusoids, and fixed phagocytes called Kupffer cells.

The hepatocytes secrete bile into small canals, the canaliculi, which empty into small bile ductules that emerge to form the common hepatic duct. The common hepatic duct joins the cystic duct from the gall bladder to form the common bile duct. About 1 L of bile is secreted each day and it is made up of water, bile salts, cholesterol, lecithin, bile pigments, and several ions. Bile is the major way of excreting excess cholesterol and bilirubin from the haem component of phagocytosed red blood cells.

The liver has two blood supplies. The hepatic artery supplies oxygenated blood for cell function and the hepatic portal vein supplies absorbed nutrients, drugs, microbes, and toxins from the GI tract. Products manufactured by the hepatocytes and nutrients are secreted into the blood via the central vein, which feeds into the hepatic vein. In this way the liver controls what enters the central circulation. Portal hypertension is a common complication of liver disease and can lead to a distended liver, ascites, and enlargement of the oesophageal varices.

Functions of the liver

Carbohydrate metabolism

The liver is essential for maintaining a normal blood glucose level of between 4 and 6 mmol/L. When blood glucose is high the liver converts glucose to glycogen and triglyceride for storage. In this way, excess dietary carbohydrate can lead to excessive triglyceride production (Box 6.1). When blood glucose is low the liver can break down glycogen to glucose and convert certain amino acids and lactic acid to glucose. It can also convert other sugars such as galactose and fructose to glucose.

Lipid metabolism

The hepatocytes synthesize very low-density lipoproteins (VLDL) and high-density lipoproteins (HDL) to transport fatty acids, triglycerol, and cholesterol to and from the liver. Altered

Box 6.1 Patients at risk of fatty liver disease

Patients who are being artificially fed via a parenteral route are at risk of developing fatty liver disease, as triglyceride is synthesized and stored in the liver. Liver function tests are recommended twice weekly when patients are fed via a parenteral route (NICE 2012).

Other patients at risk are those who are overweight and those who consume large quantities of alcohol.

Symptoms of fatty liver disease

- A third of patients have no symptoms.
- Liver is enlarged and may be tender.

blood lipids are risk factors for coronary heart disease. Cholesterol is synthesized by the liver. When cellular cholesterol stores are full, excess is excreted in bile salts.

Protein metabolism

Hepatocytes deaminate, removing $^{-}NH2$ from amino acids (Box 6.2), so that the amino acid can be used for adenosine triphosphate (ATP) production or converted to carbohydrate or fats. The resulting ammonia, NH_3, is converted to urea, which can then be excreted in urine. Hepatocytes also synthesize most plasma proteins, including albumin, C-reactive protein, prothrombin, and fibrinogen.

Drugs and hormones

During metabolism of drugs the metabolites can be active or toxic, as in the case of paracetomol (Box 6.3). If the toxic metabolite exceeds the liver's capacity to detoxify it then

Box 6.2 Amino acids

There are 20 amino acids which are found as constituents of proteins. These are essential for metabolism but only eight amino acids are essential and must be consumed in the diet:

- leucine, isoleucine, valine, phenyalanine, threonine, methinonine, tryptophan, and lysine.

In times of acute illness, the rate of synthesis of plasma proteins such as prothrombin and fibrinogen will exceed the availability of amino acids, and prothrombin and fibrinogen levels will fall. This increases the risk of bleeding. During acute illness the amino acid glutamine is considered to be conditionally essential.

Box 6.3 Liver disease and drug metabolism

Liver disease can affect the way drugs are metabolized. This may:

- increase the availability of an active drug, increasing the risk of toxic effects.
- decrease the availability of the active drug.
- increase the time taken for a drug and its metabolites to be excreted, increasing the risk of toxic effects.

damage to the hepatocytes can occur. The liver detoxifies substances such as alcohol and hormones and can excrete drugs such as penicillin and erythromycin.

Excretion of bilirubin

Bilirubin is the end product of haem metabolism. Initial bilirubin is unconjugated and insoluble in water. After uptake by hepatocytes the bilirubin is conjugated, made water-soluble, and excreted into the biliary tract for storage in the gall bladder. Alterations in the metabolism of bilirubin can lead to jaundice (Box 6.4).

Other functions of the liver

- Synthesis of bile salts: bile salts act like biological soap and solubilise ingested fat and fat-soluble vitamins, facilitating their digestion and absorption.
- Storage of glycogen and vitamins such as B12, A, D, E, K. Glycogen stores are sufficient to provide glucose for approximately 24 h in the absence of dietary intake (see section on energy balance). Stores of vitamins in the liver ensure their availability when dietary intake is compromised.

Box 6.4 Jaundice

Jaundice is a common sign associated with disease of the liver, gall bladder, or head of the pancreas (blocking the hepatopancreatic duct). It can also occur if the red blood cells die too quickly—haemolytic anaemia.

Jaundice associated with the gall bladder or obstruction of the hepatopancreatic duct will be caused by the decreased excretion of conjugated bilirubin, and the stools will be pale and clay-like; the urine will be much darker. The patient may complain of generalized pruritis.

Jaundice associated with liver disease will lead to an increase in unconjugated bilirubin in the plasma. The stools will be pale and clay-like. The urine will not be as dark but the level of jaundice can be severe.

- Activation of vitamin D: fat-soluble vitamin D is essential for calcium metabolism. Biologically inactive once synthesized in the epidermis or ingested as part of the diet, it must be activated by the liver.
- Phagocytosis of bacteria, aged red blood cells and white blood cells by Kupffer cells.

Gall bladder

The gall bladder stores bile, and in the presence of cholecystokinin the gall bladder contracts and the hepatopancreatic sphincter (sphincter of Oddi) opens, allowing bile to enter the duodenum.

In some patients gall stones will form in the gall bladder. These can pass through the biliary tract, causing biliary colic (see section on abdominal pain).

The pancreas

The pancreas is a gland that is about 15 cm long and 1 cm wide and lies posterior to the greater curvature of the stomach. It is divided into three regions: the head, the body, and the tail, and is usually connected to the duodenum by two ducts: the accessory duct and the hepatopancreatic duct.

The pancreas is both an exocrine and endocrine gland. The larger exocrine portion is made up of small clusters of glandular epithelial cells known as acini, which secrete up to 1.5 L of fluid containing a mixture of inactive and active digestive enzymes, sodium bicarbonate, and some salts. These active enzymes include pancreatic amylase, pancreatic lipase, ribonuclease, and deoxyribonuclease. In addition, the inactive trypsinogen comes into contact with a brush border enzyme, enterokinase, which splits the trypsinogen to active trypsin, activating the remaining inactive pancreatic enzymes, chymotrypsinogen, procarboxypeptidase, and proelastase. These enzymes are inactive to prevent auto digestion of pancreatic cells. The acinar cells also produce a trypsin inhibitor should any active trypsin be produced.

The remaining cells of the pancreas form islets called pancreatic islets (islets of Langerhan), which produce the hormones glucagon, insulin, somatostatin, and pancreatic polypeptide, which are secreted into the bloodstream (see section on blood glucose regulation).

Supporting patients with alterations to gastrointestinal tract functioning

In this section, common signs and symptoms associated with altered GI tract function will be explored in conjunction with the relevant disease processes.

Patients presenting with an altered swallow—dysphagia

The most common causes of dysphagia in an acute care setting are related to altered neurological function due to trauma or illness such as stroke, or general anaesthesia. Patients with a reduced level of consciousness will automatically have a reduced ability to swallow and this should be considered within the general management of the patient (see Chapter 4). Patients with altered cognitive functioning such as dementia may also have difficulties in swallowing as they no longer respond to the triggers for the swallowing reflex or even recognize when to swallow.

Swallowing

Early recognition of the signs and symptoms associated with a reduced ability to swallow (Box 6.5) will help to prevent aspiration of gastric secretions or food and reduce the risk of aspirate pneumonia developing.

Nursing assessment of a patient with dysphagia

Formal assessment of the swallow is normally completed by the speech and language team (SALT), but it is important that appropriately qualified nurses complete a basic assessment if there is a change in the patient's condition, the patient complains of having difficulty in swallowing, or there are concerns about a patient's ability to eat. The assessment is as follows:

- Check to see if dysphagia is due to airway obstruction.
- Observe for obstruction such as enlarged tonsils.
- Ensure patient has a clean, moist mouth, and, if present, correctly fitting dentures. This will aid the formation of a bolus which will assist swallowing.
- Evaluate swallowing reflex by placing your fingers along the thyroid notch and instruct the patient to swallow. If you feel the larynx rise, the reflex is functioning. If uncertain, follow local protocol and refer to SALT for swallowing assessment.
- Ask patient to cough to assess the cough reflex.

Box 6.5 Signs and symptoms of a dysphagia

- Difficulty in coordinating breathing with eating or drinking
- Wet 'gurgly' voice when speaking
- Dribbling of saliva from the mouth
- Frequent coughing
- Unexplained weight loss, altered diet, or loss of appetite
- Recurrent chest infections
- Difficulty with chewing with prolonged meal times
- Aspiration of food or liquid
- Laboured breathing
- Difficulty in speaking

Royal College of Physicians 2016 National clinical guideline for stroke. Prepared by the Intercollegiate Stroke Working Party

Source data from Royal College of Physicians. (2016). National clinical guideline for stroke, 5th edn. Prepared by the Intercollegiate Stroke Working Party.

- If certain that both the swallowing and cough reflex are present, assess the gag reflex. This can be achieved by touching the pharyngeal mucosa with a tongue depressor.
- Look at the face and listen to the speech for signs of muscle weakness. Does the patient have aphasia or dysarthria? Is the voice nasal, wet, hoarse, or breathy? Can the patient poke out their tongue?
- Ask whether solids or liquids are more difficult swallow.
- Ask whether the symptoms disappear after trying to swallow a few times. Is the swallow affected by the position in bed or chair?
- Is it painful to swallow?

Nursing management of a patient with dysphagia

Dysphagia will not only compromise food and fluid intake, increasing the risk of malnutrition and dehydration, but will also increase the risk of oral infections and mouth discomfort, as the secretions remain in the oral cavity or are lost through the mouth. NICE guidance supports the importance of good oral care in nursing and residential care homes (NICE 2016) and is extending this to patients in hospital (NICE 2017). Oral infections increase the risk of infections in the heart and lungs, and the possibility of septicaemia, bacteraemia, and endocarditis developing. In the critically ill patient oral hygiene is essential for patients who are ventilated (Sands *et al.* 2014) and its importance in the acutely ill patient is being explored. The following steps should be taken:

- Inspect the oral cavity and ensure frequent oral hygiene is performed.
- Monitor prescribed medications that reduce secretions.
- Use suctioning as required.
- Provide nutritional support (see section on nutritional support).

Clinical link 6.1 (see Appendix for answers)

Rosie Hubbard, 84, has been admitted into hospital following a right-sided stroke. She is conscious and a computerized tomography (CT) scan has confirmed she has had a bleed. She has been seen by the physiotherapist who has confirmed that she can sit unaided. An intravenous infusion has been commenced; she is currently receiving 1 L of dextrose saline over 8 h. You notice she has difficulty in drinking and water is dribbling down her chin.

- What would your priorities be for this patient?
- What actions will you take to ensure her nutritional and fluid needs are met?
- What signs might indicate that she has a problem with swallowing?

The patient with abdominal pain

Abdominal pain can be acute or chronic and is one of the most common symptoms expressed by patients and can account for up to 50% of surgical emergencies (Macaluso and

McNamara 2012). Acute and severe abdominal pain is almost always as a result of intra-abdominal disease.

As pain is experienced very differently by individuals it can be described in many ways, and identifying where the pain comes from can be difficult (see Table 6.4).

Pathophysiology of abdominal pain

Visceral pain

Pain that originates from the internal abdominal organs is known as visceral pain and is innervated by the autonomic nerve fibres, which respond mainly to sensations of distension and muscular contraction, but not to cutting, tearing, or local irritation. This type of pain is

Table 6.4 Abdominal pain

Pain description	Common causes
Pain after meals or on an empty stomach Pain can occur at night and may be relieved by antacids or food	Peptic ulcer
Pain is severe, lasting from 1 to 12 h Pain is sporadic and is located in the right epigastrum, the right upper quadrant and or right scapula	Biliary colic If the pain lasts longer than this it may be indicative of pancreatitis or cholecystitis. Following the episode of pain the patients feels generally well. If the common bile duct is obstructed this can also lead to fever (cholangitis) and jaundice.
Pain is often described as steady and radiating through to the back	Pancreatitis A patient can have several episodes and at its most severe can lead to shock. The patient may also suffer from nausea, vomiting, and weakness. Drinking alcohol can exacerbate the condition.
Waves of abdominal pain, often after eating	Ischaemic bowel disease can be caused by Crohn's disease, neoplasm, or volvulus. Patients who have a history of atherosclerosis have an increased risk of myocardial infarction, aortic abdominal aneurysm, and mesenteric ischaemia. The patient may also present with pyrexia, weight loss, nausea, vomiting, and fear of eating.
Severe left lower quadrant abdominal pain	Diverticular disease may lead to the development of peridiverticular abscess. Patient may also have a raised temperature. Diverticular disease is often asymptomatic.
Severe flank pain radiating to the groin	Renal colic, due to a stone passing through the ureter, may be accompanied by haematuria. Although not chronic it may be recurrent.
Recurring abdominal pain	In women, pelvic inflammatory disease or endometriosis may account for recurring abdominal pain. Patient is well between bouts of pain.

Source data from Jones, A., Turner, K., and Handa, A. Surgical emergencies: Acute abdominal pain. *Student BMJ*. 2000; 8: 56–7, and Lakshay, C., *et al.* Clinical profile of non-traumatic acute abdominal pain presenting to an adult emergency department. *Journal of Family Medicine and Primary Care*. 2015; 4(3): 422–5.

carried by the sympathetic autonomic nerves and enters the spinal cord from T6 to L2. The parasympathetic system also carries pain sensation from the pelvic organs via S2, 3, and 4.

Visceral pain is often described as 'vague, dull, and nauseating' and poorly localized, which means that the patient cannot always describe where it is. In general:

- pain in the upper abdomen is caused by distension or muscular contraction of the stomach, duodenum, liver, and pancreas structures.
- pain in the periumbicular region is caused by distension or muscle contraction of the small intestines, proximal colon, and appendix.
- lower abdominal pain is triggered by distension or muscular contraction of the distal colon, and genital urinary tract.

Somatic pain

Somatic pain comes from the parietal peritoneum, which is innervated by somatic nerves and responds to irritation from infectious, chemical, or other inflammatory processes. Somatic afferents supplying the abdominal wall enter the spinal cord between T5 and L2. Additionally, the undersurface of the diaphragm has innervation from the phrenic nerve (C3, 4, and 5). Thus, irritation of the diaphragm may refer pain to the shoulder. Somatic pain is sharp and well localized.

Referred pain

Referred pain is perceived some distance from its origin due to convergence of sensory neurons at the spinal cord. Common examples of referred pain include:

- pain in the scapula due to biliary colic.
- pain in the groin due to renal colic.
- pain in the shoulder due to blood or infection irritating the diaphragm.

Abdominal pain

Abdominal pain can also be caused by conditions not associated with the abdomen, including:

- herpes zoster
- alcoholic ketoacidosis
- diabetic ketoacidosis
- porphyria
- sickle cell disease
- myocardial infarction
- pneumonia
- pulmonary embolism
- opioid withdrawal

Nursing assessment of the patient with abdominal pain

The initial assessment of the patient, including presenting history is important. Signs of anxiety, pale skin, and increased sweating (diaphoresis) can all be indicative of a serious problem.

Baseline observation, including blood pressure, pulse, state of consciousness, and altered peripheral perfusion, must all be recorded

Patients with abdominal pain may present with concomitant symptoms such as nausea, vomiting, diarrhoea, constipation, jaundice, melaena, haematuria, haemetemesis, gastro-oesophageal reflux, mucus or blood in the stool, and weight loss.

Accurate recording of fluid loss and faecal loss, including consistency and odour, is important to aid diagnosis and to plan care (see Chapter 7).

Certain findings should be reported immediately:

- severe pain
- signs of shock (e.g. tachycardia, hypotension, diaphoresis, confusion)
- signs of peritonitis—see next section
- abdominal distension

Nursing management of patients with abdominal pain

Careful questioning can provide essential information that will help in pain management (see Table 6.5). Using a simple pain scale to score the pain will enable the effectiveness of interventions to be monitored.

Management of symptoms

- Pain caused by indigestion or trapped wind may respond to antacids and peppermint water.
- Severe pain will respond to opioid analgesia such as morphine. Pain associated with renal colic will respond well to diclofenac. There is some concern that administering analgesia may mask other symptoms but a Cochrane review supports the use of analgesia (Manterola *et al.* 2011).
- Symptomatic control of nausea and vomiting using anti-emetics.

The patient with intestinal obstruction

Intestinal obstruction is a common cause of pain. Patients who have had previous surgery are more at risk of obstruction due to adhesions. As the GI tract becomes obstructed, increased peristalsis occurs as the GI tract attempts to clear the blockage. This increased peristalsis can heard through a stethoscope, has a high-pitched sound and is known as borborygmi. If the obstruction is not cleared then peristalsis will stop and the patient will have a 'silent abdomen'. During this time the patient will be in severe pain, and reluctant to move.

Mechanical obstruction is divided into obstruction of the small bowel (including the duodenum) (Box 6.6) and obstruction of the large bowel (Box 6.7). Obstruction may be partial or complete. About 85% of partial small-bowel obstructions resolve with non-operative treatment, whereas about 85% of complete small-bowel obstructions require operation.

Pathophysiology

In simple mechanical obstruction, blockage occurs without vascular compromise. Ingested fluid and food, digestive secretions, and gas accumulate above the obstruction. The proximal

Table 6.5 Questions related to abdominal pain assessment

Question	Potential responses	Indication
Where is the pain?		Location of the pain: visceral, somatic, referred
What is the pain like?	Acute waves of sharp constricting pain that 'take the breath away'	Renal or biliary colic
	Waves of dull pain with vomiting	Intestinal obstruction
	Colicky pain that becomes steady	Appendicitis, strangulating intestinal obstruction, mesenteric ischaemia
	Sharp, constant pain, worsened by movement	Peritonitis
	Tearing pain	Dissecting aneurysm
	Dull ache	Appendicitis, diverticulitis, pyelonephritis
Have you had it before?	Yes	Suggests recurrent problems such as ulcer disease, gallstone colic, diverticulitis, or mittelschmerz
Was the onset sudden?	Sudden: 'like a light switching on'	Perforated ulcer, ruptured aneurysm, torsion of ovary or testis, renal stones
	Less sudden	Most other causes
How severe is the pain?	Severe pain	Kidney stone, peritonitis, pancreatitis
	Pain out of proportion to physical findings	Mesenteric ischaemia
Does the pain travel to any other part of the body?	Right scapula	Gall bladder pain
	Left shoulder region	Ruptured spleen, pancreatitis
	Pubis or vagina	Renal pain
	Back	Ruptured aortic aneurysm
What relieves the pain?	Antacids	Peptic ulcer disease
	Lying as quietly as possible	Peritonitis
What other symptoms occur with the pain?	Vomiting precedes pain and is followed by diarrhoea	Gastroenteritis
	Delayed vomiting, absent bowel movement, and flatus	Acute intestinal obstruction
	Severe vomiting precedes intense epigastric, left chest, or shoulder pain	Emetic perforation of the intra-abdominal oesophagus

Box 6.6 Signs and symptoms associated with obstruction of the small intestine

- Abdominal cramps centred around the umbilicus or in the epigastrium.
- Vomiting.
- Complete obstruction—constipation or severe constipation (obstipation).
- Partial obstruction—diarrhoea.
- Severe, steady pain suggests that strangulation has occurred. In the absence of strangulation, the abdomen is not tender.
- Hyperactive, high-pitched peristalsis with rushes coinciding with cramps is typical.
- With infarction, the abdomen becomes tender and auscultation reveals a silent abdomen or minimal peristalsis.
- Shock and oliguria are serious signs that indicate either late simple obstruction or strangulation.

bowel distends and the distal segment collapses. The normal secretory and absorptive functions of the mucosa are depressed, and the bowel wall becomes oedematous and congested.

Strangulating obstruction is obstruction with compromised blood flow; it occurs in nearly 25% of patients with small-bowel obstruction. Venous obstruction occurs first, followed by arterial occlusion, resulting in rapid ischaemia of the bowel wall. The ischaemic bowel becomes oedematous and infarcts, leading to gangrene and perforation.

The patient with peritonitis

The most serious cause of peritonitis is perforation of the GI tract, which produces immediate chemical inflammation followed shortly by infection from intestinal organisms. Peritonitis is inflammation of the peritoneal cavity and the most common symptom is pain, which may be localized or diffuse. Peritonitis can also result from any abdominal condition that produces marked inflammation (Dever and Sheikh 2015), including:

- appendicitis, diverticulitis, strangulating intestinal obstruction, pancreatitis, pelvic inflammatory disease, mesenteric ischaemia.

Box 6.7 Signs and symptoms associated with obstruction of the large intestine

- Symptoms that develop more gradually than those caused by small-bowel obstruction.
- Increasing constipation leads to obstipation and abdominal distention.
- Vomiting may occur several hours after onset of other symptoms and may smell faecal-like but is not common.
- Lower abdominal cramps unproductive of faeces occur.
- Distended abdomen with loud borborygmi.
- Systemic symptoms are relatively mild, and fluid and electrolyte deficits are uncommon.

- intraperitoneal blood from any source (e.g. ruptured aneurysm, trauma, surgery, ectopic pregnancy).
- barium, which causes severe peritonitis and should never be given to a patient with suspected GI tract perforation.
- peritoneo-systemic shunts, drains, and dialysis catheters in the peritoneal cavity, which all predispose a patient to infectious peritonitis, as does ascitic fluid (rarely, spontaneous bacterial peritonitis occurs, in which the peritoneal cavity is infected by blood-borne bacteria).

Constipation is normally present unless a pelvic abscess develops, when the patient will present with diarrhoea. Peritonitis causes fluid shift into the peritoneal cavity and bowel, leading to severe dehydration and electrolyte disturbances. The immediate management will involve maintenance of oxygenation, fluid resuscitation, analgesia, antibiotics, and positioning of a nasogastric tube to drain stomach contents to alleviate vomiting.

In severe cases adult respiratory distress syndrome can develop rapidly. Kidney failure, liver failure, and disseminated intravascular coagulation can then follow. The patient's face becomes drawn into the mask-like appearance typical of hippocratic facies: a pinched expression of the face, with sunken eyes, concavity of cheeks and temples, and relaxed lips. This is often associated with impending death.

The patient with nausea and vomiting

Nausea and vomiting are common symptoms experienced by patients. Nausea and vomiting are also common symptoms associated with treatments such as chemotherapy and radiotherapy, with as many as 25% of patients refusing chemotherapy treatments because of the discomfort they may feel (Longo *et al.* 2016).

Vomiting (emesis) is multifactorial and can be caused by a range of stimuli, including medical interventions. In addition to poisoning and gastroenteritis, emetic stimuli include motion, surgery, GI tract obstruction, pregnancy, drugs, radiation, fear, and pain. As a reflex it can be classified into three phases: nausea, retching, and vomiting.

Nausea is described as an unpleasant sensation that immediately proceeds vomiting. A cold sweat, pallor, salivation, a noticeable disinterest in the surroundings, loss of gastric tone, duodenal contractions, and the reflux of intestinal contents into the stomach often accompany nausea.

Retching follows nausea and comprises laboured spasmodic respiratory movements against a closed glottis with contractions of the abdominal muscles, chest wall, and diaphragm, without any expulsion of gastric contents. Retching can occur without vomiting but normally it generates the pressure gradient that leads to vomiting.

Vomiting is caused by the powerful sustained contraction of the abdominal and chest wall musculature, which is accompanied by the descent of the diaphragm and the opening of the gastric cardia. This is a reflex activity that is not under voluntary control. It results in the rapid and forceful evacuation of stomach contents up to and out of the mouth.

Neuronal pathways, transmitters, and receptors involved in nausea and vomiting

There are two types of receptors involved in nausea and vomiting:

- Mechanoreceptors are tension receptors that initiate emesis in response to distension and contraction (e.g. from bowel obstruction). They are located in the stomach, jejunum, and ileum.
- Chemoreceptors respond to a variety of toxins in the intestinal lumina.

A third trigger for nausea and vomiting unrelated to disorders of the gastrointestinal tract include infections of the inner ear such as labyrinthitis, and pregnancy.

Once stimulated, nerve impulses are transmitted through common afferent neuronal pathways from the abdomen to the vomiting centre in the medulla, where the vomiting reflex is initiated. The vomiting centre controls the act of vomiting and instead of being a discrete site is a series of interrelated neural networks. Inputs include the vagal sensory pathways from the GI tract, neuronal pathways from the labyrinths, higher centres of the cortex, intracranial pressure receptors, and the chemoreceptor trigger zone (CTZ). The CTZ acts as an entry point for emetic stimuli and is in the area of the fourth ventricle known as the prostrema. It is outside the blood–brain barrier, and therefore responds to stimuli from either the cerebrospinal fluid (CSF) or the blood.

When activated, the vomiting centre induces vomiting via stimulation of the salivary and respiratory centres and the pharyngeal, GI, and abdominal muscles.

Schematically the major factors influencing nausea and vomiting can be illustrated as shown in Figure 6.2.

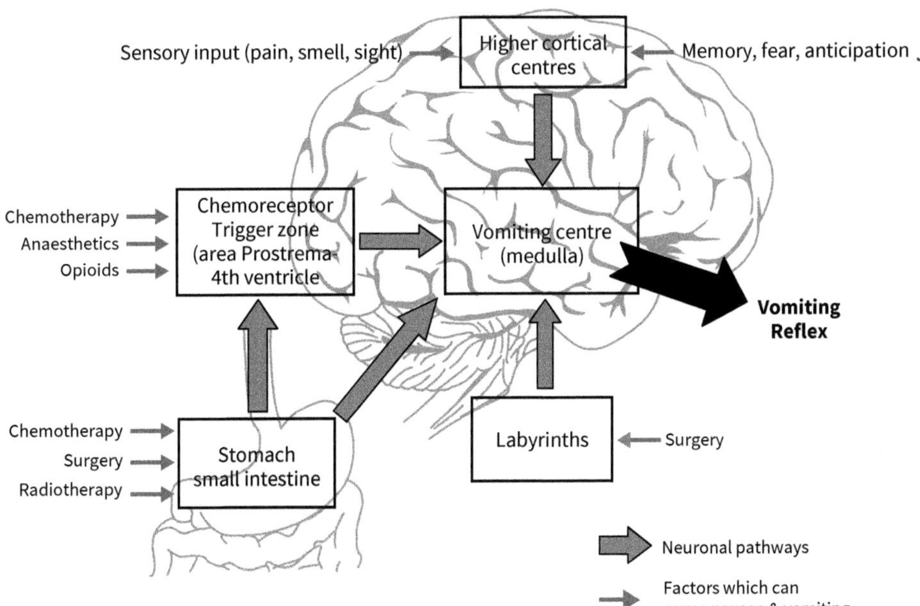

Figure 6.2 Factors influencing nausea and vomiting.

In the brain, a wide variety of receptor types and neurotransmitters are thought to have an impact on vomiting. The neurotransmitters include histamine, acetylcholine, dopamine, noradrenaline, adrenaline, 5-hydroxytryptamine (5HT), and Substance P. In support of their role in emesis, it has been shown that antagonists of receptors for each of these transmitters have anti-emetic effects.

The management of nausea and vomiting

It is important to care for the well-being and comfort of the patient, since poor management of this can lead to delayed recovery, poor clinical outcome, and aversion to future treatment.

The management of patients with nausea and vomiting should address a number of important issues:

- identification and elimination of the underlying cause if possible;
- control of the symptoms if it is not possible to eliminate the underlying cause;
- correction of electrolyte, fluid, or nutritional deficiencies;
- managing risk of bleeding or aspiration pneumonia.

Controlling symptoms: Drug treatment of nausea and vomiting

A wide range of drugs have been shown to have effects on nausea and vomiting. These include antihistamines, anticholinergics, dopamine receptor antagonists, $5HT_3$ receptor antagonists, cannabinoids, benzodiazepines, corticosteroids, and gastroprokinetic agents. Each of the drugs affects different receptors, and some act at a number of different sites. This determines their different clinical profiles.

The main classes of anti-emetic drugs commonly used are shown in Table 6.6, although it should be appreciated that many drugs have multiple mechanisms of action.

Table 6.6 Prescribed anti-emetics

Class	Drug	Comments
Anti-cholinergic	Scopolamine (hyoscine)	
Anti-histamine	Cinnarizine	Useful for post-operative nausea and vomiting
	Cyclizine Promethazine	Useful for motion sickness and nausea and vomiting associated with opioids
Dopamine antagonists	Metoclopramide Domperidone	Useful for nausea associated with enteral tube feeding as prokinetic
	Haloperidol	Patients with suspected bowel obstruction *should not* be prescribed prokinetic drugs
Cannabinoid	Nabilone	
Corticosteroid	Dexamethasone	
Histamine analogue	Betahistine	
$5HT_3$-receptor antagonist	Granisetron Ondansetron	Useful for chemotherapy and radiotherapy-induced nausea and vomiting

Based on data from the British National Formulary (2016). Available at: http://www.bnf.org/bnf/

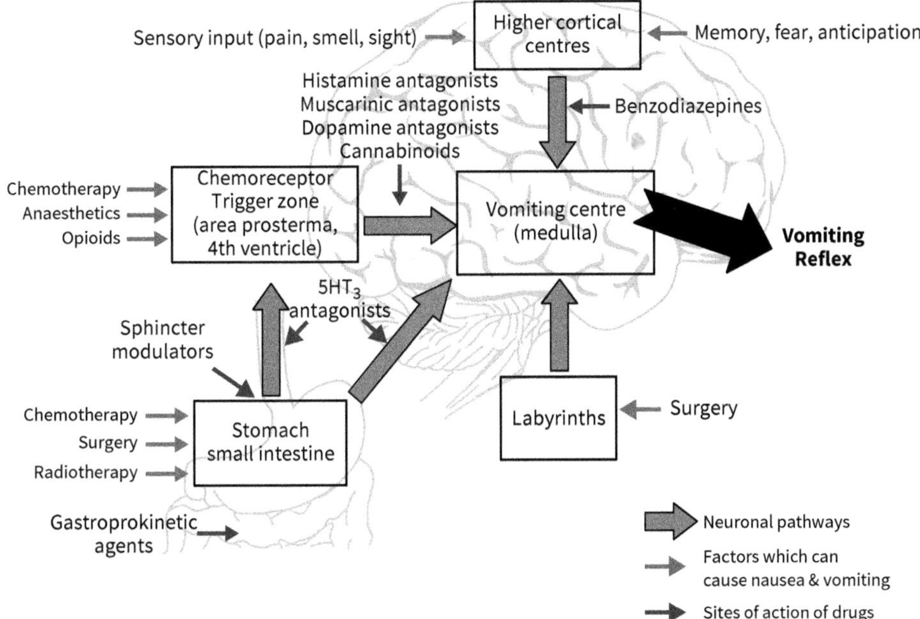

Figure 6.3 Drugs used to control nausea and vomiting and their sites of action.

A multidrug approach to the treatment of different types of nausea and vomiting is often used in clinical practice, based on knowledge of the causes of the underlying nausea and vomiting and the sites of action of each of the available drugs (Figure 6.3).

Nursing management of nausea and vomiting

Vomiting is very unpleasant and will leave a bitter taste in the mouth. Offering regular mouth care and sips of fluid will be comforting.

Management of nausea and vomiting:

- Measure and record all vomitus on a fluid chart and calculate fluid balance. The GI tract can secrete as much as 7 L of fluid into the lumen each day, which is normally reabsorbed as the gastric contents move from the stomach through to the colon. Excessive vomiting can deplete the stomach of HCl, leading to a metabolic alkalosis. The loss of sodium and water will also lead to dehydration.
- Ensure antiemetic medication is given in a timely fashion when patients undergo treatments that are known to induce nausea and vomiting.

Vomiting and nausea associated with gastrointestinal tract obstruction

- Nausea and vomiting caused by obstruction in the small intestines will contain bile, which can stain the mouth, and have an offensive smell depending on where the obstruction occurs. Patients with GI tract obstruction may require the insertion of nasogastric tube for drainage of stomach contents.

Vomiting associated with enteral tube feeding

The most common factors that contribute to nausea and vomiting associated with enteral tube feeding are reduced gastric emptying, infection, and intolerance to the feed.

- When enteral tube feeding, ensure the patient is inclined at no less than 30°.
- Gastric motility can be enhanced through the use of prokinetic anti-emetics (see Table 6.6).
- Ensure hands are washed before preparing a feed and that feeding tube is changed every 24 h (NICE 2017).
- Avoid use of milk-based feeds if patient is lactose intolerant.

The patient with diarrhoea

Diarrhoea is characterized by the passage of frequent, watery stools, which may have an offensive odour. Normally it will last for one to two days but if it persists can lead to dehydration and electrolyte imbalances (see Chapter 7). Chronic diarrhoea can lead to weight loss and malnutrition. In serious cases diarrhoea is often accompanied with other symptoms, including fever, cramps, dyspepsia, and intestinal bleeding.

Diarrhoea can be caused by several different mechanisms: osmotic diarrhoea, motility diarrhoea, and secretory diarrhoea.

Osmotic diarrhoea can be caused by carbohydrate malabsorption as sugars such as glucose, fructose, lactose, and sorbitol draw water into the colon and increase faecal water content. This can occur as a result of lactose intolerance, excessive sorbitol consumption, excessive fructose consumption in the form of fruits, and high concentrated formulated feeds.

Motility diarrhoea speeds up peristalsis and can accelerate entry of fluids into the colon. This can occur following gastric surgery and removal of the lower part of the ileum and caecum or the ileocaecal valve.

Secretory diarrhoea is often caused by bacterial food poisoning or enteritis. In hospital infections, *Clostridium difficile* can be the major cause of diarrhoea. Patients suffering from inflammatory bowel disease (Crohn's, ulcerative colitis) may also suffer from chronic diarrhoea or acute episodes of diarrhoea during exacerbations of their condition.

Nurses' role in managing diarrhoea

During episodes of diarrhoea it is important that personal hygiene is maintained and the skin around the anal sphincter is protected from excoriation. Recording faecal loss to maintain an accurate fluid balance chart and to ensure appropriate oral intake is maintained. In acute cases of diarrhoea, fluid loss can be excessive and intravenous rehydration will be required (see Chapter 7).

Treatment of diarrhoea is based on treating the underlying cause and, if food-related, omitting the dietary source. If the diarrhoea is caused by the administration of enteral feeds it is important that the feed is not stopped. Advice should be sought from the dietician, who may recommend that the rate of the feed is reduced or may prescribe fibre-containing feeds to increase the faecal bulk and reduce gastric transit time.

The patient with constipation

Many patients in hospital may complain of constipation. This may occur as a result of medication that slows down peristalsis such as opioids. During acute illness, becoming constipated may also exacerbate the management of other conditions as people strain to empty their bowels. In addition, constipation may exacerbate confusional states, especially in the elderly or, post-operatively, as toxins from the colon enter the bloodstream.

Dietary management of constipation is focused on ensuring that adequate fluids and fibre-containing foods are consumed. In the management of the acutely ill patient, laxatives, suppositories, and enemas may be required as dietary intake is reduced (see Table 6.7).

The patient with raised blood glucose

In health, blood glucose is maintained between 4 and 6 mmol/L by the action of the pancreatic hormones, insulin and glucagon, and the function of the liver. Following a carbohydrate containing meal, blood glucose will rise and this will stimulate the release of insulin to promote the cellular uptake of glucose by the liver and skeletal muscle. This anabolic response enables excess glucose to be stored in the form of glycogen and triglycerol. During periods of starvation, such as during the night, blood glucose will begin to fall and glucagon is released. This catabolic response will stimulate the release of glucose from glycogen and fatty acids from the lipids. If starvation is prolonged then fatty acids from adipocytes and amino acids derived from skeletal muscle will be used by the liver to synthesize new glucose in a process known as gluconeogenesis.

Table 6.7 Laxatives

Laxative type	Active ingredient	Method of action	Cautions
Fibre	Methylcellulose, psyllium	Increase stool weight and aid in formation of soft bulky stools	May increase flatulence. Psyllium may cause an allergic reaction
Emollient	Docusate sodium	Detergent action promotes mixing of water with stools	Limited effect
Osmotic laxative	Lactulose	Unabsorbed carbohydrate attracts water in large intestine	May cause flatulence and cramp
Saline laxatives (osmotic laxatives)	Magnesium hydroxide, sodium sulphate	Unabsorbed salt attracts and retains water in large intestine	May cause bloating and watery stools. Should be used with caution
Stimulant	Senna, bisacodyl, cascara, castor oil	Act as local irritants to colonic tissue; stimulates peristalsis and mucosal secretions	May alter fluid and electrolyte balance

Based on data from the British National Formulary (2016). Available at: http://www.bnf.org/bnf/

Acute illness and increased blood glucose

An increase in blood glucose can also be observed in acute illness, when dietary intake is often suppressed. This increase in blood glucose occurs due to:

- the presence of acute phase catabolic hormones (adrenalin and cortisol);
- the presence of circulating cytokines (chemicals), which increase glucose synthesis;
- the development of insulin resistance (see section on energy balance).

Monitoring the blood glucose of an acutely ill patient is important as uncontrolled blood glucose will lead to fluid and electrolyte imbalance. It has been demonstrated that tight glycaemic control with minimal fluctuations in patients following a myocardial infarction or stroke can reduce morbidity and mortality (Shu-hua *et al.* 2017). Research is now focusing on whether improved glycaemic control will have similar benefits in other acutely ill patients (Egi *et al.* 2016).

Patients with type 1 and type 2 diabetes can find their blood glucose is unstable and less easy to manage when they are acutely ill. It is important that they continue with their oral hypoglycaemics or insulin, even if they are not eating, and, additionally that their blood glucose levels are closely monitored.

Fluid and electrolyte disturbances when blood glucose is raised

If the blood glucose concentration is higher than 10 mmol/L, the capacity for reabsorption of glucose in the proximal convoluted tubule in the kidney is exceeded and glucose remains in the lumen of the nephron. The excretion of excess glucose in urine (glycosurea) by the nephrons is one way in which blood glucose is regulated.

The fluid in the lumen of the nephron is now more concentrated than the surrounding blood and water is 'trapped' due to the process of osmosis. The osmotic diuresis caused leads to a water loss in excess of sodium loss, increasing the sodium concentration of the blood; hypernatraemia can occur.

As blood glucose increases, the concentration (osmolality) of blood increases and water is drawn from the cells into the circulatory system through the process of osmosis. This shift of fluid into the vascular system can create hyponatraemia as the blood is diluted. As the cells become dehydrated, antidiuretic hormone (ADH) is released from the posterior pituitary gland and the thirst centre is triggered. ADH binds to receptors at the distal convoluted tubule of the nephron and triggers the reabsorption of water. Monitoring fluids and electrolytes is essential in the management of patients with raised blood glucose (see Chapter 7).

In patients with hyperglycaemia it is important that the patient is monitored and that nurses recognize the point at which additional support is required. Monitoring should include the following:

- bedside capillary blood glucose and ketone testing
- fluid balance charts
- assessment of consciousness level (ACVPU)

All patients who are acutely ill can present with, or develop, raised blood glucose.

Diabetes mellitus

Impaired regulation of blood glucose is commonly known as diabetes mellitus. In this condition insulin is either not produced or is not effective. Type 1 diabetes can occur at any age but is commonly first seen in younger people, whilst type 2 diabetes is usually associated with older people, although it is increasingly seen in younger overweight individuals. Without insulin the body is unable to regulate blood glucose levels and the glucose in the blood is not able to enter the cells.

For patients who have type 1 or type 2 diabetes acute illness can lead to the development of diabetic ketoacidosis or non-ketotic hyperosmolar states. These metabolic complications are potentially life-threatening and can lead to admission into critical care units

Diabetic ketoacidosis

The most common causes of diabetic ketoacidosis (DKA) are pneumonia, urinary tract infection, sinusitis, sepsis, and meningitis. In critically ill patients it can also be precipitated by trauma, myocardial infarction, surgery, pancreatitis, and failure to take insulin. DKA is a complex metabolic disorder that occurs when there is a relative insulin deficiency and increase in counter-regulatory hormones such as glucagon and cortisol. This imbalance leads to an increase in hepatic gluconeogenesis and glycogenolysis resulting in severe hyperglycaemia. Free fatty acids released due to lipolysis are then metabolized as an energy source increasing the production of ketones through ketogenesis. The increase in ketone bodies (predominantly 3-beta-hydroxybutyrate) leads to metabolic acidosis. In addition, there is fluid depletion due to osmotic diuresis secondary to hyperglycaemia, vomiting, and an inability to drink fluids. Osmotic diuresis also leads to electrolyte depletion and risk of hyperkalaemia or hypokalaemia developing. The signs and symptoms of developing DKA include the following (Karlya 2015; see Box 6.8):

- altered mental status
- deep and rapid breathing pattern—Kussmauls's respirations
- 'fruity' breath
- nausea and vomiting
- abdominal pain
- diffuse weakness

Box 6.8 **Diagnosis of DKA**

Ketonaemia > 3.0 mmol/L *or* significant ketonuria (more than 2+ on standard urine sticks)
Blood glucose > 11.0 mmol/L or known diabetes mellitus
Bicarbonate (HCO_{3-}) < 15.0 mmol/L ***and/or*** venous pH < 7.3

Reproduced with permission from Joint British Diabetes Societies Inpatient Care Group. (2013). *The Management of Diabetic Ketoacidosis in Adults*, 2nd edn.

- hypothermia secondary to acidosis induced peripheral vasodilation

Bedside monitoring

It is essential that the diabetes specialist team is always involved in the care of patients admitted with DKA. Patients who present with DKA should be managed based on bedside monitoring of blood glucose, blood ketones, electrolytes including bicarbonate and venous pH (JBDS 2013). The medical management of DKA will include aggressive fluid management using prescribed intravenous fluids followed by insulin administration (Box 6.9).

Nurses' role in managing patients who have DKA

Patients with DKA can rapidly deteriorate and haemodynamic monitoring during medical interventions is essential. The nurse should monitor using early warning scores and maintain accurate records of all fluids, insulin and electrolytes administered, to monitor urine output, and complete fluid balance charts. The presence of one or more of the following may indicate severe DKA:

- Blood ketones over 6 mmol/L
- Bicarbonate level below 5 mmol/L
- Blood pH below 7.0
- Hypokalaemia on admission (under 3.5 mmol/L)
- GCS less than 12
- Oxygen saturation below 92% on air (assuming normal baseline respiratory function)
- Systolic BP below 90 mmHg
- Pulse over 100 or below 60 bpm

Box 6.9 Management of DKA

- Crystalloid fluids such as 0.9% sodium chloride to restore of circulatory volume, clear ketones and correct electrolyte. It is recommended that 0.9% sodium chloride solution with potassium 40 mmol/L (ready-mixed) is prescribed when the serum potassium level is below 5.5 mmol/L and the patient is passing urine. If the serum potassium level falls below 3.5 mmol/L the potassium regimen needs review.
- A fixed rate intravenous insulin infusion (FRIII) calculated on 0.1 units/per kilogram body weight using short-acting insulin to normalize blood glucose levels
- Introduction of 10% glucose is recommended when the blood glucose falls below 14.0 mmol/L. Alongside FRIII to suppress ketogenesis. IV Glucose should continue until the patient is eating and drinking normally. It is important to continue 0.9% sodium chloride solution to correct circulatory volume. It is quite often necessary to infuse these solutions concurrently (JBDS guidelines 2013)

Source data from Joint British Diabetes Societies Inpatient Care Group. (2013). *The Management of Diabetic Ketoacidosis in Adults*, 2nd edn.

- Anion gap above 16

[Anion Gap = $(Na^+ + K^+)$—$(Cl^- + HCO_3^-)$]

If the patient exhibits any of these signs they should be reviewed by a consultant physician and considered for referral to a level 2 environment. In addition, the nurse should provide continuing care of the airway, mouth care, personal hygiene, catheter care if *in situ*, and pressure area care.

Hyperosmolar hyperglycaemic states

Hyperosmolar hyperglycaemic states (HHS) are more common in frail, elderly patients who suffer from type 2 diabetes and are unable to take adequate oral fluids. It can be precipitated by infection, medications such as diuretics, or during the perioperative period. Mortality in HHS is greater than that with DKA (Bhansali and Sukumar 2016). Symptoms of HHS developing include:

- confusion
- seizures
- focal deficits such as hemiplegia

Patients with HHS will develop profound dehydration, hyperosmolarity, and hyperglycaemia (Box 6.10). The poor tissue perfusion and dehydration leads to lactic acidosis. The dehydration, haemoconcentration, and hyperviscosity can result in the development of thrombi, which can adversely affect patient survival.

As with DKA, fluid replacement is the most important therapy and should commence with normal saline and continue until the patient is no longer hypotensive and urine output is increased. Patients with HHS are complex and often have multiple comorbidities so they require intensive monitoring. The JBDS (2012) suggests that the presence of one or more of the following may indicate the need for admission to a level 2 environment:

Box 6.10 **Definition and diagnosis of HHS**

- Hypovolaemia—patient can lose 100–220 ml/kg per day
- Marked hyperglycaemia (30 mmol/L or more) without significant hyperketonaemia (< 3 mmol/L) or
- acidosis (pH > 7.3, bicarbonate > 15 mmol/L)
- Osmolality usually 320 mosmol/kg or more (JBDS 2012)

Adapted with permission from Joint British Diabetes Societies Inpatient Care Group. (2012). *The management of the hyperosmolar hyperglycaemic state (HHS) in adults with diabetes.*

- Osmolality greater than 350 mosmol/kg
- Sodium above 160 mmol/L
- Blood pH below 7.1
- Hypokalaemia (less than 3.5 mmol/L) or hyperkalaemia (more than 6 mmol/L) on admission
- Glasgow Coma Scale (GCS) less than 12
- Oxygen saturation below 92% on air (assuming normal baseline respiratory function)
- Systolic blood pressure below 90 mmHg
- Pulse over 100 or below 60

The nursing role is to provide continuing care to ensure patient comfort during this episode and to monitor the haemodynamic status of the patient strictly. The poor tissue perfusion resulting from the severe dehydration and the frail nature of the patients who develop HHS will increase the risk of pressure ulceration, and attention to pressure areas is essential.

Hypoglycaemia

Although in most cases acutely ill patients have hyperglycaemia, hypoglycaemia can also occur. Hypoglycaemia is defined as a blood glucose < 2.8 mmol/L. The signs and symptoms associated with hypoglycaemia are neuroglycopenic:

- confusion
- irritability
- fatigue
- headache
- somnolence

There are also adrenergic responses:

- anxiety
- restlessness
- diaphoresis
- tachycardia
- arrhythmias
- hypertension
- chest pain

In severe cases hypoglycaemia can lead to seizures, coma, and death. Recognizing the potential for hypoglycaemia should be considered in any patient who develops new neurological symptoms.

Hypoglycaemia can occur quickly in patients receiving exogenous insulin, have impaired gluconeogenesis, or insufficient carbohydrate intakes. When patients are receiving artificial nutritional support, blood glucose levels should be routinely measured to avoid the development of rebound hypoglycaemia if feeding is suddenly discontinued.

Treatment of hypoglycaemia is dependent upon level of consciousness. Patients who are conscious and able to swallow should receive an appropriate quick-acting oral carbohydrate bolus. Patients with reduced consciousness or uncooperative patients will require intramuscular (IM) or IV therapy to correct hypoglycaemia; these patients require urgent medical attention. JBDS (2013) recommends that hypoglycaemia boxes are available in in-patient areas.

Nutrition and the acutely ill patient

Acute and critically ill patients have complex nutritional needs (Service and Anwar 2016). The key to nutritional management during the acute phase of an illness is ensuring that the patient is able to achieve energy balance, to minimize protein losses, and to ensure fluid balance is maintained (NICE 2012). It is important that when planning nutritional support, the patient is assessed accurately.

Maintaining energy balance

It is estimated that as many as one-third of patients will be malnourished on admission into hospital (Elia 2015).

During periods of illness there is a natural reduction in dietary intake or loss of appetite. The body's response to this is to mobilize stores of energy through hormonal and chemical signals: a stress response. These stores are mobilized by the action of glucagon, cortisol, and adrenaline. Once the glycogen stores have been utilized there is a metabolic shift towards using stored lipids and functional proteins such as skeletal muscle. The release of fatty acids and amino acids into the bloodstream provide substrates for the liver to synthesize glucose.

Unlike periods of starvation during health, when there is conservation of body mass, during the acute phase of an illness there is continued use of both lipids and proteins to meet energy demand. During acute illness, hyperglycaemia as a result of the stress response and increased gluconeogenesis is not uncommon and must be managed (see section on raised blood glucose). The continued loss of muscle mass can also lead to complications such as respiratory infections, urinary tract infections, increased risk of pressure sores, and reduced mobility due to lethargy.

Calculating energy requirements

The Harris–Benedict equation is commonly used to estimate the basal energy expenditure and this is then multiplied by a stress factor to estimate the energy needs of the acutely ill patient. This predictive calculation is commonly performed by the dieticians in high dependency areas. Alternatively, a more pragmatic approach is to multiply the patient's weight by a factor appropriate for the patient's condition or to use standard figures (Box 6.11).

Box 6.11 Estimating energy and protein requirements for patients who are not severely ill or injured

Energy for a patient with sepsis: 25–30 kcal/kg body weight/day

Protein intake: 0.8–1.5 g/kg body weight/day

Adapted from © NICE (2006) Nutrition Support for Adults Oral Nutrition Support, Enteral Tube Feeding and Parenteral Nutrition. NICE. 2006 Feb. [https://www.nice.org.uk/guidance/cg32/evidence/full-guideline-194889853] Accessed 07/06/19.

Protein requirements

During acute illness, and where protein loss is exacerbated with complex wounds or high losses of exudates, protein requirement can increase from 0.75 g/kg body weight/day to as much as 2.0 g/kg body weight/day.

Hypermetabolism and negative nitrogen balance

Metabolic stress causes hyper metabolism. Patients suffering from sepsis, head injuries, multiple fractures, malignant tumours, and burns can have a dramatically increased metabolic rate, which can exacerbate weight and lean tissue loss during the acute phase as energy and protein requirements are not met by dietary intake (Puthucheary *et al.* 2013). Negative nitrogen balance indicates that dietary protein intake (proteins contain nitrogen) is less than nitrogen loss.

Planned nutritional care for the acutely ill patient

Nutritional care plans based on screening of patients using a validated screening tool is essential to minimize risk of illness-induced malnutrition and to support patient recovery. Patients should be screened on admission and weekly thereafter. (NICE 2006, 2012). The Malnutrition Universal Screening Tool (MUST) tool has been developed to provide a quick and reliable screening tool for use by nurses to establish the risk of malnutrition in hospital. It identifies three simple steps to identify nutritional risk (Table 6.8). Completion of this tool, as part of planned nutritional support, will enable appropriate referral to the dietetic department expert guidance.

Clinical link 6.2 (see Appendix for answers)

Eva, 84 years old, has been admitted with a fracture of the left neck of femur and the left radius following a road traffic accident. She weighs 59 kg. She is 1.45 m tall.

- What actions will you take in order to plan the nutritional support for Eva during the acute phase of her illness?

After Eva returns from theatre she is confused and disorientated. She has had 3 units of packed cells whilst in theatre and there was an intravenous infusion of 1 L of normal saline running over 4 h. She is still not eating or drinking well 24 h later. No further intravenous fluids have been prescribed. She has a cannula *in situ*.

- What actions will you take to ensure that Eva's nutritional status is not compromised during this period?

NICE (2012) recommends that nutrition support should be considered in people who are malnourished, as defined by any of the following:

- a BMI of less than 18.5 kg/m^2.
- unintentional weight loss greater than 10% within the last three to six months.
- a BMI of less than 20 kg/m^2 and unintentional weight loss greater than 5% within the last three to six months.

Table 6.8 'MUST': 'Malnutrition Universal Screening Tool'

Step	Scoring	
Step 1	BMI > 20	Score = 0
	BMI 18.5–20	Score = 1
	BMI < 18.5	Score = 2
		Refer to BMI reckoner if needed
Step 2	In the past 3–6 months, has the patient experienced unplanned weight loss?	
	< 5% loss	Score = 0
	5–10% loss	Score = 1
	> 10% loss	Score = 2
	Refer to weight loss reckoner if needed	
Step 3*	Is the patient acutely ill and:	
	has had no nutritional intake for more than 5 days?	
	is likely to have no nutritional intake for more than 5 days?	
	If the answer to either of these questions is 'yes', score = 2	
	If the answer to both of these questions is 'no', score = 0	
	Refer to guidance notes in ward nutrition folder	
Step 4	Overall score	
	(Add the scores for Steps 1, 2, and 3)	

The 'Malnutrition Universal Screening Tool' ('MUST') is reproduced here with the kind permission of BAPEN (British Association for Parenteral and Enteral Nutrition). Copyright © BAPEN 2012. For further information on 'MUST' see http://www.bapen.org.uk. If unable to obtain height and weight, see MUST Explanatory Booklet for alternative measurements and use of subjective criteria.

*Step 3 is unlikely to apply outside a hospital.

Patients who have diseases where nutritional support is part of the clinical management will normally be referred to the dietetics department. This includes patients who have:

- DKA or HHS
- liver failure
- pancreatitis
- renal failure
- inflammatory bowel disease—Crohn's disease
- burns

NICE (2012) recommends that nutrition support should be considered in people at risk of malnutrition, as defined by any of the following:

- have eaten little or nothing for more than five days and/or are likely to eat little or nothing for the next five days or longer.
- have a poor absorptive capacity, and/or have high nutrient loses, and/or have increased nutritional needs from causes such as catabolism.

Compromise of patient nutritional status

Factors that will compromise a patient's nutritional status whilst in hospital include the following.

Nil by mouth

Prolonged periods spent 'nil by mouth' during diagnosis, investigations, or surgical procedures can compromise a patient's nutritional status (see Box 6.12). To avoid unnecessary delays with eating and drinking it is important that:

Box 6.12 Guidance for preoperative fasting in adults undergoing elective surgery: The '2 and 6' rule

Adults and children should be encouraged to drink clear fluids (including water, pulp-free juice and tea or coffee without milk) up to **2 h** before elective surgery (including caesarean section)
Solid food should be prohibited for **6 h** before elective surgery in adults and children
Patients with obesity, gastro-oesophageal reflux, and diabetes, and pregnant women not in labour can safely follow all the above guidelines.
Patients should not have their operation cancelled or delayed just because they are chewing gum, sucking a boiled sweet, or smoking immediately prior to induction of anaesthesia. Patients should be encouraged to drink when ready, providing there are no complications.

Adapted with permission from Smith, I., *et al.* Perioperative fasting in adults and children: Guidelines from the European Society of Anaesthesiology. *Eur J Anaesthesiol*, 28(8): 556–69. © 2011 European Society of Anaesthesiology. doi: 10.1097/EJA.0b013e3283495ba1.

- a nutritional screen is completed and discussed with the multidisciplinary team in order for a nutritional plan to be devised that will indicate when eating and drinking will resume.
- drinks and snacks are available in the clinical setting for when meals are missed.
- if investigations or operations are delayed, nurses and clinicians assess whether fluids and/or food can be given.
- if a patient is nil by mouth for more than 24 h, the dietetic team is informed, and nurses and clinicians discuss whether alternative routes for providing nutritional support are required, and they complete a nutritional plan.

Other factors

Various other factors can compromise patient nutritional status:

- uncontrolled vomiting or nausea—see section on nausea and vomiting
- uncontrolled faecal loss—see section on diarrhoea
- confusion and disorientation associated with infection, dehydration, or post anaesthesia
- uncontrolled pain—see section on abdominal pain
- increased breathlessness
- prolonged infection
- multiple pathology

Nutritional support

It is important when managing the care of the patient that food as well as fluid intake is monitored and recorded. Patients must have a balanced diet that meets their needs, and nutritional support should be planned, documented, and evaluated.

Enteral feeding

If the GI tract is functioning but the patient is unable to meet their nutritional needs with oral intake, then feeding using a fine-bore feeding tube is required. The decision to commence feeding must follow a clear assessment of the risks and benefits by two competent healthcare professionals, including the senior doctor in charge of the patients care (NPSA 2011). Enteral feeding *should not be considered* if the patient has a non-functioning GI tract.

Parenteral nutrition

NICE (2012) recommends that parenteral nutrition is considered in people who are malnourished or at risk of malnutrition due to:

- inadequate or unsafe oral/enteral nutritional intake.
- a non-functioning, inaccessible, or perforated GI tract.

Clinical link 6.3 (see Appendix for answers)

George is 38 years old and has had multiple fractures following a road traffic accident. He is on traction and is immobile. Prior to his injury he ate a normal diet. A nasogastric tube has been inserted and a lactose-free standard formula feed has been prescribed. He is prescribed 2200 mL/24 h.

- Critically discuss the actions will you take prior to commencing the feed.

Eight hours later George complains of feeling sick and nauseous.

- What actions will you take?

Nursing management of parenteral nutrition

Parenteral nutrition should be managed using strict asepsis and can cause alterations to biochemistry and fluid balance due to the increased osmolar load (see Chapter 7). The patient should be monitored for:

- hyperglycaemia
- liver dysfunction
- refeeding syndrome

Refeeding syndrome

Severely malnourished patients or those that have had little or no food intake prior to their illness may suffer from complications associated with refeeding due to over-rapid or unbalanced nutrition (Crook 2014). This can occur with oral, enteral, and parenteral feeding.

Patients at risk of developing refeeding syndrome include:

- those who have had very little to eat for > five days
- those with a BMI of 16 kg/m^2 or less
- those who have had unintentional weight loss of > 15% within the previous six months
- those with low levels of potassium, phosphate, or magnesium prior to any feeding (Crook 2014)

Nutritional support of patients with disorders of the gastrointestinal tract

Patients admitted with acute illnesses that affect the GI tract should be referred to the dietician for full assessment and nutritional management. The nurse's role is to ensure that:

- nutritional status is assessed, documented, and care is planned.
- food and fluid intakes are monitored and recorded.
- all feeds prescribed are administered and recorded.
- all prescribed vitamin, mineral, and electrolyte supplements are administered and recorded.

It is beyond the scope of the book to discuss detailed nutritional assessment but it is important to note that specialized assessment may be required in some groups of patients and specialist dietetic advice should be sort in patients presenting with:

- liver disease
- pancreatic disease
- malabsorption
- food allergies
- food intolerances

End of chapter test

The following assessment will enable you to evaluate your theoretical knowledge of GI assessment and management as well as your ability to apply this theory to clinical practice. You should undertake the following assessment with an appropriately trained member of staff in clinical practice. If you are unable to answer any questions it may be helpful to revisit the relevant section in this chapter.

Knowledge assessment

With the support of your mentor/supervisor from practice, work through the following prompts to explore your knowledge level about the GI system and nutritional support.

- Describe the structure and function of the GI tract.
- Discuss the role of the liver and pancreas as accessory organs of digestion.
- Describe the three stages of the swallowing reflex.
- Discuss the impact diet has on gastric emptying.
- Discuss the factors that stimulate nausea and vomiting.
- Describe the components of pancreatic secretions and their involvement in digestion of nutrients.
- Describe the role of bile salts in the digestion of fats.
- Describe the structure of the villus.
- Name the brush border enzymes and the substrates on which they act.
- Critically discuss the importance of fluid balance in relation to the function of the small intestine.
- Describe the difference between somatic and visceral pain.
- Explain why patients with disorders of the GI tract may have 'referred pain'.
- Explain why malabsorption of carbohydrate may contribute to diarrhoea developing.
- Describe why the stomach and the ileum are important for the absorption of vitamin B12.
- Explain the aetiology of jaundice and what physical findings you might observe.
- Explain the difference between DKA and HHS.
- Explain why acutely ill patients develop hypermetabolism.
- Explain why blood glucose can increase when you are acutely ill.
- Explain why insulin therapy may be required in the acutely ill patient.

- Critically discuss how hypermetabolism and starvation differ.
- Discuss what criteria you would use to decide whether a patient requires nutritional support.

Skills assessment

Under the guidance of your mentor/supervisor, undertake a nutritional screen, pain assessment, and swallowing assessment followed by appropriate interventions for any significant abnormality. Your mentor/supervisor will be able to assess your ability and provide feedback based on the following skills:

- Conducts a full patient history with a systems review considering key points that are relevant for a nutritional assessment.
- Demonstrates the use of a nutritional screening tool to identify the risk of malnutrition.
- Identifies what physical observations would raise concern about a patient's ability to swallow.
- Identifies what actions should be taken if a patient if a patient is 'nil by mouth' for more than 6 h.
- Completes a nutritional plan for a patient who requires enteral nutrition.
- Demonstrates ability to commence enteral feeding safely.
- Reviews current medications and intravenous therapy, rationalizing impact on pain and nausea.
- Interprets all subjective and objective findings from the nutritional screening tool, rationalizes possible causes for these abnormalities, and plans appropriate actions.
- Explains clinical reasoning and provides justification for all interventions of the nutritional management plan.
- Interprets all subjective and objective findings from the pain assessment, rationalizes possible causes for these abnormalities, and plans appropriate actions.
- Explains clinical reasoning and provides justification for all interventions of the pain management plan.
- Liaises with other members of the healthcare team as necessary, including nurse in charge, doctor, dietician, pharmacist, physiotherapist, and healthcare assistant.
- Demonstrates an ability to follow infection control guidelines while undertaking enteral feeding.
- Documents the nutrition management plan, completed actions, and evaluation of actions as per local policy.

References

Bhansali, A., Sukumar, S.P. (2016) Hyperosmolar hyperglycemic state. *World Clin Diabetol*, 2(1):1–10.

British National Formulary (2016) Available at: http://www.bnf.org/bnf/; accessed 9 December 2019.

Chanana, l., Jagari, M., Kalaaniwala, A., *et al.* (2015) Clinical profile of non-traumatic acute abdominal pain presenting to an adult emergency department. *J Family Med Prim Care*, 4(3):422–5.

Crook, A.M. (2014) Refeeding syndrome: Problems with definition and management *Nutrition*, 30(11):1448–55.

Dever, J.B., Sheikh, M.Y. (2015) Review article: Spontaneous bacterial peritonitis—bacteriology, diagnosis, treatment, risk factors and prevention. *Aliment Pharmacol Ther*, 41:1116–31. doi:10.1111/apt.13172.

Egi, M., Krinsley, J.S., Maurer, P., *et al.* (2016). Pre-morbid glycemic control modifies the interaction between acute hypoglycemia and mortality. *Intensive Care Med*, 42:562–71. doi:http://dx.doi.org.ezproxy.brighton.ac.uk/10.1007/s00134-016-4216-8.

Elia, M. (2015) The cost of malnutrition in England and potential cost savings from nutritional interventions. Maidenhead: NIHR Southampton Biomedical Research Centre Malnutrition Action Group of BAPEN Maidenhead.

HSCIC (2017) The Health and Social Care Information Centre, Hospital Episode Statistics for England, Accident and Emergency (A&E) statistics, 2014–15. Available at: http://content.digital.nhs.uk/searchcatalogue?productid=20143&q=title%3a%22accident+and+emergency+attendances%22&topics=0%2fHospital+care&sort=Relevance&size=10&page=1#top; accessed 9 December 2019.

JBDS (2012) The management of the hyperosmolar hyperglycaemic state (HHS) in adults with diabetes. August 2012 JBDS 06. Available at: https://www.diabetes.org.uk/Professionals/Position-statements-reports/Specialist-care-for-children-and-adults-and-complications/Management-of-the-hyperosmolar-hyperglycaemic-state-HHS-in-adults-with-diabetes/; accessed 9 December 2019.

JBDS (2013) Joint British Diabetes Societies Inpatient Care Group The Management of Diabetic Ketoacidosis in Adults. September 2013 JBDS 02. Available at: https://www.diabetes.org.uk/Documents/About%20Us/What%20we%20say/Management-of-DKA-241013.pdf; accessed 9 December 2019.

Jones, A., Turner, K., Handa, A. (2000) Surgical emergencies: Acute abdominal pain. *Student BMJ*, 8:56–7.

Karlya, T. (2015). Parents, professionals need better awareness of DKA and diabetes symptoms. *Endocrine Today*, 13:16.

Longo, D.L., Navari, R.M., Aapro, M. (2016). Antiemetic prophylaxis for chemotherapy-induced nausea and vomiting. *New Engl J Med*, 374:1356–67.

Macaluso, C.R., McNamara, R.M. (2012) Evaluation and management of acute abdominal pain in the emergency department. *Int J Gen Med*, 5:789–97.

Manterola, C., Vial, M., Moraga, J., *et al.* (2011) Analgesia in patients with acute abdominal pain. *Cochrane Database Syst Rev*, Jan 19 (1):CD005660. doi: 10.1002/14651858.CD005660.pub3.

NICE (2006) *Nutrition Support for Adults Oral Nutrition Support, Enteral Tube Feeding and Parenteral Nutrition* CG32. London: National Institute for Health and Care Excellence. Available at: https://www.nice.org.uk/guidance/cg32; accessed 9 December 2019.

NICE (2012) *Nutrition Support in Adults* QS24. London: National Institute for Health and Care Excellence. Available at: https://www.nice.org.uk/guidance/qs24; accessed 9 December 2019.

NICE (2016) *Oral Health for Adults in Care Homes* NG48. London: National Institute for Health and Care Excellence. Available at: https://www.nice.org.uk/guidance/ng48; accessed 9 December 2019.

NICE (2017) *Healthcare-associated Infections: Prevention and Control in Primary and Community Care* CG139. London: National Institute for Health and Care Excellence. Available at: https://www.nice.org.uk/guidance/cg139/ifp/chapter/enteral-feeding; accessed 9 December 2019.

NPSA (2011) Reducing the harm caused by misplaced nasogastric feeding tubes in adults, children and infants. Available at:
https://improvement.nhs.uk/documents/194/Patient_Safety_Alert_Stage_2_-_NG_tube_resource_set.pdf accessed 13 January 2020.

Puthucheary, Z.A., Rawal, J., McPhail, M., *et al.* (2013). Acute skeletal muscle wasting in critical illness. *JAMA*, 310(15):1591–600.

RCP (2016) National clinical guideline for stroke. Prepared by the Intercollegiate Stroke Working Party. London: RCP. Available at: https://www.strokeaudit.org/SupportFiles/Documents/Guidelines/2016-National-Clinical-Guideline-for-Stroke-5t-(1).aspx; accessed 13 January 2020.

Sands, K.M., Williams, D.W., Wilson, M.J., *et al.* (2014) Oral hygiene in critically ill patients. *Br J Intensive Care*, 24:51–7.

Service, E., Anwar, F. (2016) Nutritional management in critically ill trauma patients is challenging *Trauma*, 18:231–6.

Shu-hua, M., Gong, S., Hong-xia, Y., *et al.* (2017). Comparison of in-hospital glycemic variability and admission blood glucose in predicting short-term outcomes in non-diabetes patients with ST elevation myocardial infarction underwent percutaneous coronary intervention. *Diabetology and Metabolic Syndrome*, 9. doi:http://dx.doi.org.ezproxy.brighton.ac.uk/10.1186/s13098-017-0217-1.

Smith, I., Kranke, P., Murat, I., *et al.* (2011) Perioperative fasting in adults and children: Guidelines from the European Society of Anaesthesiology. *Eur J Anaesthesiol*, 28:556–69.

7
Fluid assessment and associated treatment

Heather Baid

Chapter contents

Evaluating a patient's fluid status is an integral aspect of any nursing assessment because an abnormally high or low fluid balance significantly influences a variety of body systems, including cardiovascular, respiratory, renal, neurological, gastrointestinal, and metabolic. The purpose of this chapter is to examine:

- the anatomy and physiology of fluid balance
- pathophysiological changes of fluid balance in acute care
- assessment of fluid status
- management of the patient with fluid excess
- management of the patient with fluid deficit
- administration of intravenous fluids and blood products

Learning outcomes

This chapter will enable you to:

- describe the normal anatomy of fluids in the body, including the intravascular, interstitial, and intercellular fluid compartments
- explain the physiology of how the body maintains normal fluid homeostasis
- identify causes for an abnormal fluid balance with acute care patients
- explain how the body responds and compensates for an abnormal fluid balance
- discuss how normovolaemia can be maintained including measures to prevent an abnormal fluid balance
- explore a systematic approach to assessing a patient's fluid status
- critically analyse normal and abnormal findings of a fluid assessment
- evaluate the nursing management of a patient with an abnormal fluid imbalance
- differentiate between crystalloid, colloids, and blood products
- discuss the nursing responsibilities for intravenous therapy

Introduction

Water is the most abundant substance in the body, contributing to 55–60% of total body weight. Because there are continual losses of water as part of normal physiological function, an intake of water is required to achieve an equal net fluid balance. Acute care nurses require a thorough understanding of their patients' fluid status to identify an altered fluid balance and manage this in relation to acute illness. This chapter will review the anatomy and physiology of fluid status, how to conduct a systematic fluid assessment, and the fluid management for common abnormalities in acute care.

Normal anatomy and physiology

The majority of the water in the body is located inside the cells, with the remaining found in extracellular areas. Of this extracellular fluid (ECF), 80% is interstitial and 20% in the intravascular space is plasma. If one area has an increase or decrease in water content, fluid will shift across to maintain the normal distribution of two-thirds intracellular fluid (ICF) and one-third ECF. Fluid homeostasis is then maintained with a constant ratio of water across these three fluid compartments (see Figure 7.1).

There are a variety of physiological pressures preventing fluid from leaking out of its designated area otherwise the normal distribution of water between the intracellular, interstitial, and intra-vascular spaces would be lost. These pressures include *osmotic pressure, hydrostatic pressure*, and *oncotic pressure*.

Osmotic pressure pulls water across a semi-permeable membrane towards an area of greater solute concentration. As there is a higher amount of sodium in the ECF, sodium creates an osmotic pressure in the extracellular compartment. Similarly, potassium contributes to the osmotic pressure that maintains fluid within the cells.

Hydrostatic pressure is the pressure a fluid places onto the wall of a vessel and acts as a 'pushing force' because it pushes water out of the blood vessels into the interstitial space. Oncotic pressure keeps fluid inside vessels from the presence of large plasma proteins and is therefore a 'pulling force' pulling fluids into the blood from the interstitium. If the hydrostatic pressure is greater than the oncotic pressure, fluid leaves the intravascular space, resulting in a higher interstitial volume. Similarly, if the oncotic pressure rises more than the hydrostatic pressure, there is an increased movement of fluid into the intravascular space.

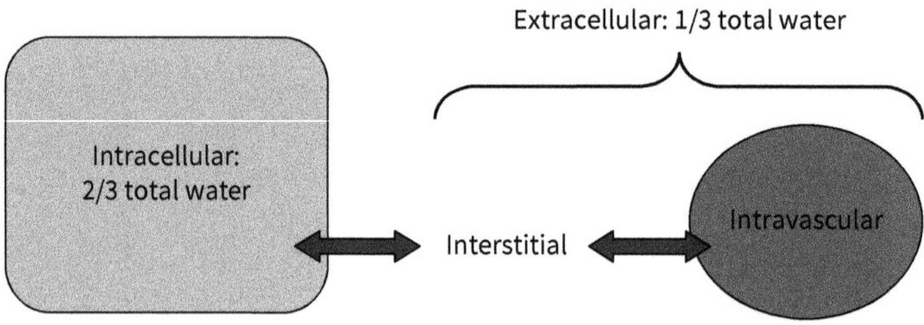

Figure 7.1 Fluid homeostasis.

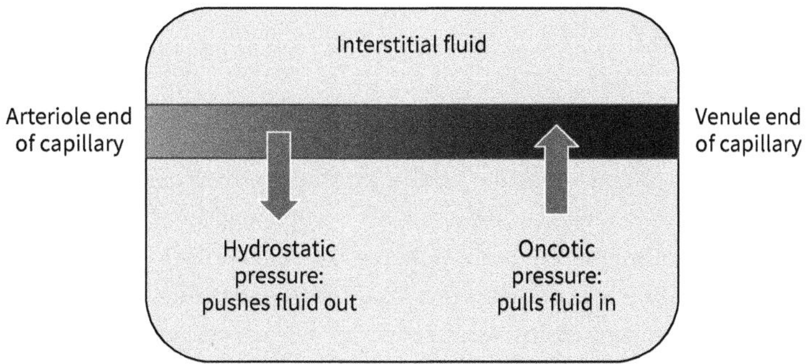

Figure 7.2 Fluid pressures.

This interplay between hydrostatic and oncotic pressure occurs naturally in the body within the capillaries where at the arteriole side, hydrostatic pressure is greater than oncotic pressure, allowing fluid to move into the interstitial space. As the blood flows through the capillary, the amount of water in the blood then decreases by the time the fluid reaches the venule end. Large molecules such as albumin are not able to cross the capillary membrane with the escaping water, leading to an increase in oncotic pressure that pulls fluid back into the capillary. The end result is equilibrium because of the overall net balance of water remaining equal as the hydrostatic and oncotic pressures counterbalance each other (see Figure 7.2).

There are further extracellular areas in the body such as fluid in the cerebral spinal space, pleural cavity, peritoneum, joints, and eyes. These are known as *transcellular fluids* but are not normally altered by significant daily losses or gains.

Normally, the amount of water gained during a day equals the amount of water lost, leaving the body with a net fluid balance of zero. Eating and drinking comprises the majority of water intake, with a small amount of water also produced through metabolic processes. In addition to water lost as urine, there are also insensible losses through the skin, lungs, and gastrointestinal tract. See Table 7.1 for a breakdown of water gain and water loss for an average adult (Marieb and Hoehn 2015).

Table 7.1 Water gain and water loss

Water gain		Water loss	
Oral fluids	1500 mL	Urine	1500 mL
Oral food	750 mL	Skin and lungs insensible loss	700 mL
Metabolic water	250 mL	Sweat	200 mL
	2500 mL	GI tract	100 mL
			2500 mL

GI, gastrointestinal.

Data from Marieb, E.N. and Hoehn, K.N. (2015). *Human Anatomy and Physiology*, 10th edn. Pearson, Boston.

Pathophysiology

Fluid deficit

A shortage of fluid in the intravascular and interstitial compartments occurs when there is a reduced amount of water and/or sodium due to abnormal losses, an inability to replace normal losses, or a combination of both. If there is an equal proportion of water and sodium lost, the extracellular fluid remains isotonic. Water then redistributes between the intra- and extracellular spaces, resulting in an overall reduction in each compartment. If mostly water is lost, the extracellular fluid becomes hypertonic, drawing water in from the ICF and causing *cellular dehydration*. Intravascular volume may initially improve from the fluid shift but will eventually drop if the water loss continues. If there is predominantly a reduction in serum sodium, the subsequent hypotonicity of the extracellular fluid encourages water to shift into the cells, leaving the extracellular space volume depleted.

Reduced fluid in the intravascular space is clinically significant because a normal blood volume (*normovolaemia*) is essential for adequate tissue perfusion, transport of substances throughout the body, and functioning of all body systems. *Hypovolaemia* refers to an ineffective volume of circulating blood because of actual fluid loss or from fluid shifting out of the intravascular space to another compartment.

Hypovolaemia typically takes place when there is a reduction in total extracellular volume (intravascular + interstitial). However, there can be hypovolaemia with normal or increased extracellular volume if the amount of interstitial fluid is high while the intravascular volume is low. The total amount of water in the patient appears to be increased with a positive daily fluid balance but the abnormal fluid distribution leaves the vascular space relatively dry. There is thus a large amount of fluid in the body but it is in the wrong place to be effective. An example would be with oedema where the total amount of extracellular fluid is high from excess fluid in the interstitial space although there is relative hypovolaemia due to a low intravascular volume. See Table 7.2 for causes of hypovolaemia with decreased interstitial volume compared with hypovolaemia with increased/normal interstitial volume.

When fluid builds up in the interstitium or another potential space that is not normally filled with fluid, it is referred to as *third-space fluid*. Third-space areas include:

- interstitium (peripheral/pulmonary oedema)
- peritoneum (ascites)
- pleural space (effusion)
- ileus (fluid accumulates within obstructed intestine)

Fluid deficit response

There is a variety of compensation mechanisms that take place in response to hypovolaemia to prevent detrimental effects from a low blood volume. Baroreceptors detect the reduction in pressure from the low volume and send a message to the central nervous system. The sympathetic nervous system is then stimulated, which increases the heart rate and force of myocardial contraction and causes vasoconstriction.

Table 7.2 Hypovolaemia

Hypovolaemia with decreased interstitial volume	Hypovolaemia with increased/normal interstitial volume
Fluid loss: • gastrointestinal—diarrhoea, vomiting, nasogastric suction • skin—sweating, burns, wounds • haemorrhage	Increased hydrostatic pressure: • chronic heart failure (increased hydrostatic pressure in veins) • liver failure (increased hydrostatic pressure in portal system)
Reduced intake of sodium and water: • poor oral intake of food and water • nil by mouth without intravenous replacement of sodium and water	Decreased colloid osmotic pressure: • low albumin Increased capillary permeability: • sepsis, shock, burns, trauma
Impaired retention of sodium and water: • diuretics • renal sodium wasting • adrenal insufficiency • osmotic diuresis	Impaired lymphatic drainage

The kidneys also sense a decreased glomerular filtration rate and activate the renin–angiotensin–aldosterone system. This begins when hypotension causes the kidneys to produce renin, which acts on circulating angiotensinogen to produce angiotensin I. Angiotensin-converting enzyme then transforms angiotensin I into angiotensin II and the following is a summary of the effects of angiotensin II:

- vasoconstriction
- increased reabsorption of sodium, chloride, and water in the proximal convoluted tubule
- adrenal cortex stimulated to release aldosterone that enhances sodium and water reabsorption in collecting ducts
- thirst sensation

An increase in plasma osmolarity stimulates the pituitary gland to release antidiuretic hormone (ADH), also known as vasopressin. ADH enhances water reabsorption in the collecting ducts that concentrates the urine and increases the amount of water in the blood.

The goal of these compensation mechanisms is to have a net result of improving cardiac output and tissue perfusion that were compromised from the reduction in circulating blood volume. If hypovolaemia continues to the point where the compensation mechanisms fail, *hypovolaemic shock* develops. This is the most common type of shock, resulting from a reduction in volume within the vascular compartment. Clinically, patients will present with hypotension, tachycardia, oliguria, decreased oxygen saturation, anxiety, disorientation, and confusion. Inadequate tissue perfusion then impairs the ability of the cells to conduct aerobic metabolism, leading to anaerobic metabolism. If left untreated, the anaerobic metabolism will eventually result in acidosis, cardiac depression, intravascular coagulation, increased capillary permeability, and release of toxins.

Fluid excess

An overall gain in extracellular fluid results in increased water in the vascular and interstitial spaces. *Hypervolaemia*, commonly called 'fluid overload', occurs when there is a high amount of circulating blood volume which may be due to:

- increased retention of sodium and water
  - heart failure
  - liver failure
  - nephrotic syndrome
  - excessive administration of glucocorticosteroids
  - Syndrome of inappropriate ADH
- reduced excretion of sodium and water
  - renal failure
- iatrogenic excessive administration of intravenous therapy
  - crystalloid/colloid infusions
  - blood transfusion
  - total parenteral nutrition
- fluid shifting from interstitial space into the blood
  - redistribution of oedema
  - excessive administration of hypertonic solutions

Although there are a variety of causes of hypervolaemia, a frequent reason seen in acute care is heart failure. Whether there is chronic heart failure present or a new acute cardiac problem causing the heart as a muscle to fail, blood is not ejected properly from the ventricles and becomes congested in the pulmonary and systemic regions (see Chapter 3).

A further consideration is the underlying processes involved with chronic heart failure. One of the normal compensation mechanisms for chronic heart failure is to increase the total blood volume, which allows for a greater stretch of ventricle wall thereby improving the force of contraction for each beat (Starling's Law). However, hypervolaemia develops over time from the overall rise in blood volume and leads to fluid leaking out of the vascular space into the interstitial space. As the heart continues to fail, blood also starts to back up, causing pulmonary oedema with left ventricular failure and peripheral oedema with right ventricular failure.

Renal dysfunction can also result in hypervolaemia. Clearly, if there is fluid intake through drinking or an intravenous infusion but the kidneys are not excreting adequate amounts of sodium and water, then the total blood volume will continue to rise. See Chapter 5 for an extensive overview of renal abnormalities.

An intravenous infusion may be necessary for a patient who is not taking in oral fluids, has recently had surgery, or requires total parenteral nutrition. If the infusion rate or total amount of fluid being delivered is excessive, iatrogenic hypervolaemia may result. This occurs when the heart and kidneys are not able to maintain normal homeostasis during the intravenous infusion.

Similarly, a blood transfusion will cause hypervolaemia if the resulting vascular volume is increased to a level where the heart has difficulty pumping effectively or the kidneys do not draw off enough fluid to maintain a normal quantity of plasma. Patients with heart failure are particularly at risk for hypervolaemia after a blood transfusion, which is why they are often prescribed a diuretic after receiving a transfusion.

Intracellular fluid excess

An abundance of ICF develops when the extracellular fluid is hypotonic because the subsequent osmotic gradient pulls water out of the extracellular space into the cells. As the cells become infused with water, they lose their ability to function normally and tissues begin to swell. The brain is particularly sensitive to swelling because the skull constricts the ability of the brain to expand. ICF excess due to *water intoxication* or *hyponatraemia* is life-threatening when the central nervous system is affected and may present with changes to level of consciousness, seizures, or other abnormal neurological signs. Attempts to correct a low sodium level should be made slowly to prevent rapid fluid shifts and subsequent damage to the brain tissue that can occur if the hyponatraemia is resolved too quickly.

Fluid excess response

The body compensates for excessive water and solutes in the body by increasing their excretion in the urine. The regulation of sodium in the kidney is influenced by angiotensin II, aldosterone, and atrial natriuretic peptide. An increase in blood volume stimulates these hormones to reduce the reabsorption of sodium and water in the kidney tubules. As more sodium is then lost in the urine, water follows through the process of osmosis. In addition, the decreased osmolarity with a diluted high volume of blood causes less ADH to be secreted, with a net result of further water loss in the urine. See Chapter 5 for a detailed explanation of the renal system's involvement in maintaining body water balance.

If these compensation mechanisms are insufficient because of underlying renal dysfunction or the high volume of intravascular fluid is simply too much for the kidneys to keep up with, there is a potential for cardiogenic shock to occur (see Chapter 3). Failure of the heart can therefore both cause hypervolaemia and result from a high volume of intravascular fluid. As the intravascular volume progressively increases, the excess fluid will redistribute, leaking out into other compartments (intracellular, interstitial, and other third-space areas) (see Figure 7.3).

Prevention of altered fluid balance

Prevention of an altered fluid balance is an essential aspect of acute care nursing. Close monitoring and ongoing assessment of the patient will detect early changes seen with fluid excess or a fluid deficit. If a patient is nil by mouth, a crystalloid infusion will be necessary to maintain adequate amounts of fluid and electrolytes in the body. An intravenous infusion or enteral feeding may also be necessary if a patient is taking some oral food and fluid but not in adequate amounts. Patients at risk for a negative fluid balance but who can drink should have oral fluids encouraged and fluid restriction may be required for patients at risk of

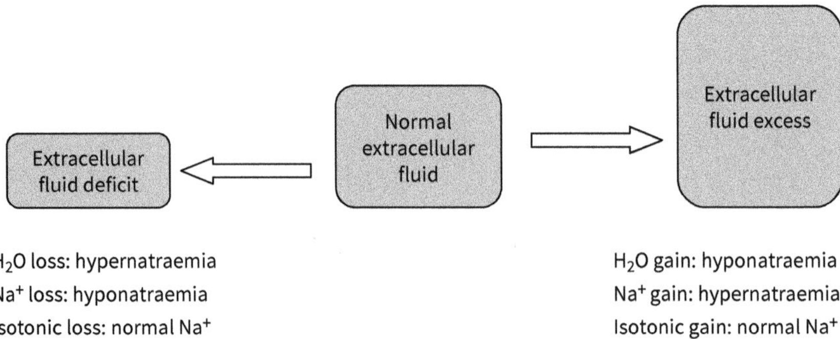

Figure 7.3 Influence of sodium on fluid shifts.

hypervolaemia. Close attention should be given to those patients who are particularly at risk of developing an abnormal fluid status.

Risk factors for fluid imbalance

Elderly

- decreased skeletal muscle mass/increased adipose tissue = reduced total water
- decreased renal and cardiovascular function
- decreased mobility and cognition may impair drinking
- decreased thirst mechanism
- decreased skin elasticity prevents skin turgor from indicating hydration status

Acute illness

- surgery (nil by mouth pre-/post-operative, peri-operative fluid losses, bleeding)
- nausea and vomiting
- diarrhoea
- nasogastric suction/drainage
- fever
- excessive sweating
- shock (septic, hypovolaemic, cardiogenic, anaphylactic, neurogenic)

Chronic illness

- impaired bodily functioning from illnesses affecting body systems
- renal insufficiency
- malnutrition influencing electrolytes and albumin
- reduced appetite and desire to drink water
- depression

Patient assessment

Assessing fluid status benefits from a holistic approach incorporating a history and physical examination of all body systems because water is an integral aspect of each system's normal functioning. A comprehensive fluid assessment utilizing a systematic structure will consider whether the following signs and symptoms of normovolaemia are present.

Breathing

- respirations regular and easy without shortness of breath
- oxygen saturation and respiration rate within normal limits
- clear breath sounds
- no cough

Cardiovascular

- systolic blood pressure >100 mmHg
- heart rate < 90 bpm
- mucous membranes pink and moist
- peripheries pink, warm, capillary refill ≤ 2 s, pulses palpable
- normal skin moisture (no sweating but not excessively dry), no oedema
- normal turgor (skin snaps back to normal position when pinched)
- clear yellow urine > 0.5 mL/kg/h
- neutral daily fluid balance

Disability

- alert and oriented to person, place, and time
- normal strength and sensation to arms and legs

Exposure

- skin intact without wounds or drains
- abdomen flat and soft (no evidence of ascites or internal bleeding)
- normal bowel functioning, normal eating and drinking/thirst

Central venous pressure

The central venous pressure (CVP) is measured by a central venous catheter located in the vena cava; the CVP is equal (or equivalent) to the right atrial pressure. During diastole when the tricuspid valve opens, the pressure in the right atrium then correlates to the pressure in the right ventricle if there is a normally functioning tricuspid valve. CVP is therefore used as an indirect assessment of right ventricular pressure. As volume and pressure are directly proportional to each other, CVP as a pressure reading is then interpreted as the 'volume' status of the right side of the heart. A high CVP suggests a high blood volume and a low CVP suggests a low amount of circulating blood. The range for a normal CVP is 2–8 mmHg if transducing a central venous catheter or 5–10 cm H_20 if obtained from a manometer.

As well as hypervolaemia, other factors contributing to an increased CVP include decreased cardiac output (low heart rate or ventricular failure causing blood to back up into veins), venous constriction (activation of sympathetic system or vasoconstricting medications), and increased intrathoracic pressure such as through the Valsalva manoeuvre (compression of vena cava). These last two factors influence the CVP from primarily a change in venous compliance rather than venous blood volume.

With intravascular fluid deficit, the response of the CVP to a fluid challenge is more clinically significant than the actual CVP number. Fluid responsiveness is evaluated by assessing whether a rise in CVP following the rapid intravenous infusion of 250–500 mL of fluid is sustained for at least 10 min otherwise it is likely there is hypovolaemia and a need for further intravenous fluid replacement. However, a systematic review by Marik and Cavallazzi (2013) demonstrated there is a very poor correlation between CVP and blood volume, indicating CVP monitoring is unreliable for predicting a haemodynamic response to fluid challenges. For this reason, some practitioners choose not to use CVP measurements to guide fluid management. Others recognize that although CVP is also influenced by other factors besides blood volume, the trend may still hold value as a clinical indicator of fluid status.

Jugular venous pressure

The jugular venous pressure (JVP) can be assessed externally without any invasive monitoring by identifying the level of venous distension in the neck. JVP is also referred to as jugular venous pulsation, jugular venous pulse, and jugular venous distension (JVD). The key land-marking area for the JVP is the triangular region between the two heads of the sternocleidomastoid muscle with these distinguishing features which are different from an arterial pulse:

- flickering, multiphasic pattern (two waves in the JVP for each cardiac cycle)
- non-palpable (should not have a palpable pulse like the carotid artery)
- variation with movement (JVP should decrease if the patient sits up)
- variation with respiration (JVP decreases with deep inspiration)

The JVP should be visible less than 4 cm above the sternum if the patient is lying supine and head of bed elevated to 30–45°. A high JVP greater than 4 cm with the patient in this position or a visible JVP while the patient is sitting fully upright could be caused by hypervolaemia, right ventricular failure, constrictive pericarditis, tricuspid stenosis, or superior vena cava obstruction. A low or absent JVP may indicate hypovolaemia, although the JVP can be difficult to find in many patients with normovolaemia therefore it has limited use in assessing for intravascular dehydration. A further limitation is that JVP measurements tend to underestimate the actual fluid status of the patient (Elder *et al.* 2016).

Patient weight

Weight is a significant aspect of a fluid assessment because it can indicate whether a patient is experiencing a deficit or excess of fluid. As with any objective number, the actual value of weight as a once-off reading does not contribute much to assessment findings. The trend of the weight as rising or falling is more clinically significant than the number itself because it can suggest whether total body fluid has been gained or lost. Typically, a change in 1 kg of body weight equates to 1 L of water. In acute care, the patient's pre-hospital weight should be recorded if available to help interpret daily weight within the context of a baseline number.

Although trends in a patient's weight may be useful for some clinical situations, caution should be taken while interpreting changes in weight because this may not be an accurate indicator of intravascular fluid volume. For example, if there is an increase in third-space fluid through the accumulation of peripheral oedema, the rise in the patient's weight could be incorrectly viewed as fluid overload if there is a low effective circulating blood volume.

Fluid balance

Maintaining an accurate fluid balance chart is an important aspect of the assessment of acute care patients to determine whether fluid input equals fluid output (McGloin 2015). A positive fluid balance indicates excessive water intake or a reduction in water excretion which will lead to hypervolaemia if sustained. Conversely, hypovolaemia and cellular dehydration will eventually develop if a negative fluid balance continues from poor intake or increased fluid loss. However, it is always important to assess the trend of a daily fluid balance rather than interpret one number in isolation in case the high or low fluid balance is an attempt to compensate for previous abnormality. A fluid balance chart is thus aided by a cumulative balance over time.

If a patient displays an alteration in fluid balance or has any type of organ dysfunction (particularly renal and cardiac), clinical judgement is used to determine the frequency of fluid measurements and fluid balance calculation ranging from hourly to daily. A fluid balance will never be absolutely accurate because of the inability to measure water loss from the skin, respiratory tract, and GI system, although metabolic water production typically evens out the deficit created from these insensible losses. Other questions to consider when evaluating fluid balance are whether the patient was already experiencing an abnormal fluid status before coming to acute care and if there are further immeasurable factors (e.g. losses during surgery or from a fever). As with all numerical observations though, it is not a 'correct' fluid balance that is valuable to know. Rather, it is the relevance of the number as a trend and how it relates to the overall clinical picture that makes a fluid balance significant.

A summary of abnormal patient assessment findings is found in Table 7.3.

Clinical investigations

There are a variety of laboratory tests that may be of use while undertaking a comprehensive fluid assessment including:

- Urine
  - specific gravity
  - sodium
  - osmolarity
- Blood
  - urea, creatinine, electrolytes (Na^+, Cl^-, K^+, Mg^{2+}, Ca^{2+})
  - haemoglobin, albumin
  - osmolarity
  - arterial blood gas: pH, HCO_3^-, base excess, lactate

Table 7.3 Fluid assessment findings

	Fluid deficit	Fluid excess
Tongue	Dry, coated	Moist
Thirst	Increased	May not be significant
Pulse	Rapid, thready radial pulse, absent/ weak pedal pulses	Rapid, normal strength (unless cardiogenic shock)
Blood pressure	Low Orthostatic hypotension	Normal or high (unless cardiogenic shock)
Respirations	Increased rate	Increased rate, short of breath, productive cough (frothy)
Weight	Loss	Gain
JVP/CVP	Low	Elevated
Peripheries	Pale, cool, capillary refill > 2 s, decreased skin turgor	Oedema
Urine output	Reduced (except with conditions causing polyuria, e.g. DKA)	Normal
Breath sounds	Clear	Bilateral fine crackles
Abdomen		May develop ascites

JVP, jugular venous pressure; CVP, central venous pressure; DKA, diabetic ketoacidosis.

In addition, if fluid overload is suspected, a chest X-ray will aid in the medical diagnosis of pulmonary oedema. See Tables 7.4 and 7.5 for a summary of typical findings from urine and blood tests with fluid deficit and fluid excess.

Fluid excess—diuresis

The care of a patient with symptomatic hypervolaemia (see Table 7.3) involves reducing the amount of circulating blood volume and taking measures to ensure normal functioning of the cardiovascular, respiratory, and renal systems. Sodium and water restriction will decrease the amount of water coming into the body. Diuretics will help to increase water loss in the urine, with common examples summarized in Table 7.6.

Evaluating the impact of a diuretic should include assessing whether it has increased urine output and resolved the hypervolaemia. Side effects of the medication such as the loss of electrolytes should also be observed. In particular, potassium levels need to be closely monitored

Table 7.4 Urine investigations

Urine test	Normal range	Fluid deficit	Fluid excess
Specific gravity	1.020–1.030 g/mL	High	Low
Sodium	50–200 mmol/24 h	Low/high	Low/high
Osmolarity	300–1200 mOsm/L	High	Low

Table 7.5 Blood investigations

Blood test	Normal range	Fluid deficit	Fluid excess
Urea	< 7.5 mmol/L	High	Low
Sodium	135–145 mmol/L	Isotonic: normal Hypotonic: low Hypertonic: high	Isotonic: normal Hypotonic: low Hypertonic: high
Haematocrit	Male: 0.42–0.52 Female: 0.36–0.48	High	Normal/low
Osmolarity	280–300 mOsm/L	Isotonic: normal Hypotonic: low Hypertonic: high	Isotonic: normal Hypotonic: low Hypertonic: high

and replaced as necessary. The diuresis should not go so far as to cause hypovolaemia therefore a comprehensive fluid assessment is necessary to establish the fluid status of the patient after administration of the diuretic. Diuretic medications depend on the kidneys responding to the medication and hypervolaemia will continue if renal dysfunction prevents an increase in urine production despite administering diuretic therapy. Ongoing hypervolaemia that is resistant to diuretics and compromising cardiorespiratory function will eventually need dialysis to remove excess intravascular fluid.

Fluid deficit—intravenous fluid therapy

Intravenous infusions are used to replace fluid and electrolytes losses in the body, maintain and prevent further loss, and repair acid–base imbalances. The type of intravenous solution needed and rate of infusion will depend on the severity of fluid deficit, fluid compartment affected, serum electrolyte levels (particularly sodium), and serum osmolarity. A fluid management plan should be in place for all patients receiving intravenous fluid therapy including a prescription for fluids and electrolytes over the next 24 hours and clear details about ongoing patient assessment and monitoring of the plan (NICE 2014a). A structured approach to planning intravenous fluid therapy can come from the following four Ds model (Malbrain *et al.* 2015):

Table 7.6 Diuretics

Classification	Action in body	Examples
Loop diuretics	Inhibit water reabsorption from ascending limb of the loop of Henlé	Furosemide Bumetanide
Thiazides and related diuretics	Inhibit sodium reabsorption at beginning of the distal convoluted tubule	Bendroflumethiazide Metolazone
Potassium sparing diuretics	Aldosterone antagonist	Spironolactone Eplerenone

- Drug—viewing intravenous fluid like it is a drug.
- Dosing—type of intravenous fluid and amount over a period of time.
- Duration—how long the patient will be receiving intravenous fluid therapy.
- De-escalation—reducing and eventually stopping intravenous fluid therapy.

It is important to give intravenous fluid only if necessary and to provide the right type of fluid for the right amount of time because the inappropriate use of intravenous fluids increases the risk of iatrogenic organ dysfunction and mortality (Hoste *et al.* 2014). Algorithms for best practice with intravenous fluid therapy are provided by NICE (2013) with guidance specifically for fluid resuscitation, routine maintenance, and replacement and redistribution (see Table 7.7).

Crystalloids

Crystalloids are clear solutions made up of water and electrolytes which are both able to cross the semi-permeable membrane between fluid compartments. The fluid and solute in crystalloids will therefore shift between the intracellular and extracellular spaces depending on the concentration of the solution. If the crystalloid is isotonic, the fluid stays extracellular including in intravascular and interstitial spaces. Hypotonic solutions distribute through both intracellular and extracellular areas. The high osmolarity of hypertonic fluids draws fluid out of the cells and interstitium into the intravascular space. Hypertonic saline infusions (sodium chloride 3%, sodium chloride 7.5%) are not used outside critical care areas because of the high risk of severe cellular dehydration. They can be used in neurological intensive care to reduce cerebral oedema if other interventions are ineffective in treating a high intracranial pressure (Mangat *et al.* 2015). See Tables 7.8 for a comparison of isotonic, hypotonic, and hypertonic solutions, and Table 7.9 for the contents of crystalloid solutions commonly used for acutely ill patients.

Table 7.7 Intravenous fluid therapy (based on NICE 2013)

Fluid resuscitation	• Source and treat cause of hypovolaemia. • Fluid bolus 500 mL crystalloid over 15 m and assess for responsiveness and improvement. • Further 250–500 ml crystalloid boluses up until 2000 mL but if shock persists, expert help should be sought. • Na^+ in intravenous fluid should be within 130–154 mmol/l range.
Routine maintenance	• Daily needs: 25–30 mL/kg/day of water, 1 mmol/kg/day K^+, Na^+, and Cl^-, and 50–100 g/day glucose. • For patients who are obese, use ideal body weight. • Less fluid should be considered for: elderly, renal dysfunction, heart failure, or risk of refeeding syndrome from malnutrition. • Administer during daytime if possible to promote sleep at night.
Replacement and redistribution	• Replace existing and ongoing fluids and electrolytes deficits. • Expert help should be sought for guidance on redistribution with: oedema, sepsis, hyper/hyponatraemia, renal dysfunction, liver failure, cardiac impairment, post-operative, and malnutrition.

Adapted from © NICE (2013) Intravenous fluid therapy in adults in hospital. NICE. 2003 Dec 10. [https://www.nice.org.uk/guidance/cg174/resources/intravenous-fluid-therapy-in-adults-in-hospital-pdf-35109752233669] Accessed: 07/06/19.

Table 7.8 Types of crystalloid solutions

Isotonic solutions	Hartmann's Lactated Ringer's Ringer's acetate Plasma-Lyte Sodium chloride 0.9% Sodium chloride 0.9% + glucose 5%
Hypotonic solutions	Sodium chloride 0.45% Sodium chloride 0.45% + glucose 5% Sodium chloride 0.18% + glucose 4% Glucose 5%
Hypertonic solutions	Sodium chloride 3%, 5%, 7.5%

Combined water and sodium loss

Isotonic dehydration where water and sodium are lost in the same proportion is the most common type of fluid deficit. This results in a reduction of plasma volume but does not have a change in blood osmolarity. An isotonic intravenous infusion is then needed as the replacement solution (see Table 7.8). Isotonic solutions remain mostly in the extracellular areas with very little entering the cells because the concentration of dissolved substances in the intravenous fluid is similar to that in plasma. Even if the isotonic fluid is meant to reverse hypovolaemia by adding volume to the vasculature, the water from the fluid is distributed throughout the extracellular space with 70% ending up in the interstitial space and only 30% left in the circulating blood volume (see Figure 7.4).

Sodium chloride 0.9% is a commonly used isotonic crystalloid; however, with 154 mmol/L of chloride, it can contribute to hyperchloraemic metabolic acidosis (Reddy *et al.* 2016). A compound sodium lactate solution (commonly called 'balanced' solution) is not only isotonic but also designed to be more physiologically equivalent to plasma with 111 mmol/L of chloride (Langer *et al.* 2015). The lactate in a sodium lactate solution (Hartmann's, Lactated Ringers) is converted into bicarbonate by the liver which then prevents an acidosis from developing as a direct result of the intravenous fluid therapy. Balanced solutions containing lactate should be used cautiously with patients who have liver dysfunction and avoided if the liver failure is severe. There are also some balanced solutions (Ringer's acetate, Plasma-Lyte) which include acetate and gluconate instead of lactate as a way of indirectly providing bicarbonate. Balanced solutions also contain other electrolytes such potassium, calcium, and magnesium. Electrolyte levels and renal function should therefore be checked prior to administering a balanced solution to avoid exacerbating high amounts of serum electrolytes.

Primarily water loss

If there has been more water lost relative to sodium loss, the extracellular fluid becomes hypertonic which then draws water in from the cells creating a fluid deficit in the intracellular compartment. Initially, this creates an increase of water in the extracellular area. With continual water loss, however, the extracellular spaces eventually become depleted of fluid as well because there is not enough water shifting in from the cells to maintain a normal blood

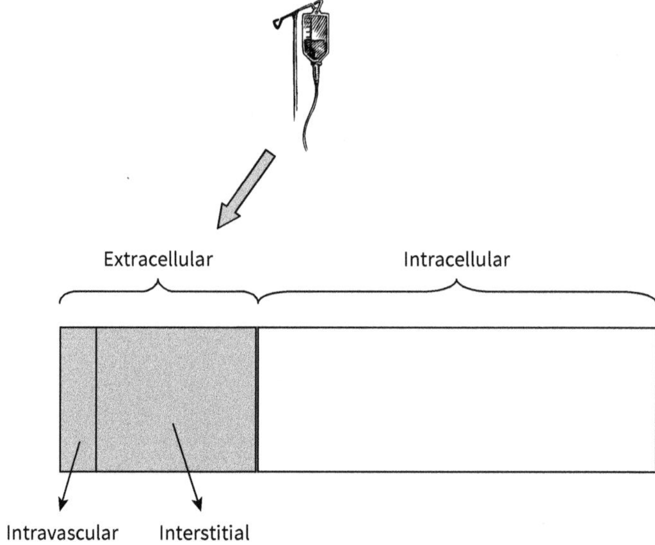

Figure 7.4 Isotonic crystalloid.

volume. The end result is a lack of fluid in both the intracellular and the extracellular spaces and hypertonic blood (high sodium level). Ultimately, the cellular dehydration and depletion in blood volume requires replacement of free water to correct the underpinning fluid deficit. In this instance, a hypotonic intravenous infusion will distribute water evenly throughout the intracellular and the extracellular areas and help to correct the blood's hypertonicity (see Figure 7.5).

Pure water cannot be administered as an intravenous infusion because the osmotic gradient it creates pulls water in from the red blood cells until they burst (haemolysis). Although glucose 5% is technically isotonic as it exists in the bag, the glucose is quickly

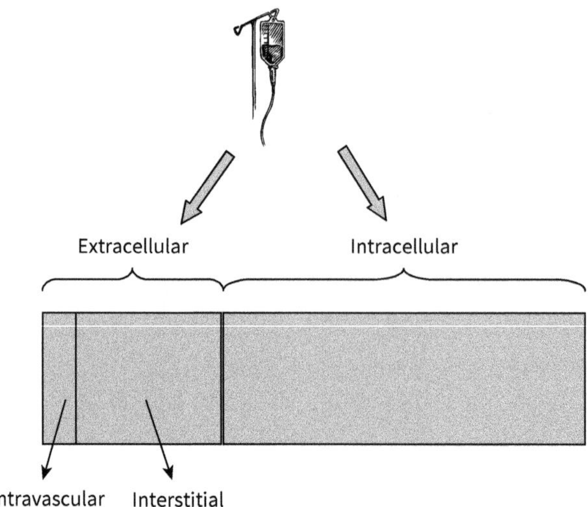

Figure 7.5 Hypotonic crystalloids.

metabolized once the fluid has been administered which then just leaves the remaining water from the solution without causing haemolysis. This means that glucose 5% essentially functions like a hypotonic solution. As glucose 5% increases interstitial and intracellular water, it should be avoided with any patient who has a high intracranial pressure to avoid swelling of the cells and interstitial space in the brain. Similarly, the technical osmolarity of solutions containing dextrose and sodium chloride may be isotonic (sodium chloride 0.18% + glucose 4%) or hypertonic (sodium chloride 0.45% + glucose 5%, sodium chloride 0.9% + glucose 5%) in the bag. The physiological impact is then the basis for how the solution is classified according to the concentration of the solution's sodium chloride content (see Table 7.9).

Primarily sodium loss

A loss of more sodium than water creates relatively hypotonic blood and fluid moves from the extracellular space to the intracellular space. This type of fluid deficit is uncommon but can be caused by diuretics, salt-wasting renal disease, or when isotonic dehydration is replaced with a hypotonic intravenous solution. Sodium chloride 0.9% is the preferred solution to provide replacement for the salt loss.

Colloids

Colloids contain macromolecules that normally stay within the plasma for a number of days because they are too large to pass through the vascular endothelial membrane and are metabolized slowly. The increased oncotic pressure from these added substances encourages the water to remain inside the intravascular space as well as draw off further fluid from the interstitium (see Figure 7.6). Compared with crystalloids then, colloids have an enhanced ability to expand plasma volume because much of the water from crystalloids ends up distributed across the extracellular area rather than remaining strictly in the plasma.

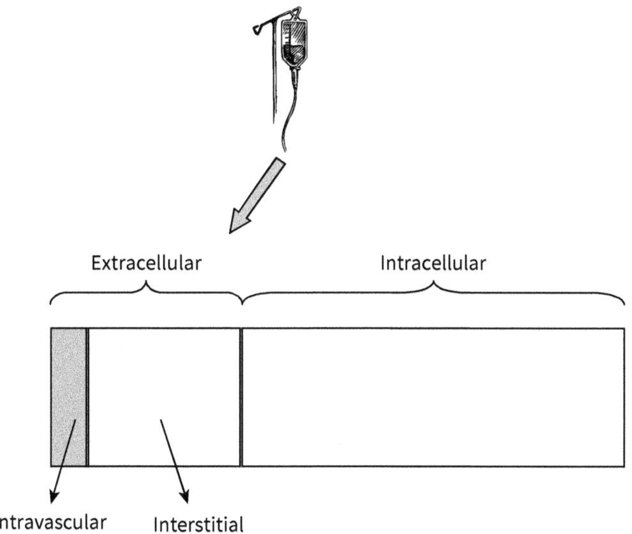

Figure 7.6 Colloids

Table 7.9 Components of crystalloid solutions. Reproduced from https://www.nice.org.uk/guidance/cg174/resources/composition-of-commonly-used-crystalloids-table-191662813

Content	Plasma	Sodium chloride 0.9%	Sodium chloride 0.18%/4% glucose[a]	0.45% NaCI/4% glucose[a]	5% glucose[a]	Harmann's	Lactated Ringer's (USP)	Ringer's acetate	Alternative balanced solutions for resuscitation**	Alternative balanced solutions for maintenance**
Na^* (mmol/I)	135-145	154	31	77	0	131	130	130	140	40
CI^- (mmol/I)	95–105	154	31	77	0	111	109	112	98	40
$[Na^+]$: $[CI^-]$ ratio	1.28–1.45:1	1:1	1:1	1:1	—	1.18:1	1.19:1	1.16:	1.43:1	1:1
K^+ (mmol/I)	3.5–5.3	*	*	*	*	5	4	5	5	13
HCO_{3-}/ Bicarbonate	24–32	0	0	0	0	29 (lactate)	28 (lactate)	27 (acetate)	27 (acetate) 23 (gluconate)	16 (acetate)
Ca^{2+} (mmol/I)	2.2–2.6	0	0	0	0	2	1.4	1	0	0
Mg^{2+} (mmol/I)	0.8–1.2	0		0		0	0	1	1.5	1.5
Glucose (mmol/I)	3.5–5.5	0	222 (40 g)	222 (40 g)	278 (50 g)	0	0	0	0	222 (40 g)
pH	7.35–7.41	4.5–7.0	4.5		3.5–5.5	5.0–7.0	6–7.5	6–8	4.0–8.0	4.5–7.0
Osmolarity	275–295	308	284		278	278	273	276	295	389

* These solutions are available with differing quantities of potassium already added, and the potassium-containing versions are usually more appropriate for meeting maintenance needs.

** Alternative balanced solutions are available commercially under different brand names and composition may vary by preparation.

A The term dextrose refers to the dextro-rotaory isomer of glucose that can be metabolized and is the only form used in IV fluids. However, IV fluid bags are often labelled as glucose so only this term should be used. Traditionally hospitals bought a small range of fluids combining saline (0.18–0.9%) with glucose but several recent NICE/NPSA documents have recommended specific combination, which are now purchased to enable guideline to be enable guidelines to be followed. Lucose-saline combinations now come in 5 different concentrations, and the addition of variable potassium content expands the pre-mixed range to 13 different products. Prescribers must therefore specify the concentration of each component; the term dextrose-saline (or abbreviation D/S) is meaningless without these details. What is specified also impacts significantly on the cost of the product.

Note: Weight-based potassium prescriptions should be rounded to the nearest common fluids available (for example, a 67 kg person should have fluids containing 20 mmol and 40 mmol of potassium in a 24-hour period). Potassium should not be added to intravenous fluid bags as this is dangerous.

Source: This table was drafted based on the consensus decision of the members of the Guideline Development Group.

As a result, a smaller volume of colloid fluid needs to be infused and there is reduced peripheral and pulmonary oedema. The colloid will leak out of the plasma to cause oedema if the capillary endothelium is not intact such as with sepsis, acute respiratory distress syndrome, or blunt trauma. Other potential complications of colloids are coagulopathy and anaphylaxis although both are quite rare. With large doses, some colloids cause pruritus and impair renal function particularly with septic patients where 'leaky capillaries' allow the macromolecules to settle in the skin and kidneys.

Despite their theoretical advantage as a better plasma expander, there is no evidence that colloids improve outcomes compared to crystalloids, and colloid solutions containing hydroxyethyl starch may even increase mortality (Perel *et al.* 2013). Colloids are also more expensive than crystalloids which, along with a lack of research to support their widespread use, has led to their decreasing popularity. However, it is difficult to make generalizations about the ideal fluid replacement solution for all patients because of individual variables and the unique aspects of each clinical context (Myburgh and Mythen 2013). The debate about colloid use continues with some gelatin-based colloids (gelofusine, haemaccel) prescribed by some clinicians for fluid resuscitation despite not being promoted by NICE's (2014a) guidelines for intravenous fluid therapy. There may also be a role for isotonic albumin (4–5%) for patients with sepsis (Muacevic and Adler 2016) or burns (Navickis *et al.* 2016) who have refractory hypotension because they remain hypovolaemic even after large volumes of crystalloid fluid resuscitation. There is no evidence to confirm albumin should be used for these conditions though, or the best timing and dosage, thus research remains ongoing. There is consensus that concentrated albumin (20%) is indicated after draining off large volumes (> 5 l/day) of ascitic fluid because giving albumin post-paracentesis of tense ascites reduces morbidity and mortality (Widjaja *et al.* 2016).

Blood products

Transfusion of blood products is indicated when there are specific deficiencies within the blood requiring replacement. Components of blood which may be transfused include packed red blood cells, platelets, and fresh frozen plasma. It is important to ensure the blood product infused is compatible with the patient's blood type by following local safety guidelines and checking procedures. There are also differences in how various blood products are stored and administered, which can be guided by protocols and clinical guidelines from the UK Blood Transfusion and Tissue Transplantation Services (2013). See Table 7.10 for details about the indication, storage, shelf life, and transfusion time of different types of blood products.

Packed red blood cells are transfused for anaemia or if the patient is actively bleeding. A dose of 4 mL/kg packed red blood cells will typically raise the haemogloblin level by 10 g/L. If there is no evidence of haemorrhage, the vital signs are stable, and the patient is otherwise asymptomatic, a low haemoglobin level may not require a transfusion. Dilutional anaemia from large amounts of intravenous crystalloid fluids lowering the haemoglobin concentration could also be monitored without specifically treating. The transfusion trigger (haemogloblin level prompting packed red blood cells to be prescribed) will be based on the context of trends and an individual patient's condition and will typically be between 70 g/L and 80 g/L. Patients with ischaemic conditions such as acute coronary syndrome, stroke,

Table 7.10 Blood products

Packed red blood cells	
Indication	Low haemoglobin from anaemia or bleeding
Storage	Blood fridge at 4°C
Shelf life	35 days
Transfusion time	Administer quickly if bleeding, otherwise each unit is typically prescribed to be given over 2–3 hours using caution with heart failure but a maximum of 4 hours/unit
Fresh frozen plasma	
Indication	Clotting disorders
Storage	Blood fridge at 4°C once thawed
Shelf life	2 years at −30°C
Transfusion time	Administer as soon as possible 10–20 mL/kg/hour
Platelets	
Indication	Very low platelet count
Storage	22°C—never refrigerate
Shelf life	5 days
Transfusion time	Administer as soon as possible over 30–60 min

or traumatic brain injury may benefit from a higher transfusion trigger level but should be evaluated on an individual basis (Norfolk 2014).

Acute transfusion reactions (< 24 hours of transfusion)

- Febrile non-haemolytic reaction—typically mild.
- Allergic reaction—can be mild (urticaria) to severe (angio-oedema, anaphylaxis).
- Acute haemolytic reaction—blood type (ABO) incompatibility.
- TACO—transfusion-associated circulatory overload.
- TRALI—transfusion-related acute lung injury.
- Blood product contaminated with micro-organism.

Intravenous therapy

In addition to crystalloids, colloids, and blood products, other indications for intravenous therapy include administration of medications, electrolytes, and total parenteral nutrition. Intravenous therapy can be delivered peripherally in a small vein or centrally if a central venous catheter has been inserted into a larger vein (e.g. internal jugular, subclavian, or femoral). The most common type of central catheter used in acute care is a short-term non-tunnelled catheter, although some patients may come into hospital with a long-term tunnelled catheter such as a Hickman, Groshong, or Port-a-cath. A peripherally inserted central catheter could also be used which has a reduced risk of infection because the insertion site is farther away from the central cardiovascular system.

Regardless of the type of fluid or catheter being used, there are core principles of intravenous therapy that are necessary for all nurses to follow, including use of non-touch aseptic technique throughout preparation and administration, ongoing assessment of the intravenous site, which should be free of complications and covered with a clear, intact dressing, and removal of the intravenous cannula if it is no longer necessary. Infection prevention and control measures are particularly important while caring for a patient with vascular access device with guidance provided by the National Clinical Guideline Centre (2012) and NICE (2014b).

Potential complications of intravenous therapy

- infection—localized, systemic
- phlebitis—mechanical, chemical, infective
- infiltration
- extravasation
- particulate contamination
- embolism—air, clot, foreign body
- fluid overload
- anaphylaxis
- speedshock
- sharps injury

Common fluid disorders

Fluid deficit: Severe hyperglycaemia

Diabetic ketoacidosis (DKA) and hyperglycaemic hyperosmolar syndrome (HHS) are both metabolic emergencies that can develop with diabetic patients (see Chapter 6). With DKA, ketogenesis occurs as fatty acids are used for energy instead of glucose that cannot be utilized without insulin. Ketone bodies are produced which acidify the blood, bringing about a metabolic acidosis and increase in the serum osmolarity. In addition, the large glucose molecules enhance the high osmolarity even further, which draws water out of the cells creating intracellular dehydration. As the glucose molecules build up in the blood, they begin to spill over into the urine. Water follows in an osmotic diuresis, which also brings about severe fluid deficit in all fluid compartments. There are absent ketones with HHS but the hyperglycaemia, hyperosmolarity, and fluid deficit are even greater, which leads to a high mortality with this particular clinical situation.

The care of the patient with DKA/HHS focuses on intravenous therapy, including crystalloids, potassium, and insulin. If large amounts of potassium are needed, continual electrocardiogram (ECG) monitoring and central venous access will be needed. The goal of the insulin is to lower the blood sugar slowly otherwise a sudden drop can create cerebral oedema. The insulin infusion is kept until ketoacidosis and osmolality return to normal (10% glucose may be needed to maintain blood glucose).

Fluid deficit: Haemorrhage

A patient who is actively bleeding will eventually begin to show signs of hypovolaemia because of the decreased effective circulating blood volume. Obvious signs of bleeding may be apparent when the skin integrity is broken, a patient has recently come back from surgery with an open wound/drains, or when blood is found in fluids being drained from the body such as urine from a foley catheter or pleural fluid from a chest tube. Internal haemorrhage should also be considered, which may not be seen on inspection but suspected from the patient's history.

Up to 10–15% of total blood volume can be lost without clinical significance because of the body's compensation mechanisms to maintain adequate tissue perfusion. This involves normal hypovolaemia responses such as peripheral vasoconstriction, increase in heart rate, increase in cardiac output, secretion of ADH, and activation of the renin–angiotensin–aldosterone system. In addition, the liver acts as a reservoir as it holds up to 15% of the total blood volume at any given time and releases blood during haemorrhage to improve the effective circulating blood volume. As the amount of blood loss increases, so does the compensation, which then becomes evident in the patient's vital signs. Further bleeding will then overwhelm the body, causing the failure of the compensation mechanisms and leads to severe complications or death if left untreated.

The American College of Surgeons Committee on Trauma (2018) has traditionally classified blood loss according to a severity scale:

- Class I (< 15% blood volume): no changes to vital signs
- Class II (15–30% blood volume): tachycardia, narrow pulse pressure, pale, cool, respiratory rate 20–30 breaths/min
- Class III (30–40% blood volume): tachycardia, narrow pulse pressure, hypotension, capillary refill > 3 s, cold, clammy, respiratory rate > 30 breaths/min, oliguria, anxiety, confusion
- Class IV (> 40% blood volume): compensation mechanisms fail with severe tachycardia and hypotension, respiratory rate > 35 breaths/min, anuria, altered mental status

Adapted with permission from Advanced Trauma Life Support (ATLS®) Student Course Manual. 10th edition. 2018. American College of Surgeons. Chicago.

This scale highlights how blood pressure may remain normal despite a moderate amount of blood loss. Abnormality in the strength of peripheral pulses, systolic blood pressure, and mental status are late clinical signs of central hypovolaemia, and tachycardia in the supine position may be absent until quite severe blood loss. This haemorrhage classification scale has limitations though because young, previously well patients may be able to compensate for long periods of time because of their large physiological reserves. In addition, elderly patients may have chronic treatments such as β-blockers which influence the body's ability to compensate normally (El Sayed and Noureddine 2014).

Although haemoglobin level is useful to measure in the patient with haemorrhage, it is expressed as a concentration, meaning that the total blood volume influences the numerical result. In an actively bleeding patient, it takes time for the fluid compartments to adjust to the decrease in intravascular volume therefore the haemoglobin level as a concentration may be misleading. Crystalloid infusions dilute the blood which further complicates the interpretation of a haemoglobin level after the initial fluid resuscitation. Transfusing one unit of packed red blood cells typically increases a haemoglobin level by 10 g/L in the absence of bleeding although if the bleeding continues, it is difficult to assess the exact effect of a transfusion on the blood volume through the haemoglobin level. Haemoglobin or haematocrit (percentage of red blood cells in the blood) are useful investigations to measure in the patient with blood loss but the values must be considered within the context of when the haemorrhage occurred as well as the types and amount of fluid replacement used.

Clinical link 7.1 (see Appendix for answers)

You are caring for a patient who returned from surgery 4 h ago from a right hemicolectomy. Initially, the vital signs were stable, pain was well controlled with an epidural, abdominal dressing was dry and intact, and there was minimal drainage from the nasogastric tube and abdominal drain. While doing a routine set of vital signs, you notice that the patient appears anxious, has cool peripheries, is tachycardic (115 bpm), hypotensive (80/45 mmHg), and has a high respiratory rate (25 breaths/min).

- What would be your immediate actions and why?
- What other signs and symptoms would indicate post-operative bleeding is occurring?
- If active bleeding was ruled out, what other reasons could be causing these abnormalities?
- If active bleeding was confirmed, how would you coordinate care of the patient, including interaction with the nurse in charge and surgical team?

Nursing management

If a patient was previously bleeding or appears to be having continual blood loss, care should focus on identifying the source and liaising with the medical and the surgical teams for interventions that will stop the haemorrhage. In the meantime, ongoing assessment of vital signs, physical assessment signs of hypovolaemia, and blood results (haemoglobin, haematocrit, and lactate) will provide information for establishing trends and allow an estimation of whether the bleeding is resolving or getting worse (see Table 7.11).

Fluid deficit: Vomiting and diarrhoea

Large amounts of gastrointestinal fluid can be lost from the body through nasogastric drainage/suction, vomiting, and diarrhoea. In addition to the water loss, this also depletes the patient of hydrogen ions, sodium, chloride, and potassium. Gastric secretions contain very little magnesium, although prolonged vomiting for a number of weeks can result in hypomagnesaemia. As a result of the acidic nature of gastric fluid, continual loss eventually leads

Table 7.11 Nursing care of hypovolaemia from blood loss

Potential problem	Nursing care
External bleeding	Monitor for evidence of external bleeding from skin, wounds, drains, intravenous sites, or body orifices (eyes, nose, ears, tracheostomy, anus, urethra, vagina) Report increase in bleeding to doctor Apply pressure if possible to site of bleeding Document estimated amount of bleeding on fluid balance Monitor vital signs and Hb regularly
Internal bleeding	Consider patient history while assessing for possible internal bleeding Monitor bodily fluids for signs of bleeding (urine, stool, sputum, gastrointestinal drainage/emesis) Assess abdomen: inspection, palpation, percussion, auscultation Liaise with doctor about further investigations (ultrasound, CT scan, X-ray) Document bodily fluids with signs of blood on fluid balance Monitor vital signs and Hb regularly
Decreased Hb and oxygen carrying capacity	Monitor haemoglobin level until stable Transfuse packed red blood cells as prescribed Consider the impact of crystalloid intravenous infusions on haemoglobin level Monitor for signs of poor oxygenation (shortness of breath, cyanosis, low PaO_2, high lactate) Maintain O_2 saturations 94–98% or 88–92% if at risk of hypercapnic respiratory failure O_2 saturation may be normal (i.e. Hb molecules fully saturated) but total amount of Hb is low from the blood loss making it difficult to use O_2 saturation as clinical sign of oxygenation
Hypotension	Monitor blood pressure regularly Administer intravenous fluids as prescribed
Tachycardia	Monitor heart rate regularly Monitor ECG Monitor electrolytes
Impaired tissue perfusion	Assess peripheral pulses and capillary refill regularly Assess skin colour, warmth, movement, and sensation regularly Monitor lactate
Altered level of consciousness	Monitor Glasgow Coma Scale regularly Assess ability to maintain airway Report any change in level of consciousness to medical team
Fluid deficit	Establish intravenous therapy and administer crystalloids and blood products as prescribed Fluid balance chart 24-hour balance Monitor clinical signs and symptoms of fluid deficit/excess

(continued)

Table 7.11 *Continued*

Potential problem	Nursing care
Acute kidney injury	Monitor urine output regularly Report to doctor if urine output drops below 0.5 mL/kg/h Monitor urea, creatinine, and electrolytes Administer intravenous therapy as prescribed to maintain adequate blood pressure
Reaction to blood transfusion	Monitor vital signs as per local protocol for administration of blood products Assess for signs and symptoms of acute or delayed reaction, post transfusion purpura, and acute lung injury If reaction suspected, stop transfusion and report to doctor and blood bank as per local protocol

to metabolic alkalosis. The loss of bicarbonate from the lower gastrointestinal tract contributes to the development of metabolic acidosis. There are numerous causes for both vomiting and diarrhoea, including infection, side effects from medication, and gastrointestinal illness.

Clinical link 7.2 (see Appendix for answers)

An 80-year-old male patient was originally admitted to hospital 10 days ago due to confusion, reduced mobility, and the inability of his wife as the main care giver to cope with caring for him. He is now experiencing yellow, watery stools, which are increasing in frequency and amount. Although he had been eating and drinking well up until two days ago with encouragement and assistance, today he has only agreed to minimal oral intake. At 15:30, you realize he has not had any urinary output since the beginning of your shift at 07:30 and there was no fluid balance chart recorded for the previous day. The patient is not catheterized and when you question him whether he needs a urinal, his answer is vague and not appropriate.

- Identify all the potential causes for fluid and electrolyte deficit with this patient.
- How would you manage the diarrhoea?
- How would you manage improving the fluid input?
- What investigations and treatments does this patient appear to need?

As a result of the loss of electrolytes, hydrogen ions, or bicarbonate, the patient is also at risk of:

- hyponatraemia
- hypocholeraemia
- hypokalaemia
- hypomagnesenaemia
- metabolic acidosis or alkalosis

For nursing care associated with vomiting and diarrhoea, interventions will be in response to any abnormalities identified from monitoring blood pressure, electrolytes, metabolic acid–base balance, level of consciousness, renal function, and the overall gastrointestinal function. It is also important to evaluate the patient's nutritional needs and refer to the doctor and dietician as need be if vomiting and diarrhoea persist. Further care of a patient with abnormality of the gastrointestinal tract is discussed in Chapter 6.

Fluid excess: Liver failure

The liver has a number of different functions including synthesizing albumin, which is a large plasma protein. Because of its size, albumin creates an oncotic pressure that helps to maintain fluid within the intravascular space. With liver failure, the ability to produce albumin is impaired, which decreases the oncotic pressure and allows water to redistribute to the interstitial area.

A further influence on fluid status for patients with liver failure is the ascites that develops as fluid collects in the peritoneal cavity. The underlying contributing factors for ascites include sphlanchnic vasodilation, arterial hypotension, increased cardiac output, and decreased vascular resistance. The subsequent decrease in intravascular volume leads to impaired renal function and sodium/water retention. As water is retained proportionally more than sodium, the patient then presents with dilutional hyponatraemia. Depending on a patient's albumin and retention of sodium and water, the intravascular volume may appear to be normal, low, or high and therefore patients with liver failure could be in either fluid deficit or fluid excess.

The nursing care associated with fluid management of a patient with liver failure will depend on findings from monitoring the blood pressure, fluid balance, weight, renal function and signs of third spacing such as peripheral oedema and ascites. Actions could be intravenous fluid or diuretics depending on if the patient presents as intravascular fluid deficit or in fluid overload.

Clinical link 7.3 (see Appendix for answers)

You are caring for a 55-year-old female patient with chronic liver disease. She has been admitted to an acute ward because of severe ascites and suspected infection of unknown cause (temperature 38.3°C and white blood cells 16×10^9/L). On your initial assessment you note peripheral oedema up to her knees bilaterally and her breathing appears laboured at 25 breaths/min. Paracentesis was performed by the doctor, which drained off 6 L of clear yellow fluid. An albumin infusion was then prescribed, which you administer.

- Explain why hypotension due to hypovolaemia may occur with this patient, who has both peripheral oedema and ascites.
- What impact does the excessive fluid in the peritoneal space have on other body systems?
- Why was an albumin infusion prescribed?

Fluid excess: Iatrogenic intravenous infusion overload

Any patient with an intravenous infusion has the potential to receive an excessive total amount of fluid or to have the infusion administered too quickly for the cardiovascular system to cope. The use of a pump ensures the exact amount of fluid at the prescribed rate which decreases the chance of overloading the patient with fluid while providing an intravenous infusion. This is particularly important for patients with heart failure or renal dysfunction who are already at risk for hypervolaemia.

Whether it is a crystalloid, colloid, blood product, total parenteral nutrition, or medication, intravenous therapy can potentially deliver too much fluid, resulting in water leaking out to the interstitium. Normally, this would be prevented because the liver expands to help manage the increased level of circulating blood volume and the kidneys produce more urine. However, when there is far too much fluid for the compensation mechanisms to cope with or the function of the heart and kidneys are impaired, iatrogenic hypervolaemia would develop. This is clinically significant when oedema not only develops in the peripheries but also begins to form pulmonary oedema, which impairs gas exchange in the lungs. Management of the patient experiencing iatrogenic fluid overload is to stop the intravenous fluid therapy and administer diuretics as necessary with ongoing monitoring of the fluid status of the patient.

End of chapter test

The following assessment will enable you to evaluate your theoretical knowledge of fluid assessment and management as well as your ability to apply this theory to clinical practice.

Knowledge assessment

With the support of your mentor/supervisor from practice, work through the following prompts to explore your knowledge level about fluid assessment and management.

- Describe fluid compartments and how fluid homeostasis is maintained.
- Differentiate between osmotic, hydrostatic, and oncotic pressures.
- Identify all sources for water gain and water loss in the body.
- Define normovolaemia, hypovolaemia, and hypervolaemia.
- Explain the role of sodium in maintaining fluid homeostasis.
- Identify potential third-space areas and define the term third-space fluid.
- Explain how hypovolaemia can exist when there is excess water in the body.
- Critically analyse causes of fluid deficit along with associated compensation mechanisms.
- Define hypovolaemic shock.
- Critically analyse causes of fluid excess along associated compensation mechanisms.
- Explain your role and responsibilities as a nurse in preventing an altered fluid balance.
- Recognize risk factors for fluid imbalance.
- Critically analyse the clinical presentation of fluid deficit and fluid excess.

- Explain how blood tests, urine investigations, and chest X-ray contribute to a fluid assessment.
- Differentiate between types of diuretics, including actions on the body, indications, contraindications, and side effects.
- Compare and contrast different types of intravenous fluids including benefits, limitations, indications for use, contraindications, and side effects for each.
- Critically analyse your role and responsibilities in transfusing blood products.
- Discuss different types of blood products, including packed red blood cells, fresh frozen plasma, and platelets.
- Critically discuss nursing assessment and management of peripheral and central venous access and potential complications of intravenous therapy.
- Describe how fluid assessment and management are documented where you work.
- Explain how fluids are managed with a patient presenting with DKA or HHS.
- Recognize possible causes of internal bleeding and how you would act if you suspected a patient was experiencing internal bleeding.
- Critically analyse the progression of blood loss as it becomes more severe.
- Discuss how vomiting and diarrhoea influence fluids and electrolytes in the body.
- Explain how an alteration in fluid balance occurs with liver failure.
- Explain how an alteration in fluid balance occurs with heart failure and renal dysfunction.

Skills assessment

Under the guidance of your mentor/supervisor, undertake a full fluid assessment followed by appropriate interventions for any significant abnormality. Your mentor/supervisor will be able to assess your ability and provide feedback based on the following skills:

- Conducts a patient history, vital signs, and physical assessment considering key points that are relevant for a fluid assessment.
- Weighs the patient and explains the clinical significance of the actual number as well as any trends.
- Assesses all sources and amount of fluid intake and output from the patient.
- Calculates the current net fluid balance and explains the clinical significance of the actual number as well as any trends.
- Facilitates relevant clinical investigations such as blood, urine, and X-ray tests and evaluates results.
- Reviews current medications and intravenous therapy, rationalizing their impact on fluid status.
- Interprets subjective and objective findings from the fluid assessment, identifies significant abnormalities, explains possible causes for these abnormalities, and plans appropriate actions with rationales.
- Incorporates fluid assessment findings into an early warning sign score.
- Liaises with other members of the healthcare team as necessary, including the nurse in charge, doctor, pharmacist, physiotherapist, and healthcare assistant.

- Demonstrates an ability to follow infection control guidelines while undertaking intravenous therapy.
- Documents a fluid management plan, completed actions, and evaluation of actions.

References

American College of Surgeons Committee on Trauma (2018) *Advanced Trauma Life Support for Doctors* 10th edn. Chicago, IL: American College of Surgeons.

Elder, A., Japp, A., Verghese, A. (2016) How valuable is physical examination of the cardiovascular system? *Brit Med J*, 354: i3309.

El Sayed, M. and Noureddine, H. (2014) Recent advances of haemorrhage management in severe trauma. *Emerg Med Int*, Article ID 638956.

Hoste, E.A., Maitland, K., and Brudney, C.S. (2014). Four phases of intravenous fluid therapy: A conceptual model. *Br J Anaes*, 113(5):740–7.

Langer, T., Santini, A., Scotti, E., *et al.* (2015). Intravenous balanced solutions: From physiology to clinical evidence. *Anaesthesiol Intensive Ther*, (47):s78–s88.

Malbrain, M.L.N.G., Regenmortel, N.V., Owczuk, R. (2015) It is time to consider the four D's of fluid management. *Anaesthesiol Intensive Ther*, 47:S1–S5.

Mangat, H.S., Chiu, Y.L., Gerber, L.M., *et al.* (2015) Hypertonic saline reduces cumulative and daily intracranial pressure burdens after severe traumatic brain injury. *J Neurosurg*, 122:202–10.

Marieb, E.N., Hoehn, K.N. (2015). *Human Anatomy and Physiology* 10th edn. Boston, MA: Pearson.

Marik, P.E., Cavallazi, R. (2013) Does the central venous pressure predict fluid responsiveness? An updated met-analysis and a plea for some common sense. *Crit Care Med*, 41(7):1774–81.

McGloin, S. (2015). The ins and outs of fluid balance in the acutely ill patient. *Br J Nurs*, 24(1):14–18.

Muacevic, A., Adler, J.R. (2016) The use of fluids in sepsis. *Cureus*, 8(3):e528.

Myburgh, J.A., Mythen, M.G. (2013) Resuscitation fluids. *N Engl J Med*, 369:1243–51.

National Clinical Guideline Centre (2012) *Infection: Prevention and Control of Healthcare-associated Infections in Primary and Community Care.* London: National Clinical Guideline Centre.

Navickis, R.J., Greenhalgh, D.G., Wilkes, M.M. (2016) Albumin in burn shock resuscitation: A meta-analysis of controlled clinical studies. *J Burn Care Res*, 37(3): e268–e278.

NICE (2013) *Intravenous Fluid Therapy in Adults in Hospital* CG174. London: National Institute for Health and Care Excellence.

NICE (2014a) *Intravenous Fluid Therapy in Adults in Hospital* QS66. London: National Institute for Health and Care Excellence.

NICE (2014b) *Infection Prevention and Control* QS61. London: National Institute for Health and Clinical Excellence.

Norfolk, D. (2014) *Handbook of Transfusion Medicine*, 5th edn. Norwich: TSO.

Perel, P., Roberts, I., Ker, K. (2013) Colloids versus crystalloids for fluid resuscitation in critically ill patients. *Cochrane Database System Rev*, Issue 2. Art. CD000567. doi:10.1002/14651858.CD000567.pub6.

Reddy, S., Weinberg, L., Young, P. (2016). Crystalloid fluid therapy. *Crit Care*, 20:59.

UK Blood Transfusion and Tissue Transplantation Services (2013) *Guidelines for the Blood Transfusion Services in the United Kingdom*, 8th edn. Norwich: TSO.

Widjaja, F.F., Khairan, P., Kamelia, T., *et al.* (2016) Colloids versus albumin in large volume paracentesis to prevent circulatory dysfunction: Evidence-based case report. *Acta Med Indones*, 48(2):148–55.

8

Assessment and care of the patient with sepsis

Kevin Barrett

Chapter contents

In order to understand how to assess and manage the patient with sepsis, it is essential to have an understanding of the pathophysiology of a dysregulated inflammatory response to an infective process. This chapter will examine:

- definitions of sepsis and septic shock
- physiological changes following widespread inflammation.
- physiological changes to the cardiovascular system
- nursing assessment of sepsis
- nursing care of the patient with sepsis to include:
  - care bundles and their rationale
  - nursing management of the septic patient

Learning outcomes

This chapter will enable you to:

- to appreciate the discussion surrounding the use of qSOFA and SOFA scoring systems
- to consolidate your understanding of the normal inflammatory response
- to develop an understanding of changes to this response during sepsis
- to understand the significance of early and repeated assessment in patients with suspected sepsis
- to discuss the management of patients with sepsis
- to understand when the patient with worsening symptoms requires an escalation of support
- to use the clinical assessment framework to guide your practice

Introduction

Sepsis is defined as life-threatening organ dysfunction caused by a dysregulated host response to infection (Rhodes *et al.* 2017). In lay terms, sepsis is a life-threatening condition that arises when the body's response to an infection injures its own tissues and organs (Singer *et al.* 2016). Sepsis and its most serious consequence, septic shock, are very significant healthcare problems, affecting millions of people around the world every year. Although the mortality rate for sepsis varies globally, in England it is stated as 30% (NCEPOD 2015). However, assessing actual sepsis-related mortality is complicated, as the International Classification of Diseases, 10th Revision (ICD-10) is not clear in its coding for sepsis and sepsis-related conditions are not always used as the principle cause of death (McPherson *et al.* 2013). It is noted that sepsis is increasing in its occurrence (Sepsis Alliance 2015; APPG 2016) and that hospitalization for sepsis has more than doubled in the past decade (Nutbeam *et al.* 2016).

To date, much of the relevant research has focused on early identification and interventions for patients with sepsis in Accident & Emergency (A&E) departments and critical care areas. However, many patients actually acquire sepsis on the general wards (Bhattacharjee *et al.* 2017). Early sepsis recognition by ward nurses can both reduce progression of this lethal disease and improve survival for patients in hospital with sepsis (Torsvik *et al.* 2016). This is the focus of this chapter.

Infection is caused by microbes—most often bacteria—invading the tissues which results in a localized inflammatory response from the immune system. Sepsis is the body's *systemic*, rather than localized, inflammatory reaction to infection (Mitchell and Whitehouse 2009). This is what is referred to as 'dysregulated'; the locally mediated and contained immune system controls are lost and the response becomes disproportionate and global.

It is recognized that medical education about sepsis is variable (Health Education England 2016) and that training for registered staff varies significantly too, within the United Kingdom (APPG, 2016; Health Education England, 2016). Regrettably, instances of sepsis are still being misinterpreted by nurses and other healthcare staff with sometimes tragic consequences (Glasper 2016). It is also noted that the general public's understanding of the condition is poor in the United Kingdom; 55% of the public had not heard of the term 'sepsis' and 25% were unaware that sepsis is a medical emergency (UK Sepsis Trust 2016). This widespread lack of awareness about sepsis alone constitutes a barrier in recognizing when these patients are becoming very unwell and require an escalation of interventions to try to avoid the very serious, often fatal, consequences of the condition, whether the patient begins to deteriorate at home or in hospital.

A recent systematic review (Smyth *et al.* 2016) identified some of the difficulties for identification of sepsis in the community and there is now a clinical toolkit provided for prehospital staff supported by NICE and the College of Paramedics (Nicholls *et al.* 2016)

Epidemiology: 'The World's Oldest Killer'

The epidemiology of sepsis, which is the study of the spread of the condition throughout populations, is helpful to look at because its incidence is so pervasive. Worldwide, there are over 18 million cases of sepsis each year, equivalent to the combined populations of Ireland, Norway, Denmark, and Finland. Although the focus of this chapter is on ward-based patients, it is worth realizing that once patients with sepsis are transferred to an intensive treatment unit (ITU) setting, where they can be best supported, even then a recent global assessment of the mortality rate of these patients, treated in ITU, found that more than one-third of these patients died before leaving hospital (Vincent *et al.* 2014). In fact, it is reported that within the ITU, patients with sepsis had a 70% relative higher mortality rate compared with patients without sepsis (Melville *et al.* 2015). This is an extremely high mortality rate and recent parliamentary reports highlight that a number of deaths from sepsis are preventable (PHSO 2013).

In the United Kingdom, the estimated annual figure for deaths from sepsis is in the region of 37,000. Sepsis is more common than myocardial infarction and has a higher mortality than any cancer (Global Sepsis Alliance 2015). The most recent figures for England show the number of deaths from sepsis is increasing; the escalating trend is thought to be due to an increasingly older population becoming ill with a greater comorbidity (NHS England 2015).

Additionally, the therapies used in hospitals are often invasive and any breach in a patient's anatomical barriers to infection will increase their vulnerability to opportunistic infection (NICE 2016). Widespread use of antibiotics has resulted in many strains of micro-organisms developing resistance to antibiotic therapy and thus are becoming immune from the mainstay of treatment for infection (Sepsis Alliance 2017); consequently, the infection can become much more difficult to contain and suppress.

Sepsis also places a huge financial strain on the healthcare budget. The estimated cost of sepsis each year, including direct and indirect costs, in the United Kingdom is £7.76 billion, a sum that is likely to be a significant underestimation, given that sepsis is still under-reported (York Health Economics Consortium 2017). Much of the high expenditure results from this patient group requiring very intensive nursing care; the nurse-to-patient ratio for very dependent patient groups is high; often one to one (Intensive Care Society 2013). Sepsis is the leading cause for a need for intensive care.

The Surviving Sepsis Campaign

Appreciating the vast scale of sepsis worldwide, as well as the unacceptably high mortalities involved, an initiative to form the 'Surviving Sepsis Campaign', endorsed by many of the major critical care societies in North America and Europe, was put into effect in 2002. The initial mandate of the Campaign was to reduce mortality (Surviving Sepsis 2017). The means by which this is to be accomplished is through a seven-point strategy:

- Building awareness of sepsis: increasing the awareness of healthcare workers and government agencies that fund healthcare as well as the general public of the dangers of sepsis
- Improving diagnosis: improving early and accurate diagnosis of sepsis, partly by providing a consensus definition of sepsis that is relevant worldwide.
- Increasing the use of appropriate treatment: disseminating a range of treatment options and urging their timely intervention. Since 2004 there have been internationally accepted guidelines for the bedside management of sepsis (Dellinger *et al.* 2004).

These guidelines are periodically updated, with the most recent being in 2017 (Rhodes *et al.* 2017) and include the early stages of sepsis which nurses will be managing on the wards.

- Educating healthcare professionals: providing support and information to all professionals who manage patients with sepsis, including interventions and standards of care.
- Improving post-ICU (intensive care unit) care: providing a framework for improving and accelerating access to post-ITU care and counselling for patients who have had sepsis.
- Developing guidelines of care: recognize the need for clear referral guidelines adopted by all countries through the development of global guidelines.
- Implementing a performance improvement program

All of these points are relevant for nurses, and they are all addressed in this chapter.

New international guidelines have been published for the management of sepsis and septic shock (Rhodes *et al.* 2017). Within these new guidelines is the proposal that sepsis be identified or suspected through the use of a bedside assessment tool called 'qSOFA' or 'quick SOFA': SOFA standing for 'Sequential (Sepsis-Related) Organ Failure Assessment'. The qSOFA score is intended to be an easy to implement tool to identify patients rapidly who are more likely to have poor outcomes typical of sepsis if they have at least two of the relevant clinical criteria, which are a systolic blood pressure of less than 100 mmHg, a Glasgow Coma Score (GCS) of less than 15/15, and a respiratory rate of more than 22 breaths per minute (Singer *et al.* 2016)

However—and of particular note to nurses practising in the United Kingdom—the qSOFA score has not been recommended by the National Institute for Health and Care Excellence (NICE), the UK Sepsis Trust, or the Royal College of Emergency Medicine to become the primary bedside test for sepsis in the United Kingdom (Nutbeam *et al.* 2016). One key reason for this is that it would require the introduction of an additional scoring system for patients who are likely to have already been identified as being at risk of sepsis using track-and-trigger systems already in use such as the National Early Warning Score (NEWS2). qSOFA has not been shown to be superior to NEWS in identifying patients with infection at risk of deterioration (Nutbeam *et al.* 2016).

This point has been highlighted because although qSOFA and SOFA scoring will appear in any of the up-to-date literature you read regarding sepsis, they may well not be used in your Trust.

For your information, the more comprehensive SOFA assessment tool, which requires some invasive tests and laboratory results, is demonstrated in Table 8.1.

Sepsis and septic shock

Because sepsis can manifest in varying degrees of severity leading, in the worst instances, to a state of shock and collapse of multiple organ systems, there are terms to define the progression of the illness that aim to define the scale of the damage that sepsis is causing to the patient. The terms used are sepsis and septic shock which we will consider; they are terms which have recently been reviewed in regard to their assessment criteria and their definitions (Seymour *et al.* 2016; Shankar-Hari *et al.* 2016) (see Table 8.2).

Table 8.1 Sequential Organ Failure Assessment (SOFA) Score

System		Score				
		0	1	2	3	4
Respiratory	Pa/FiO_2 mHg (kPa)	≥ 400 (53.3)	< 400 (53.3)	< 300 (40)	< 200 (26.7) with respiratory support	< 100 (13.3) with respiratory support
Coagulation	Platelets, $\times 10^3/\mu L$	≥ 150	≥ 150	< 100	< 50	< 2 0
Liver	Bilirubin, mg/dL	< 1.2 (20)	1.2–1.9 (20–32)	2.0–5.9 (33–101)	6.0–11.9 (102–204))	> 12.0 (204)
Cardiovascular	MAP	MAP ≥ 70 mm Hg	MAP < 70 mm Hg	Dopamine* < 5 *or* Dobutamine* (any dose)	Dopamine*5.1–15 or epinephrine* ≤ 0.1 *or* norepinephrine* ≤ 0.1	Dopamine* > 15 *or* Epinephrine* > 0.1 *or* norepinephrine* > 0.1
Central nervous system	Glasgow Coma Scale	15	13–14	10–12	6–9	< 6
Renal	Creatinine, mg/dL (μmol/L)	< 1.2 (110)	1.2–1.9 (110–170)	2.0–3.4 (171–299)	3.5–4.9 (300–440)	> 5.0 (440)
	Urine output, mL/day				<5 00	<2 00

Adapted by permission from Springer Nature: *Intensive Care Medicine*, Vincent J-L., Moreno R., and Takala J. The SOFA (Sepsis.related Organ Failure Assessment) score to describe organ dysfunction/failure. 22:707–710. Copyright © 1996, SCCM and ESICM.

Abbreviations:

FiO_2, fraction of inspired oxygen; MAP, mean arterial pressure; PaO_2. partial pressure of oxygen.
* = Vasopressor doses are given as μg/kg/min for at least 1 hour. Vasopressor drugs constrict the arterial vessels to help maintain blood pressure.

It should be noted that neither the qSOFA nor SOFA scores were intended to be *definitive* of sepsis. Sepsis is a broad term applied to a process that is still only partly understood. At present, there are no unequivocal clinical criteria that exclusively identify a patient with sepsis (Seymour, *et al.* 2016). For this reason, the emphasis is put very much on *suspecting* sepsis—and indeed suspecting infection—from the outset.

One of the difficulties in recognizing sepsis in its early stages is that the patient will complain of very general symptoms which might be attributable to any number of causes; the onset of the disease can be insidious (NCEPOD 2015). Also, although there are a variety of signs that the patient is developing sepsis, none of them alone are definitive of a septic patient; it is difficult to predict how poorly someone is becoming in early sepsis. Nurses need to be able to recognize that adults with any of the symptoms or signs in Table 8.3 can be at high risk of severe illness or death from sepsis.

It is easy to see how the development of sepsis might remain unsuspected in a patient with one or two of the above signs or symptoms. What is needed is an enhanced ability to *suspect* sepsis earlier and provide an escalation of support for the patient as quickly as possible.

One term that has long been used in close association with sepsis is 'SIRS', which is worth explaining, even though the most recent definitions have recommended that the term is not used

Table 8.2 Definition of key terms

Sepsis	Life-threatening organ dysfunction caused by a dysregulated host response to infection. (Rhodes, *et al.* 2017:1).
Septic shock	Septic shock is defined as a subset of sepsis in which underlying circulatory, cellular, and metabolic abnormalities are associated with a greater risk of mortality than sepsis alone. Adult patients with septic shock can be identified using the clinical criteria of hypotension requiring vasopressor therapy to maintain mean BP 65 mmHg or greater and having a serum lactate level greater than 2 mmol/L after adequate fluid resuscitation *. (Shankar-Hari, *et al.* 2016: 775)

*Lactate is considered later in the chapter.

Table 8.3 Signs and symptoms of early sepsis

Breathing	High respiratory rate, in excess of 25 per minute, possibly with shortness of breath. Purulent sputum if associated with a chest infection
Oxygen requirements	New need for 40% oxygen or more to maintain oxygen saturation more than 92% (or more than 88% in known chronic obstructive pulmonary disease)
Heart rate	Tachycardia of 130 or more beats per minute
Blood pressure	Systolic blood pressure of 90 mmHg or less, or systolic blood pressure more than 40 mmHg below normal.
Urine output	Low urine output (oliguria): not passed urine in previous 18 hours (or, for catheterized patients, passed less than 0.5 ml/kg/hour). May be painful to pass urine or the urine is foul smelling if associated with a urinary tract infection.
Central nervous system symptoms	Objective evidence of new altered mental state—a change in GCS. Headache if associated with CNS infection (e.g. meningitis)
Skin signs	Warm to touch and/or possible non-blanching skin rash
Abdominal symptoms	Pain if associated with abdominal infections or surgery.
Temperature	High—can be with rigours: this is especially associated with early sepsis but not always found *OR* can be Low—especially in very young or elderly *OR* those patients who are immunosuppressed
General weakness	'Fluey' symptoms.
White cell count	Can be raised *OR* can be abnormally low
Microbiology report	Positive to bacteria or other organisms in biological fluids: blood, urine, sputum CSF, etc.

in relation to sepsis anymore as it does not necessarily indicate a dysregulated immune response (Singer et al. 2016). When a patient exhibits the systemic signs and symptoms of infection, but does not have a documented infection, the term 'Systemic Inflammatory Response Syndrome' (SIRS) is used. This could be caused by any event provoking inflammation in multiple sites throughout the body simultaneously, examples being burns, pancreatitis, or multiple trauma (Balk 2014). These patients can exhibit broadly similar clinical signs to sepsis but the response would not necessarily be a dysregulated one: what defines sepsis is organ failure (Singer et *al.* 2016).

One further, pre-emptive way of suspecting sepsis is to consider which patients might be at an increased risk of developing sepsis. When, for example, a change in temperature or an unexplained tachycardia is noted in such patients, it is imperative to monitor them closely and alert the shift leader or outreach team about their condition quickly. Patients that are at a high risk of developing sepsis are:

- the very young (under 1 year) and older people (over 75 years) or people who are very frail
- people who have impaired immune systems because of illness or drugs, including:
    - people being treated for cancer with chemotherapy
    - people who have impaired immune function (e.g. people with diabetes, people who have liver failure or who have had a splenectomy, or people with sickle cell disease)
    - people taking long-term steroids
    - people taking immunosuppressant drugs to treat non-malignant disorders such as rheumatoid arthritis or people who are already on antibiotics
    - people who have had surgery, or other invasive procedures, in the past six weeks
    - people with any breach of skin integrity (e.g. cuts, burns, blisters, or skin infections)
    - people who misuse drugs intravenously
    - people with indwelling lines or catheters
- women who are pregnant, have given birth or had a termination of pregnancy or miscarriage in the past six weeks
- people with complex comorbidities

Reproduced from National Institute for Health and Clinical Excellence (2016) Sepsis: recognition, diagnosis and early management. NICE. London. Available from https://www.nice.org.uk/guidance/ng51. NICE guidance is prepared for the National Health Service in England. All NICE guidance is subject to regular review and may be updated or withdrawn. NICE accepts no responsibility for the use of its content in this product/publication.

The first two groups are those with weak (or immature) immune systems and the next groups are those who have been made vulnerable or susceptible to invasion from micro-organisms. It is helpful to bear these two points in mind when caring for patients that cause concern in terms of changes in their routine observations or who begin to complain of feeling generally unwell.

In order to appreciate why a 'systemic' or 'global' response to infection is so problematical, it is important to review what the body's normal or expected response would be.

The immune system: Layers of defence

For an infective agent, be it a bacteria, fungus, or virus, to establish itself within our tissues—or 'colonize' them—it must initially bypass the body's many surface barriers. An infection occurs once our immune system cannot defend against colonizing micro-organisms and they begin to damage tissue (Chapel 2014). The surface barriers constitute the first in a series of defences against the outside world. An intact skin surface with a slightly acid pH provides an effective obstacle as there is no easy way through the skin and the pH is unsuitable for many organisms to inhabit. As the skin is keratinised and thus waterproofed, water-soluble organisms are kept at bay. A number of organisms do manage to colonize the skin surfaces but because the epidermal layers are constantly shedding, the colonies of micro-organisms are shed, too.

Generally, good personal hygiene means that the areas that are most likely to become colonized, such as the mouth, perineum, and hands, are kept clean and don't allow colonization to develop. The body cavities that are exposed to the outside world such as the respiratory, digestive, and uro-genitary tracts secrete enzyme-laden fluids which are either directly antimicrobial or are lined with mucous that obstruct the pathogen from attaching to and colonizing those areas (Hall *et al.* 2016). The gastrointestinal tract uses extreme changes in pH to kill foreign bodies. As long as these first lines of defence stay undamaged and intact, patients are protected from most invading organisms. Later in the chapter, the frequently encountered breaks to the integrity of these surface barriers found in ward patients and the significance of these breaks in relation to sepsis will be considered.

However, once a foreign body does penetrate these defences, there are two further levels of protection: the innate responses and the acquired or adaptive reactions (Rote *et al.* 2014a). The innate system, although including the surface barriers, also consists of cellular and molecular components as well as the inflammatory response. Cells that employ phagocytosis—that is, they ingest other cells—circulate in the blood, lymph, and interstitial fluids as well as inhabit tissues: macrophages and neutrophils, for example. They engulf particles that are recognized as foreign and destroy them with powerful enzymes.

Macrophages are cells that can also release powerful inflammatory mediators which are responsible for much of the classical inflammatory reaction: localized production of heat, redness, swelling, and pain. The inflammatory response is central to and definitive of the second line of defence, and it is the inflammatory response—when it becomes widespread rather than locally contained—that causes many of the problems encountered in sepsis. This is examined in the next section.

The molecular element of the innate immune system is the collection of 'chemical messengers' that control the inflammatory and clotting responses and help contain them in the area that is affected. One of the key points here is that the inflammatory reaction is carefully controlled and manifests only in a limited area. These reactions occur in relation to *any* invading organism or breach in the first line of defence. They all form part of what is termed non-specific immunity; that is, they respond in the same way to any provoking agent and are not specific to that one agent only.

The third line of defence is the adaptive immune system, the behaviour of antigen-specific B- and T-cells which bind to antigen. Antigen is what the immune system interacts with and which helps it to recognize self- and non-self molecules (Male *et al.* 2013). B-cells secrete immunoglobulins; antibodies which are antigen-specific and which kill that particular antigen. T-cells assist B-cells in making these antibodies (*Hall et al.* 2016). A key point here is that these defences are *specific* to individually identified molecules and are thus called our specific immunity.

The inflammatory response and sepsis

It is the second line of our immune system—and in particular the inflammatory reaction—that is responsible for the exaggerated physiological response and the complications that we see in sepsis. Inflammation is a rapid and coordinated reply to cellular injury (Male 2014), characterized by the classic findings of redness, heat, swelling, and pain as well as loss of function. Blood tests will reveal an increased concentration of leucocytes—white blood cells (Blann 2013). Because much of the problem with sepsis is caused by inflammatory changes, this process is reviewed in-depth below.

When tissue is damaged or becomes contaminated with invading organisms, cells that are scouting for foreign bodies—mast cells and macrophages—are activated. Mast cells located in the interstitium around the affected area will 'degranulate'—that is, release a number of chemical messengers—into the bloodstream. These chemicals will attract white blood cells—primarily neutrophils which are the most abundant white cell type—to the area to help fight the infection. They will also cause vasodilation, widening of the blood vessel, to increase blood flow to that localized area, increasing the supply of the oxygen, white cells, and nutrients needed to combat the infection. Additionally, the permeability the cells making up the lining of the capillary wall, the endothelium, is impacted upon, allowing plasma fluid and some white cells to migrate from within the capillaries to the area that has been injured or infected.

Macrophages will be also be amongst the first components of the innate response to encounter the invading organism. They will release numerous cellular messengers, collectively called cytokines, to alert other parts of the immune system of the invasion and they too, attract neutrophils to the site of infection. Cytokines will also instruct bone marrow cells to produce more neutrophils (Helbert 2017); they are sometimes referred to as the hormones of the immune system. Not all of the messengers involved are cytokines so the term inflammatory mediators can be used to address all of the different 'families' of chemicals released during inflammation.

The role of the endothelium

The inflammatory response is carefully orchestrated and something that plays a remarkable part in the coordination of events is the endothelium itself. As a single layer of cells, the capillary endothelium acts as a semi-permeable barrier between the bloodstream and the interstitium, the environment around the cells themselves (Aaronson 2013). Nevertheless, the endothelium is an extremely dynamic membrane.

- It controls exchange of proteins, hormones, minerals, and immunoglobins between the blood and the tissues.
- It secretes numerous substances that help control the degree of contraction of the muscle wall in the blood vessels, affecting blood flow and pressure
- It secretes substances to encourage and also inhibit clotting processes and ensures that clotting is contained locally.

- It responds to the mediators that are released in inflammation by becoming more permeable or 'leaky' (Pappano and Wier 2013).

It is not so important to remember the names of the various substances which are involved in the behaviour of the endothelial cells, but it is necessary to appreciate that once the endothelium is subject to widespread damage, as happens with sepsis, that all of the above controls are lost.

The role that the permeability of the endothelium plays in the normal inflammatory reaction is absolutely central (Levick 2010). For example, when neutrophils arrive at the site of inflammation, they will need to be allowed passage through the blood vessel wall to the affected tissue. The neutrophils are normally too large to squeeze through the tiny junctions between the individual cells of the capillary wall. This particular process, called diapedisis, is managed by cytokine influence on the integrity of the endothelium (Male 2014), making the endothelium 'porous' enough for the neutrophils to migrate out of the vascular space. Here the white cells can begin the process of ingesting and destroying foreign particles; it is the concentration of white cells and bacterial debris that is largely responsible for the colour of pus (Rote *et al.* 2014). This increase in permeability results in the collection of white cells found in inflamed tissue and also for the exudate of plasma fluid that results in inflammatory swelling.

This rather complex sounding series of events can be simplified through a flow chart representation shown in Figure 8.1.

The cardinal signs of inflammation are:

- redness (erythema): caused by vasodilation and the increased blood flow to the affected area.
- heat: also caused by vasodilation and increased blood flow as well as the increased metabolic activity at the area.
- swelling: caused by the collection of plasma exudate.

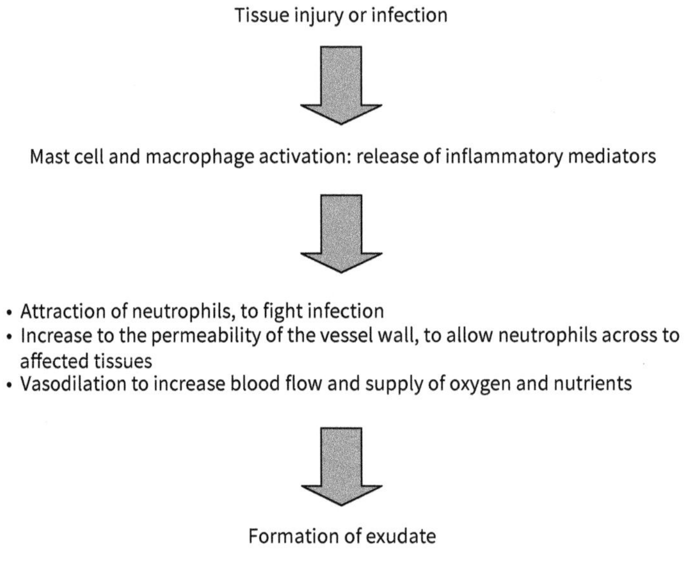

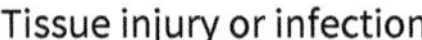

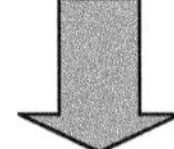

Mast cell and macrophage activation: release of inflammatory mediators

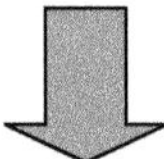

- Attraction of neutrophils, to fight infection
- Increase to the permeability of the vessel wall, to allow neutrophils across to affected tissues
- Vasodilation to increase blood flow and supply of oxygen and nutrients

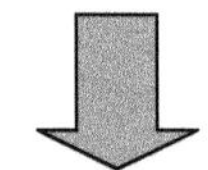

Formation of exudate

Figure 8.1 Inflammatory reaction.

- pain: caused by some inflammatory mediators (noticeably one called bradykinin).
- loss of function: caused by the localized swelling and the effects of pain.
- leucocytosis (concentration of white cells): facilitated by the permeability of the endothelium.

These inflammatory processes are controlled in what is called a positive feedback loop. In the presence of an alien organism, an increase in macrophage activity and cytokine populations signal the need for a further increase of macrophage activity and release of even more cytokines which, in turn, results in an even further increase, and so on. These processes, by virtue of being influenced by positive feedback, are very powerful and fast acting; they need to be in order to respond to infection and contain it locally (Rote and McCance 2014). When the infection becomes spread throughout the body, as happens with sepsis, these same powerful responses are activated *everywhere* which results in a massive overreaction and the body's response becomes uncontrolled and dysfunctional. The term 'Systemic Inflammatory Response Syndrome' is easier to appreciate in this light. The overwhelming inflammatory response acting globally on the epithelium actually damages it; it is not particularly the infection that is causing the damage but the patient's response to it, their own inflammatory processes. Sometimes sepsis is therefore termed a type of hypersensitivity reaction (type V hypersensitivity) (Murphy and Weaver 2017). The widespread leakiness across the endothelium throughout the body results in significant losses of circulating plasma volume, causing hypovolaemia and hypotension, and also in widespread oedema. These are frequent findings in sepsis.

The increased presence of neutrophils (their production in the bone marrow having been stimulated by cytokines) contributes to a rise in the total number of white cells in the blood generally and this becomes a marker for infection. Generally, the white cell count (WCC) is between 3.7 and 9.5×10^9/L (Blann 2013). When the WCC rises above these limits it is indicative of an infective process.

The flooding of inflammatory mediators into the bloodstream typifies the 'acute-phase response' to infection in which core temperature is increased and certain proteins in the plasma become activated (Helbert 2017). These are key findings in most patients who have sepsis; the development of a temperature is an especially important one to be vigilant about. The increase in temperature—pyrexia—is caused by the hypothalamus' reaction to the presence of specific cytokines. The autonomic nervous system (ANS) then 'resets' the body's core temperature in an attempt to make the body's internal environment hostile to the replication of invading organisms. The acute-phase proteins will be monitored by the medical team in patients suspected of having a systemic infection; the most commonly measured of these proteins is called C-reactive protein (CRP).

One further blood test may be the erythrocyte sedimentation rate (ESR). This test is also suggestive of infection if the value is prolonged. The ESR indicates that cells are taking longer to 'settle' or 'sediment' in a sample of blood than expected. This, in turn, indicates that the blood has become more viscous or sticky. The viscosity is the result of an increased presence of released cytokines and activated plasma proteins secondary to infection. CRP is a more sensitive test for infection and inflammatory processes than ESR and more likely to be done (Higgins 2013).

The infective agents that are associated with sepsis can be bacteria, viruses, fungi, and some parasites. Predominantly, it is bacteria that are the causative agents and particularly the 'Gram-negative' bacteria. Gram-negative simply describes the fact that these bacteria don't retain a stain—called the 'Gram stain'—which is applied in the laboratory to differentiate bacteria. Gram-negative bacteria contain molecules called 'endotoxins' which are responsible for much of the cardiovascular dysfunction seen in septic patients. Endotoxins are a component of the Gram-negative bacterial cell wall and directly injure the endothelial lining of capillary vessels; endotoxin will cause vasodilatation, inappropriately activate the coagulation cascade, and depress the myocardium (Cilliers *et al.* 2009). Gram-positive bacteria can also result in similar compromises.

One group of patients that require particular vigilance in terms of the development of sepsis and shock are neutropenic patients (Dunkley and McLeod 2015). Neutropenic patients are unable to mount a normal response to infection because their white cell population is very low. By definition the WCC will be less than 4×10^9/L (Gargani 2012), but it can be much lower even than this. Neutropenia may be congenital or, more likely, acquired due to infections, autoimmune disorders, or due to chemotherapeutic regimens in cancer treatment, for example (Barrett and Dikken 2010). Neutrophils have a very short life span and the stem cells that produce them in bone marrow must divide very rapidly to maintain circulating levels in the bloodstream (Coico and Sunshine 2015); for this reason, chemotherapy agents that target rapidly reproducing cells (such as tumour cells) will affect neutrophils levels too.

Neutrophils help contain infection and without them infection can spread unhindered and become systemic quickly (Nairn and Helbert 2017). An infection in the lungs, for example, will not result in localized symptoms and pus formation but can spread rapidly into the blood. The macrophage activity is still intact, however, so cytokine release will still produce a temperature and shivering responses. Sometimes this is the only warning sign in neutropenic patients that an infection is present and in these patients sepsis may develop quickly. It may be that patients simply report feeling generally poorly, which is not uncommon in chemo- or radiation therapy patients. If a temperature rise is noted in a neutropenic patient, intravenous antibiotics are indicated and should be given immediately (NICE 2012), within one hour of the pyrexia being noted, in order to combat the bacteria and the effects of its endotoxin. If a tachycardia and hypotension are noted in the patient, it signifies that sepsis and shock are already developing and these patients need an urgent medical review.

Review point 1

- Sepsis is the result of a dysregulated immune response to an infection.
- Sepsis can lead to shock states with a very high mortality.
- The inflammatory response is influenced and moderated by the endothelium. When the endothelium is damaged in a widespread fashion, this moderation is lost and inflammation becomes inappropriate.
- Neutropenic patients cannot mount a normal white cell response. These patients may only show a temperature or complain of feeling vaguely unwell. Time is of the essence in these patients, particularly in terms of having a medical review and intravenous antibiotics being administered.

- The prevalence of sepsis is very high but this is underestimated by healthcare professionals. The Surviving Sepsis Campaign aims to raise awareness of sepsis and provides treatment guidelines.

Clinical link 8.1

- Septic shock is sometimes referred to as 'distributive' shock. Why do you think this is?
- The hypovolaemia found in sepsis is sometimes referred to as 'relative' hypovolaemia. Why do you think this is?

Pathophysiology: The cardiovascular system

Sepsis will affect every system in the body to some degree, partly because the infective agent is blood-borne and thus can spread everywhere, but also because the effects upon the cardiovascular system, responsible for blood pressure and oxygen delivery to all cells, is so profoundly and immediately affected. The cardiovascular manifestations of sepsis are essentially vasodilatation, the resultant maldistribution of blood flow, and myocardial depression (Guarracino *et al.* 2016) The main cardiovascular response to sepsis is widespread vasodilation: the relaxing of the smooth muscle wall inside the blood vessels which leads to looser, wider blood vessels. This global vasodilation is caused in part by the release of a substance called nitric oxide which the endothelial cells release in response either to changes in blood flow or in response to cytokines (Levick 2010).

The main consequence of such widespread vasodilatation is that of hypotension, inadequate blood pressure to supply the tissues and cells with nutrients and, in particular, oxygen. Hypotension, if it is left unnoticed and untreated, will affect every body system simply because they all rely upon the cardiovascular system to deliver oxygen and remove waste products. The worst case scenario in terms of hypotension is shock. Shock can be defined as circulatory insufficiency (Levick 2010): the cardiovascular system cannot meet the metabolic demands of the cells and the cells begin to dysfunction. This leads, if unsuccessfully treated, to multiple organ failure, because all cells are affected, and ultimately to death.

In order to appreciate exactly why hypotension occurs in these patients it is helpful to quickly review how blood pressure is maintained in health (see also Chapter 3). The cardiac cycle is the sequence of events that the heart undergoes throughout one heart beat (McCance 2014). The heart pumps blood through the pulmonary and systemic vasculature by generating enough pressure to propel the blood that has drained into the ventricles—the 'stroke volume'—forward. This is called the systolic pressure and is produced by forceful contraction. The heart then relaxes and allows the next stroke volume to drain into the ventricles; this stage of the cycle is termed diastole. Clearly, the previous stroke volume will stop its forward movement as the propelling force from the heart comes to rest, as in diastole. There must be some other influences that support both the forward movement of blood and also maintenance of the pressure that the blood is under in order for it to reach the tissues far from the heart and at a pressure high enough to perfuse those tissues. These other influences are the behaviour of the blood vessels; there are cardiac and vascular components to blood pressure, hence the term 'cardiovascular'.

When the arterial vessels receive the stroke volume under high systolic pressure, they distend in order to accommodate the bolus of blood. They are able to do this because of the elastic nature of their walls; they have a layer of smooth muscle and elastic tissue, called the 'tunica media', which provides the ability to stretch. Whilst the heart stops contracting, the vessel wall can recoil from their stretched position, further squeezing the blood onward, and this provides some continuity of forward propulsion for the blood. The most important factor, however, in preserving the blood pressure throughout the cardiac cycle is the tension that the blood vessel wall is kept under. This accounts for the pressure of blood in the vessels during the period that the heart is resting and filling: the diastolic pressure. This is the pressure that the heart has to overcome in order to provide the next stroke volume and is termed the 'systemic vascular resistance' (SVR) (Pappano and Wier 2013). SVR is maintained by a number of factors, though primarily through the sympathetic nervous system (SNS). The SNS innervates the smooth muscle wall of the vessels and sustains a level of contraction, or muscular tone, to ensure that the lumen, or internal diameter of the vessel, is within a range of functional limits. The timing of the cardiac cycle is approximately two-thirds diastole and only one-third systole, and thus the vessel wall tone contribution to maintaining blood pressure is very significant.

With a wider lumen in the blood vessels, it is increasingly harder for the heart to maintain the blood pressure at its normal value. An analogy here would be of a hose pipe with a narrow lumen—perhaps because a thumb has been partly placed over the opening—providing a good pressure of water. Compare that with the pressure of water from the hose when the thumb is removed; the pressure drops because the lumen is wider. When the blood vessel lumen widens, the diastolic component or SVR is reduced. In response to the decreased SVR, the heart rate increases to compensate for this loss in diastolic pressure, and tachycardia is a classic finding in patients in early stages of sepsis. The bounding, fast heartbeat is indicative of the cardiovascular system adjusting for vasodilation and the patient is said to be in a 'hyperdynamic' state. At this stage of sepsis the patient has a high cardiac output but only a normal or adequate blood pressure. This hyperdynamism can only be maintained for a limited amount of time. After further vasodilation, the ability to compensate with a tachycardia alone becomes exhausted and the blood pressure becomes 'de-compensated' and falls to inadequate levels. At this point the pulse will feel 'thready' or weak. This is when shock is likely to develop very quickly. One of the reasons that patients with sepsis will be moved to a critical care unit is that their blood pressure and cardiac output can be monitored very closely and supported with powerful drugs, such as vasopressors, which are considered in Chapter 3.

Vasodilatation is also responsible for, or contributes to, some of the other frequently encountered assessment findings in the patient with sepsis. These include the heat of their skin—surface temperature, their flushed appearance, and widespread peripheral oedema—although this is most markedly noticeable in patients in the latter stages of sepsis; hopefully these patients have already been relocated to the high-dependency unit (HDU) or ITU by this point. The flushed appearance and, in part, increased skin temperature are due to the inappropriate dilation of peripheral vessels close to the skin, bringing an increased flow of blood close to the skin surface. Physiologically, the formation of oedema is more complex.

Oedema formation

In health, a constant balance of the 'escape' and return of plasma from the intravascular space into the interstitial space and back to the intravascular space is maintained. Fresh plasma fluid bathes the cells and so helps to deliver dissolved oxygen, electrolytes, and nutrients directly to respiring cells. The homeostatic mechanisms that regulate this circulation prevent any build-up of fluid in the interstitium which would interrupt the supply, for example, of fresh oxygen and the removal of waste gas. Because oedema can be global and very exaggerated in septic patients and because it can cause a number of secondary complications requiring nursing care, it is helpful to review how oedema occurs in sepsis.

Typically, blood arrives at the capillary beds from arterioles at a perfusing pressure of approximately 32 mmHg. This perfusing pressure is enough to push a small yet constant volume of the plasma, complete with all of its dissolved contents, through the microscopic junctions that exist between the single cell layer of the capillary vessels. The volume able to leave the vascular space is regulated by the perfusing pressure and the size of the cell junctions and the integrity of the vessel wall; there are only a certain number of tiny outlets for the fluid. It is also regulated by a force exerted by molecules in the capillary blood called colloid molecules; these are large molecules that are too big to squeeze through the cell junctions—red and white blood cells and proteins, for example—and create what is known as colloid or oncotic pressure. Oncotic pressure, approximately 20 mmHg in the capillaries, serves to retain most of the plasma fluid in the vascular space; it exercises a holding force on the fluid which can only escape its influence if the perfusing pressure is greater. At the arteriolar end of the capillary bed, the perfusing pressure (32 mmHg) *is* greater and plasma leaves the vascular space and becomes part of the interstitial fluid.

Once the fresh plasma has bathed the cells it will be depleted of fresh oxygen and nutrients, etc., and also will have picked up the waste products of the cells' metabolism—noticeably, carbon dioxide gas. This exchange will be due to concentration gradients of the various substances between the cell and the interstitial fluid. Unless the interstitial fluid is able to 'drain' itself back into the vascular space, there will be an accumulation of waste products and an interruption of the concentration gradients. This drainage happens because of the constant oncotic pressure in the capillary vessels provided by the presence of the large molecules: in a healthy, intact capillary vessel the large colloid molecules cannot escape through the vessel wall and this guarantees a consistent oncotic pressure along the length of the vessel. The perfusing pressure however, decreases along the length of the capillary from the arterioles (32 mmHg) to venules (12 mmHg) (Figure 8.2).

Note now that the colloid pressure (20 mmHg) exceeds the perfusing pressure at the venous end (12 mmHg). At this point the interstitial fluid can be drawn back into the vascular space, through the same epithelial wall junctions, because the 'pulling' colloid influence of all of the large molecules now exerts a stronger influence than the 'pushing' perfusing pressure. In this way there is a constant flow of fluid into and out of the interstitium. Any residual fluid that might collect in the interstitium is collected by lymphatic vessels and then drained back into the bloodstream.

Sepsis disrupts this mechanism predominantly through compromising the integrity of the vessel walls. Endotoxin injures the endothelium directly and excessive cytokine activity causes the capillary junctions to become inappropriately permeable: sepsis has 'over-induced' the inflammatory response, causing it to 'overreact' (Figure 8.3).

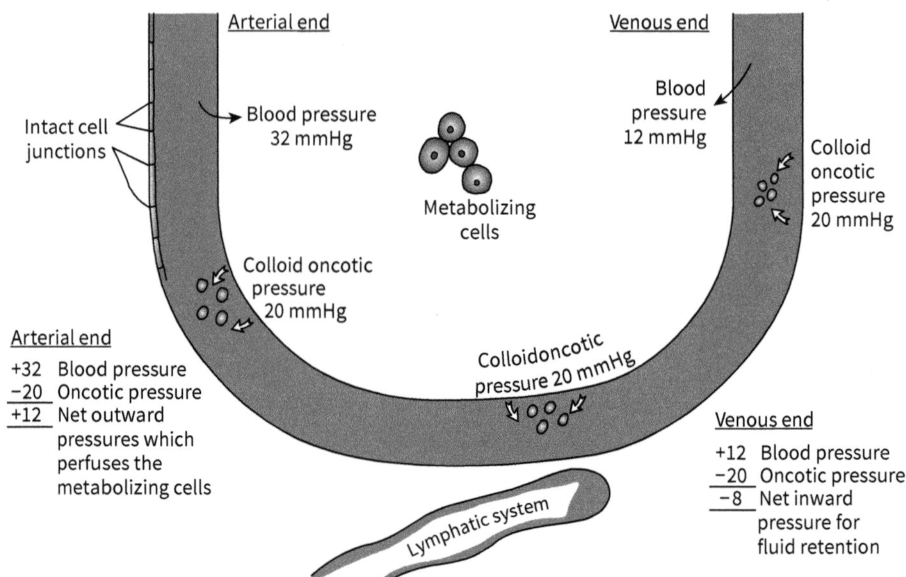

Figure 8.2 Normal tissue perfusion and drainage.

The combined effect is to let not only far too much fluid into the interstitium but also to allow some of the colloid molecules, especially the smaller proteins, to enter the interstitial space and thus ruin the oncotic pressure balance responsible for draining fluid back into the circulation. Too much fluid in to the interstitium and not enough back out results in the oedema that develops in more advanced cases of sepsis and also in the patients who have returned from ITU settings after having survived sepsis. Oedema can be

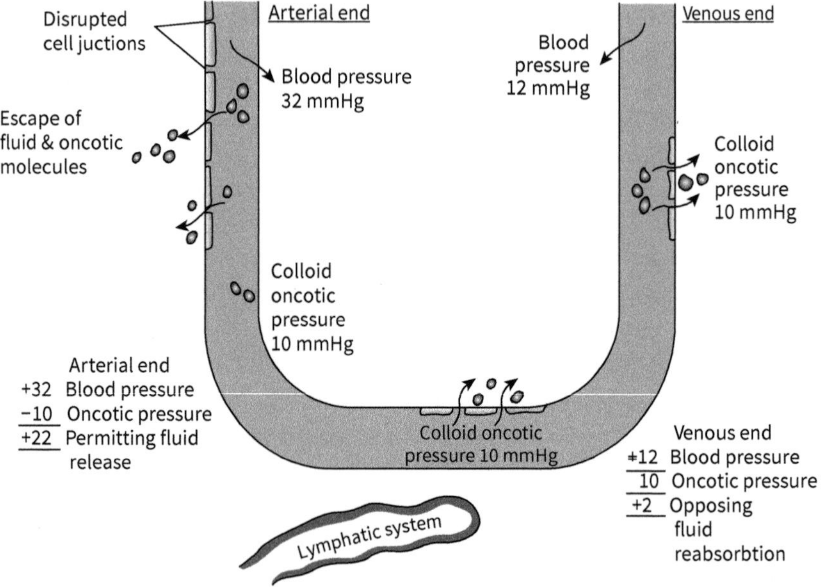

Figure 8.3 Formation of oedema.

incapacitating for patients because it may lead to blisters and rashes and cause restrictive, swollen joints and swelling of, or effusions around, vital organs (Levick 2010). The oedema experienced by patients who have had sepsis will have been profound and, as well as its debilitating physical effects on the patient themselves, it may have had a disturbing effect on relatives as the swelling of the soft facial tissue such as eyelids and lips can render people unrecognizable.

Secondary to hypotension and poor perfusion will be hypoxia of the tissues. When cells are in an 'oxygen-poor' environment, they begin to respire anaerobically, a byproduct of which is lactate. Lactate is acidic and when it builds up in the tissues it has a toxic effect on cells. Lactate levels in health are low—normal values being 0.5–2 mmol/L (Higgins 2013) and raised levels signify that tissues are being under-perfused, hence lactate has become a frequently monitored blood value at the bedside. Other clinical signs of poor perfusion are acutely diminished mental status, a slow capillary refill time when a nail bed is pressed, cool and/or pale skin (Vaughan and Parry 2016).

Another of the key features of cardiovascular compromise in sepsis is the effect upon the body's clotting mechanisms. In sepsis the epithelium has a prominent role in the derangement of clotting controls; coagulopathy (Levick 2010). Damage to the epithelium will activate the clotting cascade (Levi and Schmaier 2016); this can occur in sepsis from excessive cytokine activity or endotoxin from Gram-negative bacteria, for example. Because of the extensive nature of the injury to the endothelium in sepsis, the clotting cascade will be activated in numerous sites resulting in microthrombi which occlude vessels supplying vital organs and tissue beds. Because the clotting processes are widespread rather than locally contained and because the thrombus is formed inside blood vessels, the condition is termed disseminated intravascular coagulopathy (DIC) and is seen in up to 35% of cases of sepsis and septic shock (Okamoto *et al.* 2016). The indiscriminate nature of thrombus formation throughout the body results in the profound depletion of clotting factors and this leads, in turn, to uncontrolled bleeding or 'oozing' of blood from any puncture sites such as intravenous access or the patient's gums or invisibly as internal bleeds from ulceration points, for instance. When the occlusion of vessels is combined with poor perfusing pressure due to vasodilation and loss of circulating fluid due to oedema formation, the effects are catastrophic and patients develop refractory shock; that is, shock which is unresponsive to fluid resuscitation and the powerful drugs that constrict blood vessels to support the blood pressure. This combination of pathologies contributes to the organ failure that results in such high mortality for sepsis.

The last of the three main cardiovascular compromises is myocardial depression which is commonly met in sepsis (Lu and Wang 2016). This is caused directly by some inflammatory mediators; in fact, one is named myocardial depressant factor. The result upon the heart is a reduced contractility so that even when fluid is given to resuscitate the blood pressure, the heart fails to respond adequately (Kakihana *et al.* 2016). This reduced contractility affects the ability to generate sufficient systolic pressure. This is dangerous for the septic patient as they also have a loss of circulating volume in the form of oedema and a reduced diastolic pressure due to vasodilation. All three situations together wreak havoc with the body's ability to supply enough oxygen to cells, this is why shock states develop so frequently in sepsis and why mortality is so high. The important point is to suspect its development and act quickly with the other multidisciplinary team (MDT) members to support the patient early, and this is how septic patients are most likely to survive.

Review point 2

- Global endothelial dysfunction results in profound cardiovascular compromise which, in turn, will affect all body systems.
- Sepsis causes vasodilation due to endothelial damage and massive inflammatory mediator release, resulting in hypotension from compromise of the diastolic function.
- At a time when increased oxygen delivery is needed, the myocardium becomes 'depressed' resulting in hypotension from compromise of the systolic function.
- Widespread oedema, caused by global endothelial permeability changes, is a common finding in sepsis which effectively renders the patient hypotensive.
- Sepsis, through damaging the endothelium, can initiate the clotting cascade globally. This can result in multiple microthrombi that occlude vessels, resulting in poor perfusion of vital organs which can lead to organ failure.
- Lactate is an indicator of tissue hypoxia and shock.

Sepsis thus affects the cardiovascular system in a profound way, but all systems are affected. The respiratory system is a major indicator of physiological changes in sepsis. The increased metabolic demand for oxygen and increase in production of carbon dioxide, will result in a higher respiratory rate (tachypnoea). Tachypnoea is viewed as being a reliable marker of patient deterioration (Resuscitation Council (UK) 2017). Other signs of the patient struggling with respiratory function are use of accessory muscles which include the abdomen, shoulder girdle, and facial muscles. If the infection has come from the respiratory system, which is likely as a reported 68% of sepsis cases are from pneumonia (Royal College of Nursing 2016), there may be other signs of respiratory distress such as coughing, painful breathing, low saturation levels, or purulent sputum. Sputum samples should be sent for microbiological culture and sensitivity testing (MC&S).

The renal system relies on a perfusing pressure to filter blood plasma at the glomerulus in order to begin to form urine (Doig and Huether 2014). Without this pressure, urine production falls or ceases altogether. Urine output is a good indicator of the perfusion of the kidneys (and thus all other vital organs) and so it is important for us to have a clear indication of the patient's renal function. The minimum that a normal urine output amounts to is 0.5mL/kg, so in a person weighing 80kg, 40mL per hour is expected; anything less is termed oliguria. The complete absence of urine output, which is a serious indication of renal failure, is called anuria.

It is important to recognize if a patient is becoming oliguric before they become anuric; once organ failure is evidenced, the patient is in sepsis and beginning the decline into the awful morbidity and mortality associated with it. To this end an hourly urine output is helpful as it alerts to possibly small but consistent changes in kidney function and a catheter can facilitate these observations. However, catheters are also a frequent source of hospital-acquired infection (NICE 2015) and, thus, sepsis. Needless to say, strict asepsis is always imperative in catheter insertion (NICE 2015).

If the original infection has come from the urinary tract, the patient may complain of discomfort when passing urine and the urine itself may well be cloudy, discoloured, and foul smelling. A urine-analysis dip stick test can identify the presence of leucocytes or nitrites—both indicators of bacterial presence. Any abnormal findings from this simple and quick test need to be followed up or referred on to the senior nurses or medical team. In the case of a positive result for bacterial presence a urine sample needs to be sent for MC&S; urinary tract infections (UTI) make up 14% of infective sources for sepsis (Royal College of Nursing 2016). Other markers of renal function will be gleaned from biochemistry results such as urea and creatinine levels and are discussed in Chapter 5.

The other significant source of infection in sepsis is the gastrointestinal (GI) tract; 22% are from abdominal sources (Royal College of Nursing 2016). Abdominal pain would be an obvious cause for concern as would a distended abdomen; this may be caused by collections of gas or fluid. These collections, in turn, are due to poor perfusion of the gut causing an 'ileus' or immobile intestine, which allows fluids to collect rather than be absorbed or transported. One interesting point in relation to the GI tract is that it will allow much of its own blood supply to be diverted to the other vital organs in hypovolaemic or shock states. If the shock state is not resolved quickly, the GI tract begins to suffer the consequences of poor perfusion.

Clinical link 8.2

One way of defining different stages of sepsis is to call early sepsis 'hot' sepsis and later sepsis can be called 'cold' sepsis. Why do you think this is?

Immediate response—the 'Sepsis Six'

It is known that delayed identification and response to serious illness like sepsis results in poorer care for the patient, which will impact on their morbidity and mortality (NCEPOD 2015). It is also well known that recognition and therapeutic support given early—in the 'golden hours' of illness—provide the most benefit for patients. There are elements of evidence-based care that all patients should receive, but which are subject to variability; sometimes they are not put into effect in the same way (Williamson *et al.* 2014). To standardize care into best practice everywhere, these elements are sometimes grouped into 'care bundles', and there are two care bundles for sepsis, one for the first three hours and one for the first six hours. Both bundles have recently been refined (Surviving Sepsis Campaign 2015). Implementation of the bundles has been shown to improve survival (Levy *et al.* 2015), although in order to have their positive impact on patient care, *all* components of the bundle must be carried out.

In order to improve awareness of sepsis and the implementation of these two sepsis care bundles, the UK Sepsis Trust, a registered charity (see Resources section) has developed a number of educational resources for healthcare professionals. It has specific sections for acute hospital ward staff, recognizing that initiation of early management steps outside of designated critical care areas is an essential part of providing the best care for patients who are ill with sepsis. Some elements of the six-hour bundle do require specialist environments with specially trained staff and equipment, highlighting the need for responses to sepsis to be multidisciplinary in nature (Vaughan and Parry 2016a). Nonetheless, there are six points of care that can be initiated or requested quickly by ward nurses within the first hour of recognizing deterioration from sepsis, which have a major impact on whether the patient survives or not. These are called the 'Sepsis Six' and are outlined below as per the guidelines produced in collaboration with NICE by the UK Sepsis Trust (2016a). The Sepsis Six is one of many toolkits that are published by the Sepsis Trust; there are protocols for A&E departments and other specific areas.

1. Oxygen
   Metabolic demand for oxygen throughout the body is hugely increased by sepsis and it is essential to at least ensure the *supply* of oxygen is maximized; as discussed earlier in the chapter, delivery and uptake at cellular level may be impaired. The British Thoracic Society's Guideline for Oxygen Use in Adults in Healthcare and Emergency Settings (2017) stipulates the following:

   > In critical illness, including major trauma, sepsis, shock and anaphylaxis, initiate treatment with a reservoir mask at 15 L/min and aim at a saturation range of 94–98%. This advice also applies to patients with critical illness who have risk factors for hypercapnia pending the results of blood gas measurements and expert assessment. In patients with spontaneous circulation and a reliable oximetry reading, it may be possible to maintain a saturation of 94–98% using lower concentrations of oxygen. (The British Thoracic Society's Guideline for Oxygen Use in Adults in Healthcare and Emergency Settings, 2017:49)

   The patient will also benefit from an arterial blood gas sample being taken, so a member of the medical team will need to be involved for this. High-flow oxygen will be drying to the patient's upper respiratory tract mucosa so a humidified delivery system and frequent oral hygiene should be offered. The patient should not be left alone at this stage; reassurance is particularly important and their observations may need repeating frequently. It is also important for the mask to be kept on; if a patient is becoming hypoxic and confused they will often try and remove the mask.
2. Blood cultures
   It is imperative to identify the infecting organism and blood cultures must be taken prior to administration of antibiotics. At least two sets should be drawn: one percutaneously, from a peripheral vein, and one from each intravascular device if in for more than 24 hours. Consideration should be given to other samples, including sputum, urine, cerebrospinal fluid, and pus. Strict asepsis whilst obtaining the samples is vital (NICE 2012a). Contamination of blood results can lead to 'false positive' results suggesting infection where there is none. Typically results are ready within 48 hours and all members of the team should be involved in actively seeking the results.
3. IV antibiotics
   The early administration of broad-spectrum antibiotics is associated with significant reductions in mortality (Ferrer *et al.* 2014). Prescriptions should be reviewed once positive blood cultures are obtained to ensure that the identified organism is being targeted in as specific a fashion as possible. Most Trusts have strict protocols addressing this.
4. IV Fluids
   Patients with sepsis often require early, rapid fluid resuscitation to optimize tissue perfusion and limit subsequent shock and multi-organ dysfunction (see also Chapter 7). Fluid resuscitation is replacing some of the circulating volume that has been 'lost' because of capillary leak and oedema. Crystalloids are favoured over colloids in recent international guidelines (Rhodes *et al.* 2017) and a bolus of 500 mL is recommended and is repeatable,

although must not exceed 30 mL/Kg in total (UK Sepsis Trust, 2016a). A successful response would be indicated by a rise in blood pressure and central venous pressure, where that is being measured, and these improvements would be maintained without the need for further fluid. Patients that we must observe especially closely here are those with a history of heart failure, left ventricular failure in particular, because of the ease with which they can become fluid-overloaded and begin to develop pulmonary oedema. Elderly patients and those in renal failure must also be cautiously monitored during fluid resuscitation.

5. Serial lactate levels
   Tissue perfusion is compromised in sepsis and when cells are in a hypoxic environment they respire anaerobically resulting in lactate production. Lactate therefore provides an indication of the adequacy of tissue perfusion. Normal values are 0.5–2 mmol/L (Higgins 2013) and values above 4 mmol/L are diagnostic of shock. Lactate is important in the recognition of sepsis and is prognostic of mortality (Nutbeam *et al.* 2016), although as an isolated value is not definitive of sepsis per se (Fenwick 2016). Serial measurements may demonstrate a response or a lack of response to resuscitation. If the fluid resuscitation is raising blood pressure and improving perfusion, the cells can begin to respire aerobically once again and stop producing the lactate. Lactate can be measured using a blood gas analyser or hand-held device.
6. Measure and improve urine output
   This often requires insertion of a urinary catheter where not already in place; some patients are still able to urinate spontaneously but ideally urine output should be measured hourly to notice when it begins to fall. Urine output is a direct measure of blood flow to the kidneys and therefore an easily observable measure of cardiac output, for most people. A low cardiac output will mean poor blood supply to all organs, not just the kidneys. Early recognition of a low urine output, and taking steps to improve it, will help to reduce the likelihood of an acute kidney injury developing (NICE 2013). Fluid balance charts should be precisely maintained and certainly should be commenced for patients if they are not already on one.

A helpful, preliminary step may be to ensure that the patient has a patent intravenous access for the IV therapies mentioned above. It may be prudent to ensure two cannulae are in place so that antibiotics and fluid can run concurrently. Check if existing cannulae are patent. Check if the lumen is wide enough to run fluid in quickly, if needed. Check for signs of phlebitis at any existing cannula site and the need to change it as this can be a precursor to infection and even sepsis in itself. These checks for phlebitis can be extended to other catheters; central venous lines, for instance. A check on how long they have been *in situ* is also valuable. If a central line is in place and asymptomatic then ensuring that the ports are all patent and available for infusions, in keeping with local policy, is sensible.

The term 'Red Flag Sepsis' was introduced by the UK Sepsis Trust (2014) and a series of screening tools have been developed to support clinicians in a range of settings (UK Sepsis Trust 2016a, 2014b) to highlight the significance of some key individual physiological findings in relation to suspected sepsis. The 'red flag' indicators are:

- Systolic BP ≤ 90 mmHg
- Heart rate > 130 per minute
- Respiratory rate ≥ 25 per minute

- Oxygen saturations < 91% (it may be appropriate to accept SpO_2 < 91% in patients with known chronic obstructive pulmonary disease (COPD))
- Responds only to voice or painful stimuli or is unresponsive
- Has a purpuric rash

Adapted with permission from The UK Sepsis Trust. *Sepsis Red Flags*. https://sepsistrust.org/.

Any of these findings alone in a patient with suspected sepsis needs to be escalated to senior staff's attention.

The other essential point is that specialist help is available to commence any additional interventions or therapies. Certainly the Trust's support team such as the Critical Care Outreach team or Patient at Risk Team (PART) will be involved in the care of this patient group, and a referral to the HDU will need to have been made. This is because the continuing care for these patients does generally require specialist facilities. One area of support that can be provided for ward-based patients is blood glucose monitoring: in sepsis, the cells' ability to take up the glucose they need is impaired and there is a resultant hyperglycaemia. It may be that an intravenous insulin regime needs to be initiated to control high glucose levels because poor glycaemic control is associated with worse survival levels (NICE 2014).

Referral

It has been acknowledged that some acutely ill patients have received suboptimal care in hospitals, leading to their condition worsening unnecessarily (PHSO 2013). Errors in the early management of these patients include failure of the organization, but issues within the MDT have also been identified. There was a failure to take a timely history and make a timely patient examination, the source of infection was not identified quickly enough, and the key treatments were not initiated soon enough. Some of the organizational issues included inadequate staff education and training about sepsis and appropriate, timely senior input was not ensured (PHSO 2013).

Government documents have extolled the need for track-and-trigger systems to be in place for patients who are deteriorating in hospitals, culminating in the Royal College of Physicians' recommendations of the use of the National Early Warning Score (NEWS2) (Royal College of Physicians 2017). This scoring system is now used across NHS Trusts within the United Kingdom to identify acute deterioration in patients such as those with sepsis. Staff are encouraged to review for sepsis if the NEWS2 is greater than 5 (RCP 2017). Early escalation of concern and initiation of therapeutic support for patients suspected of developing sepsis is emphasized (Nutbeam *et al.* 2016) and these issues relate directly to the nurse's role in the management of sepsis (McClelland and Moxon 2014).

Critical Care Outreach Services are now understood as an integral aspect of the critical care specialty (Quinton and Gonzalez 2019). Essentially, the outreach team is a central means of supporting patients who are deteriorating and also of referring them on to critical care if required and the team has become a key resource for ward staff concerned about a deteriorating patient. Being willing to contact the outreach team as early as possible with concerns about suspected sepsis helps to speed up referral to definitive care.

There are issues, however, involved in what is seemingly a simple process of referral. Studies to date in the utilization of care bundles and early recognition of sepsis outside of critical care, for instance, have shown that there is a need for improvement (Levy *et al.* 2010). Some of the obstacles recorded to successful referral have been incomplete recordings of the observation charts and hesitation in escalating concerns, leading to adverse incidents that are deemed avoidable; these nursing issues are global in their occurrence (Massey *et al.* 2017). The cause for these situations was considered to be complex, a combination of confidence and communication skills amongst other factors. These issues cannot be viewed in too simplistic a manner, however. Reports from ward nurses looking after critically ill patients identify that there are not only educational issues that still need to be met but that assertiveness in professional relationships appears to be a key skill—and one that often comes with experience—in terms of ensuring that a patient is reviewed (Massey *et al.* 2017). Concerns about calling the medical team inappropriately have been voiced, as well as a need for emotional support in terms of dealing with unstable patients in a ward setting and anxieties with inter-professional issues such as appearing foolish for misinterpreting a degree of deterioration (Massey *et al.* 2014).

However, it is known that basic physiological observations are delegated to healthcare assistants in many instances and that a reliance on automated machinery to take blood pressures, for example, is commonplace. This removes nurses from core physical assessment findings that we would be exposed to if we were undertaking them; noticing that a pulse was weak by feeling it rather than reading it from a display or feeling that an arm was very cool whilst taking a blood pressure, for example. As more patients being cared for on the wards are especially unwell or prone to deterioration, the role of nurses' physical assessment abilities is vital and will have an impact on detection of abnormalities and patient well-being (Zambas *et al.* 2016).

Counselling and support

A critical illness, in its entirety, can be viewed as a continuum and ward nurses are in a position to be with the patient at the start and the end of their stay in hospital whilst having sepsis. Care needs for those patients who have survived sepsis needs further consideration.

Typically, patients with sepsis will be cared for in an ITU. For many patients and their families, leaving the perceived security of a critical care unit to anywhere else in the hospital can be anxiety provoking and it is important that counselling and support is provided for patients who survived an episode of sepsis as it is a component of the Surviving Sepsis Campaign. Patients and their loved ones begin to try and make sense of what will have been a near-death experience. Patients and families will need to construct a 'story' of what has happened to make sense of events and nurses have a key role in facilitating this (Stayt *et al.* 2016)

It is well recognized that patients experience an enduring impact after having survived sepsis (Gallop *et al.* 2015) and follow-up care afterwards is now a recognized component of critical care (NICE 2009, 2015a). NICE quality standards (2017) address the need for short- and medium-term rehabilitation goals to be agreed before discharge from critical care and for those patients transferring to a general ward to have a formal handover of their individualized rehabilitation programme, ideally. Patients discharged from hospital should be given information about what to expect afterwards and those with ongoing rehabilitation needs should have a review two to three months after their discharge from critical care (NICE 2017), and the fact that patients may need a variety of types of help for several months after discharge from critical care units should be impressed upon family members (Svenningsen *et al.* 2015). It is also noted that patients who have had sepsis are likely to be readmitted to critical care areas (Bateson and Patton 2015).

Problems encountered after a critical illness, such as sepsis, include physical, psychological, emotional, and cognitive dysfunction (NICE 2015a). Post-Intensive Care Syndrome is a term referring to new or worsening impairments in physical, cognitive, and/or mental health in patients that have required intensive care (Wolpaw *et al.* 2016). These morbidities persist beyond patients' stay in critical care areas and may be present in their stay on general wards. Patients report profound disorientation (Parker *et al.* 2013). Strahan and Brown (2005) have compiled some practical recommendations for care for patients at this phase of their recovery, which are still very relevant:

- Nursing interventions should aim at maximizing patient control and help towards reducing anxiety levels. This will entail inclusion of the patient in possible choices available for medical or nursing care and explanations of all that is being done.
- Patients should be encouraged to re-adopt their 'normal' sleep pattern.
- Education regarding rehabilitation and diet is essential—physiotherapy and dietician input is important here.
- Families should be involved in care and the rehabilitation process.
- Opportunity should be offered to discuss memories and nightmares, both real and hallucinatory. This is potentially time-consuming for nurses on a busy ward but needs to be accommodated. It may also be that specially trained personnel such as hospital counsellors are best suited to this.
- The need for patient information, explanation, and reassurance is real. One significant difference between critical care environments and wards is the staffing ratio and patients and relatives should be assured that although staff may not be constantly at the bedside, they are available and approachable.

Adapted from *Intensive and Critical Care Nursing*, 21, 3, Strahan, E.H.E., and Brown, R.J., A qualitative study of the experiences of patients following transfer from intensive care, pp. 160–71. https://doi.org/10.1016/j.iccn.2004.10.005.

The multidisciplinary approach is an important overview to keep when patients return to the ward. Relevant referrals are essential; perhaps to the Occupational Therapy department or to the chaplaincy service or other forms of spiritual support. It is possible that the mental health team might be an appropriate resource or a hospital counsellor would be able to offer practical input for the patient or family members. These referrals are within the remit of nurses to consider and put forward as practical, helpful options. Because they can entail the addressing of sensitive issues, it is advisable to broach matters privately with the patient first, if possible. Some resources for patients or relatives which can be particularly meaningful are those that share the experiences of other patients—one online example being healthtalk.org (see Resources section); there may be support groups active locally, too.

It is also appreciated that the turmoil that relatives experience during a family member's critical illness can leave them very drained physically and psychologically (O'Gara and Pattison 2015). It is also highly likely that the care of the patient at home will involve family members, and to this end it may be appropriate to engage with social services to offer them support. As before, this referral needs to be done, ideally after consultation with the family members themselves.

An important reality check for relatives to be aware of is that psycho-social recovery from this kind of extreme illness is often complex, alongside a slow recovery of physical functioning (McPeake and Quasim 2016). This point is now becoming the focus of intensive care follow-up, and guidelines to support physical and non-physical rehabilitation have recently been published (NICE 2015a). The community nursing team will benefit from a very thorough handover of the history of the patient's stay in hospital and of any referrals that have been put in place.

Clinical link 8.3

John Earle-Grey is 78 and weighs 90 kg. He was admitted to hospital with abdominal pain, which was found to be due to a duodenal ulcer and treated with a laparotomy for a repair of the ulcer. He is now day 5 post operation and has been on your ward since this morning. He is receiving 1 L of 0.9% sodium chloride ('normal saline') over six hours via peripheral cannula, but has no appetite—he reports feeling 'queasy' and 'achy', his temperature is 37.7°C. His urine output is being measured by his urinary catheter and over the past four hours has only been 35 mL per hour. The past three blood pressure recordings and heart rate taken by the healthcare assistant (HCA) are:

BP = 120/80, Heart rate = 85 bpm at 08.00
BP = 110/66 Heart rate = 98 bpm at 12.30
BP = 110/ 56 Heart rate = 120 bpm at 14.30

The last set of results have worried the HCA and you have been asked to review him as you start your shift.

Clinical scenario questions

- Which risk factors for developing sepsis does John have?
- What suggests to you that John is possibly developing sepsis? How advanced is this development?
- What possible sources for the infective agent might there be that are identified in the scenario?
- What other possible causes of infection might you follow up on?
- Which of John's recent laboratory results will the surgical team be particularly interested in, in relation to your findings?
- What would your course of action be in response to your findings for John?

Review of assessment practice

Below is a list of the main factors to consider in assessing a patient with sepsis or suspected sepsis. You can use this as a revision of the points discussed throughout the chapter and to prepare for the Skills Assessment. The assumption here is that you have only a sphygmomanometer and watch as equipment, even though you may well have access to other tools such as pulse oximetry, and are therefore employing a 'look, listen and feel' approach to your assessment.

Risk factors

- Is the patient very elderly?
- Do they have an already compromised immune system from taking immune suppressant drugs for auto-immune disorders or chemotherapy for cancer?
- Do they have addictions to drugs or alcohol?
- Do they have deep tissue wounds: for example, from burns or trauma, or have had invasive surgery?
- Do they have indwelling IV lines or catheters?

Patient history

- Do they have an identified infection (or have they had a recent infection)? Do they have a past medical history that includes sepsis?

Patient complaining of ...

- coughing phlegm, which is new for them.
- discomfort passing urine, or discoloured, malodorous urine.
- dizziness.
- vague responses when interacted with.
- feels unwell—non-specific or 'fluey' symptoms.

Skin

- Hot to touch due to:
  - vasodilatation carrying blood (and therefore) metabolic heat to peripheries
  - viral/ bacterial pathogens increasing metabolic/inflammatory response from cells
  - hypothalamus 're-setting' the internal thermostat

Blood pressure

- Hypotensive due to:
  - vasodilatation—this is seen in the diastolic pressure
  - myocardial depressant effect of sepsis—this is seen in the systolic pressure

Pulse

- Fast—tachycardic
- In early sepsis this will feel to be a 'bounding' pulse

- Compensation for relative hypovolaemia/distributive shock
- In later or decompensated sepsis and shock the pulse will be felt to be thready (due to hypovolaemia)
- Possibly difficult to find, due to oedema, and 'thready' in quality.

Pallor

- Flushed (more noticeable in Caucasians), due to
  - vasodilatation -more blood at periphery
- *OR* mottled, due to
  - patchy maldistribution of blood and poorly perfused capillary beds.
- *OR* pale, due to poor perfusion globally secondary to low cardiac output/oxygen delivery
- Also, impeded oxygen delivery due to oedema
- Poor capillary refill

Central nervous system

- Acutely altered/low GCS due to:
  - hypoperfusion
  - endotoxin
- Pupils—constricted—shock state
- Dull, responses obtunded—shock state

Kidneys

- Oliguric (poor urine output): less than 0.5 mL/kg/h

Abdomen

- Possibly distended, hard, uncomfortable/ painful
- Bowel sounds possibly absent due to:
  - ischaemia—poor GI tract perfusion—'auto transfusion' of gut blood supply to other vital organs
  - ileus—poor motility secondary to hypoperfusion

End of chapter assessment

The following assessment will enable you to evaluate your theoretical knowledge of sepsis and its management as well as your ability to apply this theory to clinical practice.

Knowledge assessment

With the support of your mentor/supervisor from practice, work through the following prompts to explore your knowledge level about sepsis and its management.

- Demonstrates an understanding of the difference between sepsis and septic shock.
- Broadly discusses the role of the inflammatory reaction and sepsis.
- Is able to identify common origins of sepsis, including those that are hospital acquired.
- Can explain the broad differences in patient presentation between 'early' and 'late' sepsis.
- The rationale behind lactate readings can be explained.
- Can demonstrate awareness of essential management responses of the 'Sepsis Six' and their underpinning rationale.
- Can discuss the notion of 'care bundles'.
- Discuss the nurse's role with microbiology samples for septic patients.
- Describe the clinical syndrome D and why it is related to septicaemia.
- Understands the local Trust's policy for taking blood cultures.
- Can identify local, national, and international strategies to address sepsis.
- Is aware of support resources available to relatives.
- Is aware of support resources and research available to nurses.

Skills assessment

Under the guidance of your mentor/supervisor, undertake a full assessment of a patient for signs and symptoms of sepsis followed by appropriate interventions for any significant abnormality. Your mentor/supervisor will be able to assess your ability and provide feedback based on the following skills:

- All universal precautions are adhered to whilst clinically interacting with the patient.
- Conduct a full patient history with a systems review considering key points that are relevant for a patient with sepsis or suspected sepsis.
- Demonstrate a comprehensive physical assessment and explain the physiological underpinnings normal/abnormal findings from the respiratory, cardiovascular, renal, gastrointestinal, skin, and neurological systems.
- Findings are related to the data already charted and trends in potential deterioration or compensation identified.
- The likely source and cause of sepsis for the patient are discussed.
- Microbiological and biochemical laboratory results are related to the patient's condition.
- Intravenous access and all invasive lines are checked for date and necessity. Line sites are assessed for signs of inflammation or infection.
- Demonstrate an ability to follow infection control guidelines while undertaking intravenous therapy including the management of the intravenous access and intravenous fluids.

- Any potentially diagnostic samples are taken and documented.
- Any outstanding and relevant laboratory results are pursued and relevant personnel informed.
- Any vulnerability to further infection is identified, in terms of threats of infection and the patient's own physiological reserve.
- If an early warning observations chart is in use, score the patient.
- Any indication from the observations gathered that member of the MDT or the Medical Emergency Team/Patient at Risk/Outreach teams need to be informed is acted upon. The shift leader for the ward is also notified.
- Ensure an estimation of when these personnel are able to review the patient is provided and follow this up if necessary.
- Document all interventions and referrals, including times as per Trust policy.
- Care for that shift is prioritized on the basis of the clinical picture gathered.

Resources

The UK Sepsis Trust: http://sepsistrust.org/

The UK Sepsis Trust seeks to save lives and improve outcomes for survivors of sepsis by instigating political change, educating healthcare professionals, raising public awareness, and providing support for those affected by this devastating condition. The website has information for healthcare professionals and for the public.

Surviving Sepsis: http://www.survivingsepsis.org/

The Surviving Sepsis Campaign is a joint collaboration of the Society of Critical Care Medicine and the European Society of Intensive Care Medicine committed to reducing mortality from severe sepsis and septic shock worldwide.

Global Sepsis Alliance

The Global Sepsis Alliance is a non-profit charity organization with the aim to raise awareness of sepsis worldwide and reduce sepsis deaths by 20% by 2020. It organizes and manages World Sepsis Day: http://www.world-sepsis-day.org/

Healthtalk: http://www.healthtalk.org/

Its mission is to help and inform patients, carers, and healthcare professionals by sharing trustworthy, personal health experiences.

Its aims are:

- To support patients and their loved ones, who may feel alone or ill-prepared for challenges ahead.
- To support healthcare professionals in providing patient-focused care.
- To promote better communication between patients and health professionals.

ICUsteps: http://www.icusteps.org/

ICUsteps is the UK's only support group for people who have been affected by critical illness and has helped many former patients, their relatives, and medical staff from organizations around the world.

References

Aaronson, P.I. (2013) *The Cardiovascular System at a Glance* 4th edn. Oxford: Wiley-Blackwell.

APPG on Sepsis (2016) *Sepsis and the NHS—Annual Review by the All-Party Parliamentary Group on Sepsis 2015/16.* London: All Party Parliamentary Group.

Balk, R.A. (2014) Systemic inflammatory response syndrome (SIRS) Where did it come from and is it still relevant today? *Virulence*, 5(1):20–6.

Barrett, K., Dikken, C. (2010) Neutropenic sepsis *JPP*, 3(3):116–22.

Bateson, M., Patton, A. (2015) Sepsis: Contemporary issues and implications for nursing. *Br J Nurs*, 24(17): 864–6.

Bhattacharjee, P., Edelson, D.P., Churpek, M.M. (2017) Identifying patients with sepsis on the hospital wards. *Chest*, 151(4):898–907.

Blann, A. (2013) *Routine Blood Results Explained* 3rd edn. Keswick: M&K Update.

British Thoracic Society Emergency Oxygen Guideline Development Group (2017) BTS Guideline for Oxygen Use in Adults in Healthcare and Emergency Settings. *Thorax*, 72(Suppl 1):i1–i90.

Chapel, H. (2014) *Essentials of Clinical Immunology* 6th edn. Chichester: Wiley.

Cilliers, H., Whitehouse, A., Tunnicliffe, W. (2009) Serious Complications of Sepsis in: R. Daniels and T. Nutbeam (eds) *The ABC of Sepsis.* Oxford: Wiley-Blackwell, pp. 15–19.

Coico, R., Sunshine, G. (2015) *Immunology: A Short Course.* Chichester: Wiley.

Dellinger, R.P., Carlet, J.M., Mansur, H. *et al.* (2004) Surviving Sepsis Campaign guidelines for management of severe sepsis and septic shock. *Intensive Care Med*, 30:536–55.

Doig, A.K., Huether, S.E. (2014) Structure and Function of the Renal and Urologic Systems in: K.L. McCance and S.E. Huether (eds) *Pathophysiology. The Biologic Basis for Disease in Adults and Children* 7th edn. St Louis, MO: Elsevier.

Dunkley, S., McLeod, A. (2015) Neutropenic sepsis: Assessment, pathophysiology and nursing care. *Br J Neurosci Nurs*, 11(2):79–87.

Fenwick, R. (2016) Lactate in the emergency department: A case-based critical reflection. *Emergency Nurse*, **24** (5): 25–9.

Ferrer, R., Martin-Loeches, I., Phillips, G., *et al.* (2014) Empiric antibiotic treatment reduces mortality in severe sepsis and septic shock from the first hour: Results from a guideline-based performance improvement program. *Crit Care Med*, 42(8):1749–55.

Gallop, K.H., Cerr, C.E.P., Nixon, A., *et al.* (2015) A qualitative investigation of patients' and caregivers' experiences of severe sepsis. *Crit Care Med*, 43:296–307.

Gargani, Y. (2012) *Crash Course: Immunology and Haematology* 4th edn. Edinburgh: Mosby Elsevier.

Glasper, A. (2016) Recognising and responding to the early signs of sepsis. *Br J Nurs*, 25(5):874–5.

Global Sepsis Alliance (2015) *Fact Sheet Sepsis* Available at: http://www.world-sepsis-day.org/CONTENTPIC/2015_WSD_FactSheet_long_English.pdf; accessed 9 December 2019.

Guarracino, F., Baldassarri, R., Pinsky, M.R. (2016) Pathophysiological Determinants of Cardiovascular Dysfunction in Septic Shock in: J.L. Vincent (ed.) *Annual Update in Intensive Care and Emergency Medicine 2016.* New York, NY: Springer, pp. 177–84.

Hall, A., Scott, C., Buckland, M. (2016) *Clinical Immunology.* Oxford: Oxford University Press

Health Education England (2016) *Getting It Right: The Current State of Sepsis Education and Training for Healthcare Staff across England Executive Summary.*

Available at: https://hee.nhs.uk/sites/default/files/documents/Getting%20it%20right%20The%20current%20state%20of%20sepsis%20education%20and%20training%20for%20healthcare%20staff%20across%20England%20-%20executive%20summary_0.pdf; accessed 9 December 2019.

Helbert, M. (2017) *Immunology for Medical Students* 3rd edn. Philadelphia, PA: Elsevier.

Higgins, C. (2013) *Understanding Laboratory Investigations: A Guide for Nurses, Midwives and Healthcare Professionals* 3rd edn. Chichester: Wiley-Blackwell.

Intensive Care Society (2013) *Core Standards for Intensive Care Units.* London: Faculty of Intensive Care Medicine/Intensive Care Society.

Kakihana, Y., Ito, T., Nakahara, M., *et al.* (2016) Sepsis-induced myocardial dysfunction: Pathophysiology and management. *J Intensive Care*, 4(22). doi:10.1186/s40560-016-0148-1.

Levi, M.M., Schmaier, A.H. (2016) Disseminated intravascular coagulation. Available at: http://emedicine.medscape.com/article/199627-overview; accessed 9 December 2019.

Levick, J.R. (2010) *An Introduction to Cardiovascular Physiology* 5th edn. London: Arnold.

Levy, M.M., Dellinger, R.P., Townsend, S.R., *et al.* (2010) The Surviving Sepsis Campaign: Results of an international guideline-based performance improvement program targeting severe sepsis. *Crit Care Med*, 38(2):367–74.

Levy, M.M., Rhodes, A., Phillips, G.S., *et al.*, (2015) Surviving Sepsis Campaign: Association between performance metrics and outcomes in a 7.5-year study. *Crit Care Med*, 43(1):3–12.

Lu, X.,Wang, H. (2016) Pathophysiology of sepsis-induced myocardial dysfunction. *Military Medical Research*, 3(30). Available at: https://mmrjournal.biomedcentral.com/articles/10.1186/s40779-016-0099-9; accessed 9 December 2019.

Male, D.K. (2014) *Immunology: An Illustrated Outline*. New York, NY: Garland Science.

Male, D.K., Brostoff, J., Roth, D.B. *et al.* (eds) (2013) *Immunology* 8th edn. Philadelphia, PA: Elsevier.

Massey, D., Chaboyer, W., Aitken, L. (2014) Nurses' perceptions of accessing a Medical Emergency Team: A qualitative study. *Aust Crit Care*, 27(3):133–8.

Available at: https://www.ncbi.nlm.nih.gov/pubmed/24290323; accessed 9 December 2019.

Massey, D., Chaboyer, W., Anderson, V. (2017) What factors influence ward nurses' recognition of and response to patient deterioration? An integrative review of the literature. *Nursing Open*, 4(1):6–23.

McCance, K.L. (2014) Structure and Function of the Cardiovascular and Lymphatic Systems in: K.L. McCance and S.E. Huether (eds) *Pathophysiology: The Biologic Basis for Disease in Adults and Children* 7th edn. St Louis, MO: Mosby Elsevier.

McClelland, H., Moxon, A. (2014) Early identification and treatment of sepsis. *Nursing Times*, 110(4):14–16.

McPeake, J., Quasim, T. (2016) The role of peer support in ICU rehabilitation *Intensive Crit Care Nurs*, 37(12):1–3.

McPherson, D., Griffiths, C., Williams, M., *et al.* (2013) Sepsis-associated mortality in England: An analysis of multiple cause of death data from 2001 to 2010. *BMJ Open*. Available at: http://bmjopen.bmj.com/content/bmjopen/3/8/e002586.full.pdf; accessed: 9 December 2019.

Melville, J., Ranjan, S., Morgan, P. (2015) ICU mortality rates in patients with sepsis compared with patients without sepsis. *Crit Care*, 19(Suppl 1):14.

Mitchell, E., Whitehouse, T. (2009) The Pathophysiology of Sepsis in: R. Daniels and T. Nutbeam (eds) *The ABC of Sepsis*. Oxford: Wiley-Blackwell, pp. 20–4.

Murphy, K.M., Weaver, C. (2017) *Janeway's Immunobiology*. New York, NY: Garland Science.

Nairn, R., Helbert, M. (2017) *Immunology for Medical Students* 3rd edn. Philadelphia, PA: Mosby Elsevier.

NCEPOD (2005) *Confidential Inquiry into Quality of Care before ITU Admission*. London: National Confidential Enquiry into Patient Outcome and Death.

NCEPOD (2015) *Just Say Sepsis! A Review of the Process of Care Received by Patients with Sepsis*. London: National Confidential Enquiry into Patient Outcome and Death.

NICE (2009) *Rehabilitation after Critical Illness in Adults*. London: National Institute for Health and Care Excellence.

NICE (2012) *Neutropenic Sepsis: Prevention and Management in People with Cancer*. London: National Institute for Health and Care Excellence.

NICE (2012a) *Healthcare-associated Infections: Prevention and Control in Primary and Community Care*. Updated February 2017. London: National Institute for Health and Care Excellence.

NICE (2013) *Acute Kidney Injury: Prevention, Detection and Management*. London: National Institute for Health and Care Excellence.

NICE (2014) *The Space Glucose Control System for Managing Blood-Glucose in Critically Ill Patients in Intensive Care. Medtech Innovation Briefing*. London: National Institute for Health and Care Excellence.

NICE (2015) *Urinary Tract Infections in Adults*. London: National Institute for Health and Care Excellence.

NICE (2015a) *Ward-based Care after Critical Care*. London: National Institute for Health and Care Excellence.

NICE (2016) *Sepsis: Recognition, Diagnosis and Early Management.* London: National Institute for Health and Care Excellence.

NICE (2017) *Rehabilitation after Critical Illness in Adults. NICE Quality Standard. Draft for consultation.* London: National Institute for Health and Care Excellence.

NHS England (2015) Improving Outcomes for Patients with Sepsis. London: NHS England.

Nicholls, T., Wenman, J., Nutbeam, T., *et al.* (2016) *Toolkit: Prehospital Management of Sepsis in Adults and Young People over 12 Years—2016.* Available at: https://sepsistrust.org/wp-content/uploads/2016/07/PH-toolkit-FINAL-2.pdf; accessed 9 December 2019.

Nutbeam, T., Daniels, R., Keep, J. (2016) *Toolkit: Emergency Department Management of Sepsis in Adults and Young People over 12 Years—2016.* Available at: https://sepsistrust.org/wp-content/uploads/2016/07/ED-toolkit-2016-Final-1.pdf; accessed 9 December 2019.

O'Gara, G., Pattison, N. (2015) Information and psychosocial needs of families of patients with cancer in critical care units. *Cancer Nursing Practice*, 14(6):26–30.

Okamoto, K., Tamura, T., Sawatsubashi, Y. (2016) Sepsis and disseminated intravascular coagulation. *J Intensive Care*, 4(23). Available at: https://jintensivecare.biomedcentral.com/articles/10.1186/s40560-016-0149-0, accessed 13 January 2020.

Pappano, A.J., Wier, W.G. (2013) *Cardiovascular Physiology* 10th edn. Philadelphia, PA: Elsevier Mosby.

Parker A., Sricharoenchai, T., Needham, D.M. (2013) Early rehabilitation in the intensive care unit: Preventing physical and mental health impairments. *Curr Phys Med Rehabil Rep*, 1(4):307–14. Available at: https://www.ncbi.nlm.nih.gov/pmc/articles/PMC3889146/; accessed 9 December 2019.

PHSO (2013) *Time to Act. Severe Sepsis: Rapid Diagnosis and Treatment Saves Lives.* London: Parliamentary and Health Service Ombudsman.

Quinton, S. and Gonzalez, I. (2019) Critical Care Outreach in *Faculty of Intensive Care Medicine/The Intensive Care Society Guidelines for the Provision of Intensive Care Services*, 2nd edn. London: Faculty of Intensive Care Medicine/The Intensive Care Society. Available at: https://www.ficm.ac.uk/sites/default/files/gpics-v2-final2019.pdf; accessed 7 January 2020.

Resuscitation Council (UK) (2017) Guidelines and Guidance: The ABCDE Approach. *Underlying Principles.* Available at: https://www.resus.org.uk/resuscitation-guidelines/abcde-approach/; accessed 9 December 2019.

Rhodes, A., Evans, L.E., Alhazaani, W., *et al.* 2017 Surviving Sepsis Campaign: International guidelines for management of sepsis and septic shock. *Intensive Care Med*, 43(3):304–77.

Rote, N., Huether, K.L., McCance, S.E. (2014) Innate Immunity: Inflammation in: K.L. McCance and S.E. Huether (eds) *Pathophysiology. The Biologic Basis for Disease in Adults and Children* 7th edn. St Louis, MO: Elsevier, pp. 190–209.

Rote, N., McCance, K. (2014) Adaptive Immunity in: K.L. McCance and S.E. Huether (eds) *Pathophysiology. The Biologic Basis for Disease in Adults and Children* 7th edn. St Louis, MO: Elsevier, pp. 220–51.

Royal College of Nursing (2016) *Sepsis: What's New and What's the Challenge?* Available at: https://www2.rcn.org.uk/__data/assets/pdf_file/0007/657934/Sepsis-event-presentation.pdf; accessed 9 December 2019.

Royal College of Physicians (2012) *Royal College of National Early Warning Score. Standardising the Assessment of Acute-Illness Severity in the NHS.* London: Royal College of Physicians.

Sepsis Alliance (2017) Sepsis and Antibiotic Resistance. Available at: http://www.sepsis.org/sepsis-and/sepsis-antibiotic-resistance/; accessed 9 December 2019.

Seymour, C.W., Liu, V.X., Iwashyna, T.J., *et al.* (2016) Assessment of clinical criteria for sepsis. *JAMA*, 315(8):762–74.

Shankar-Hari, M., Phillips, G.S., Levy, M.L., *et al.* (2016) Developing a new definition and assessing new clinical criteria for septic shock. *JAMA*, 315(8):775–87.

Singer, M., Deutschman, C.S., Seymour, C.W., *et al.* (2016) The Third International Consensus Definitions for Sepsis and Septic Shock (Sepsis-3). *JAMA*, 315(8):801–10.

Smyth, M.A., Brace-McDonnell, S.J., Perkins, G.D. (2016) Identification of adults with sepsis in the prehospital environment: A systematic review. *BMJ Open*, 2(6). Available at: http://bmjopen.bmj.com/content/6/8/e011218; accessed 9 December 2019.

Strahan, E.H.E., Brown, R.J. (2005) A qualitative study of the experiences of patients following transfer from intensive care. *Intensive Crit Care Nurs*, 21(3):160–71.

Stayt, L.C., Seers, K, Tutton, E. (2016) Making sense of it: Intensive care patients' phenomenological accounts of story construction *Nurs Crit Care*, 21(4):225–32.

Surviving Sepsis Campaign (2015) Updated Bundles in Response to New Evidence. Available at: http://www.survivingsepsis.org/SiteCollectionDocuments/SSC_Bundle.pdf; accessed 9 December 2019.

Surviving Sepsis Campaign (2017) *History*. Available at: http://www.survivingsepsis.org/About-SSC/Pages/History.aspx; accessed 9 December 2019.

Svenningsen, H., Langhorn, L., Ågård, A.S., *et al.* (2015) Post-ICU symptoms, consequences, and follow-up: An integrative review. *Nurs Crit Care*. doi: 10.1111/nicc.12165.

Torsvik, M., Gustad, L.T., Mehl, A. (2016) Early identification of sepsis in hospital inpatients by ward nurses increases 30-day survival. *Crit Care*, 20:244. Available at: https://ccforum.biomedcentral.com/articles/10.1186/s13054-016-1423-1; accessed 9 December 2019.

UK Sepsis Trust (2014a) *UK Sepsis Trust Clinical Toolkits 2014. Appendix 1: Introducing Red Flag Sepsis.* Available at: http://sepsistrust.org/wp-content/uploads/2015/08/1409314199UKSTAppendix1RFS2014.pdf; accessed 9 December 2019.

UK Sepsis Trust (2014b) *General Practice Sepsis Screening and Action Tool.* Available at: http://sepsistrust.org/wp-content/uploads/2015/08/1409322477GPScreening2014Final.pdf; accessed 9 December 2019.

UK Sepsis Trust (2016) *World Sepsis Day. New UCST Statistics Released Today.* Available at: http://sepsistrust.org/world-sepsis-day-ukst-new-statistics-released-today/; accessed 9 December 2019.

UK Sepsis Trust (2016a) *In-Patient Screening and Action Tool.* Available at: http://sepsistrust.org/wp-content/uploads/2016/07/Inpatient-adult-NICE-Final-1107-2.pdf; accessed 9 December 2019.

Vaughan, J., Parry, A. (2016) Assessment and management of the septic patient: Part 1. *Br J Nurs*, 25(17):958–64.

Vaughan, J., Parry, A. (2016a) Assessment and management of the septic patient: Part 2. *Br J Nurs*, 25(21):1196–200.

Vincent, J.L., Marshall, J.C., Namendys-Silva, S.A., *et al.* (2014) Assessment of the worldwide burden of critical illness: The Intensive Care Over Nations (ICON) audit. *Lancet Respir Med*, 2(5):380–6.

Williamson, T., Salman, B., Body, R., *et al.* (2014) *Care Bundles in Emergency Medicine.* Milton Keynes: Radcliffe.

Wolpaw, J., Cha, S., Dorman, T. (2016) Post-intensive Care Syndrome (PICS) in: N.D. Martin and L.J. Kaplan (eds) *Principles of Adult Surgical Critical Care.* New York, NY: Springer.

York Health Economics Consortium (2017) *The Cost of Sepsis Care in the UK.* Final Report. York: University of York.

Zambas, S.I., Smythe, E.A., Koziol-Mclain, J. (2016) The consequences of using advanced physical assessment skills in medical and surgical nursing: A hermeneutic pragmatic study. *International Journal of Qualitative Studies on Health and Well-being*, 11:1–13. Available at: http://dx.doi.org/10.3402/qhw.v11.32090; accessed 9 December 2019.

9
Pain assessment and management in acute care

Wendy Caddye

Chapter contents

The purpose of this chapter is to highlight the importance of recognizing, assessing, and managing patients in pain safely, in the acute care setting and particularly when they are acutely ill.

The chapter will include:

- pain theories and development to inform current knowledge of pain physiology
- pain assessment and the challenge in this group of patients
- analgesics with examples of useful adjuncts
- regional analgesic techniques; their uses and management
- non-pharmacological pain management

Learning outcomes

This chapter will enable you to:

- understand the development of pain theory and physiology
- carry out a pain assessment
- develop an understanding of the pharmacology of analgesics
- understand the rationale for a multimodal approach to the use of analgesics
- manage the care of a patient in pain using non-pharmacological techniques
- understand the safe rationale for monitoring a patient on a continuous epidural infusion; a local anaesthetic infusion and a Patient-Controlled Analgesia (PCA) machine
- understand how to manage a patient having Entonox safely and effectively
- apply this knowledge to acutely ill adults in pain where relevant

Physiology of pain and pain theories

Pain is a vital function of the nervous system providing the body with a warning of potential or actual injury. It is both a sensory and emotional experience, affected by psychological factors such as past experiences, beliefs about pain, and fear or anxiety (International Association for the Study of Pain (IASP) 2012).

Many theories have been suggested to explain pain mechanisms and an historical overview with examples of the main competing theories are presented here.

1. The 'Intensity' (Erb 1874) theory suggested that pain was a non-specific sensation and depended on high intensity stimulation. This was disproved because in conditions like, for example, trigeminal neuralgia the patient can suffer intense pain from a stimulus no greater than gentle touch.
2. The 'Specificity' theory proposed a specific pain pathway from pain receptors in the skin with messages travelling to a pain centre in the brain originally described by Descartes (1664). Muller (1840) and Von Frey (1895) developed this idea further by suggesting that pain is a modality similar to hearing or vision.
3. Strong (1895) and Hardy, Wolff, and Goodell (1940) described pain as an experience based on both the noxious stimulus and the psychological reaction or displeasure provoked by the sensation, which is similar to how we describe it today.
4. The 'Gate Control' theory (Melzack and Wall, 1965) suggested that non-painful input closes the 'gate' to painful input, which prevents pain sensation from travelling to the central nervous system. This can be demonstrated by when a child falls over and bangs their knee the mother can reduce the pain by rubbing the area affected: thereby stimulating the A-beta nerve fibres and blocking the transmission of the A-delta nerve fibres (Moayedi and Davis 2013).
5. Recent advances in neurobiology have increased the understanding of pain pathways and the physiology of pain mechanisms (Dickenson 2015), including the ideas of transduction, transmission, perception, and modulation.
   - Nociception is the process by which this painful stimulus is relayed from the site of stimulation to the central nervous system.
   - Transduction occurs when a stimulus at the site of trauma, injury, or illness causes chemical changes in peripheral nerve endings, ionic and pH changes, endothelial damage, and visceral changes, especially distension.
   - A-delta (myelinated; fast, and cause the initial 'ouch') and C-nerve fibres (unmyelinated; slow, and pain is 'dull and throbbing') send the pain signal by 'transmission' through the dorsal root ganglion, where they synapse with *neurons* in the dorsal horn of the spinal cord.
   - Perception takes place when the secondary neurons send signals up to the brain along the spinothalamic tract into the thalamus, which then travel to the sensory cortex, where the individual perceives and localizes the pain.

Central connection of this pain pathway with the limbic system (our emotional centre) will have a significant effect on the response to pain which becomes both physiological and psychological (Figure 9.1)

The 'Biopsychosocial Model' of pain (Sullivan *et al.* 2005) includes factors like culture, family, nociceptive stimuli, and environment as an influence on pain perception.

Other influences include:

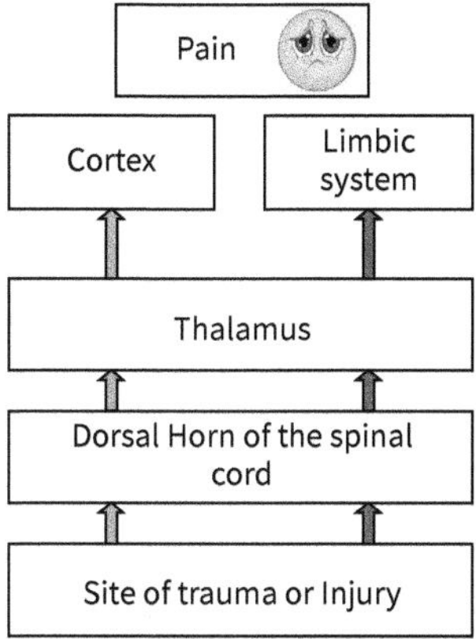

Figure 9.1 Pain pathway showing the influence of the limbic system.

- **Age**—brain circuitry generally degenerates with age, so older people may have lower pain thresholds and therefore more problems dealing with pain.
- **Gender**—women may have a higher sensitivity to pain than men but men are expected not to show or report their pain.
- **Fatigue**—we may feel more pain when our body is stressed or sleep-deprived.
- **Past experience** may influence neural responses (memory comes from the limbic system).
- **Anxiety** may have the largest psychological influence on pain scores.

Pain assessment

Pain assessment is considered a basic human right (IASP 2012) and practitioners have a professional and ethical duty to ensure that adequate pain relief is available to patients. Also, poor pain assessment can have a harmful effect on the patient.

Body systems affected by poor pain control

These include the following:

1. Respiratory: increased respiration rate, decreased deep breathing and coughing, atelectasis, sputum retention, chest infection, hypoxia.
2. Cardiovascular: tachycardia, hypertension, increased peripheral resistance, increased myocardial oxygen consumption, myocardial ischaemia, altered regional blood flow, deep vein thrombosis (DVT).
3. Gastrointestinal: delayed recovery of gastric and bowel motility.
4. Genitourinary: urinary retention.
5. Immune and endocrine: poor wound healing leading to infection, changes in endocrine function.
6. Psychological: anxiety, fear, insomnia, reduced cognitive function.
7. Musculoskeletal: reduced mobility (increasing risk of DVT), muscle spasm.

Pain is inherently subjective, so patients' self-report should be the primary basis of all pain assessments. In the acute care setting, assessment of pain should include previous experience, a description of severity, the type of pain, how the pain is impacting on mobility (so a dynamic pain score is essential), and how the patient responds to any pain management treatment, so therefore both before and after pain relief.

Also, because pain can affect core vital signs, it is imperative to document accurate pain scores using a validated and standardized pain tool, reporting any episode of unexpected severe pain (Varndell *et al.* 2017), particularly if it is sudden or associated with altered vital signs such as hypotension, tachycardia, or fever, and this should be evaluated to consider new diagnoses (e.g. patients following abdominal surgery who maybe haemorrhaging).

An example of a validated pain assessment tool is the Verbal Rating Scale (VRS) which consists of a list of adjectives describing different levels of pain intensity which should reflect extremes, so the patient reports, for example, on whether the pain is rated on a scale from 0 (no pain) to 10 (worst pain experienced) out of 10, reporting further adjectives to capture gradations of pain intensity that best describe their level of pain and include the type of pain they are experiencing (i.e. nociceptive, at the site of trauma or injury; or neuropathic, which can be described as burning, shooting, or 'like an electric shock'). Some patients find it easier to verbalize their pain as mild, moderate, or severe but a consistent approach for each patient is essential (Chou *et al.* 2016). There is inadequate evidence on the effects of different pain assessment tools on pain outcomes, so selection should be based on cognitive status, sedation, and educational level plus cultural and language differences.

However, taking a pain history, asking for location/site, character/quality, onset, and intensity rating, and repeating these questions may be challenging in this group of patients. Patients experience pain from a range of medical conditions, surgery, or trauma, and, if they are acutely ill, in association with invasive devices: they may be unable to quantify their pain because of an endotracheal tube and/or a decreased conscious state due to illness or co-administration of sedative agents (Australian and New Zealand College of Anaesthetists (ANZCA) 2015).

For these patients, Barr and colleagues (2013) recommend that pain assessment and management should include:

- routine monitoring of patients
- use of alternatives to vital signs alone
- administration of pain relief prior to painful procedures
- the use of opioids as first-line analgesia for non-neuropathic pain when indicated
- titration of sedation levels to light level
- development of a multidisciplinary team approach

Pain Assessment Tool for patients unable to self-report

Gregory and Richardson (2014) audited the evaluation of three validated pain tools by nurses using them in the acute care setting:

- The Abbey pain tool
- The Checklist of Non-Verbal Pain Indicators (CNPI)
- Pain Assessment in Advanced Dementia (PAINAD) tool

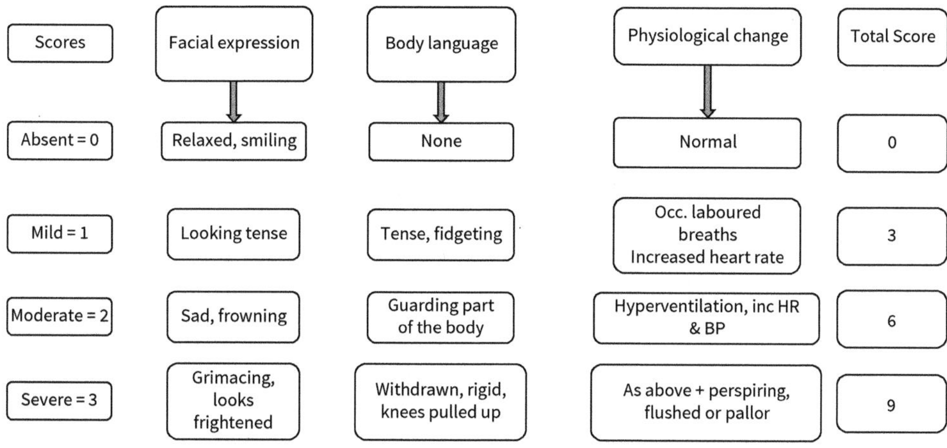

Figure 9.2 Example assessment.

Adapted from Gregory J., Vernon C., Onwudike et al. The Bolton Pain assessment tool: devising and implementing a pain assessment tool for patients unable to communicate. *Age and Ageing*, 2014, 43 (suppl_2): ii1, by permission of British Geriatrics Society and Oxford University Press.

Based on evaluation of data collected, the Bolton Pain Assessment tool was created by combining the Abbey Pain Scale with PAINAD tools. Patients are scored on: vocalization; facial expression; changes to body language; behavioural change; physiological change; physical change; and pain on movement or physiotherapy (see Figure 9.2).

Pharmacological pain management

Using analgesics in acute care needs consideration of: (a) increased drug toxicity due to acute illness, and (b) worsened acute illness due to improper analgesic selection requiring a thorough risk/benefit assessment.

The World Health Organization (WHO) ladder (1996) suggested for palliative pain management provides a framework for a pharmacological approach. However, for patients in severe acute pain from an acute injury, surgery, or illness, then the reverse ladder may need to be applied to achieve good pain control (Grisell Vargas-Schaffer 2010). Figure 9.3 illustrates both, although some steps may need to be missed out and adjuncts added considering individual patient pain assessment, past medical history, current diagnosis, and blood chemistry.

Non-opioid analgesics

The first step (mild pain) going up the ladder is *paracetamol* which is known to be an effective anti-pyretic suggesting it may work centrally in the brain by cyclooxygenase (COX) inhibition, although the precise mechanism of action is still not fully understood. The route of administration may be oral, intravenous, or rectal choice, is related to access: intravenous provides 100% bioavailability, is more effective reaching peak effect, and may be more useful in the acutely ill patient when other routes are either unavailable or unreliable.

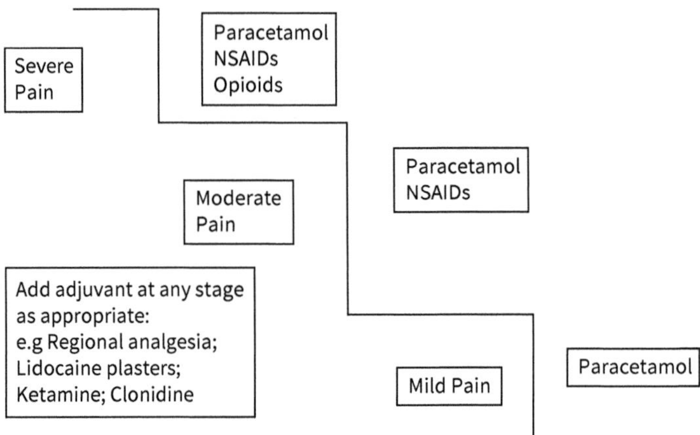

Figure 9.3 Analgesic ladder (up and down).
Adapted with permission from World Health Organization. *Cancer Pain Relief.* Copyright © World Health Organization 1986. [https://apps.who.int/iris/bitstream/handle/10665/43944/9241561009_eng.pdf] Accessed 07/06/19.

Side effects are rare but dosage must be related to the patient's weight: patients weighing greater than 50 kg are likely to tolerate 4 grams in 24 hours in divided doses, but those weighing less than 50 kg should have a reduced dose because of the risk of hepatotoxicity with higher doses. Similarly, the use of paracetamol both in liver disease or damage from alcohol abuse should involve a 50% or 75% reduction in dose or none at all (Bosilkovska *et al.* 2012).

Non-steroidal anti-inflammatory drugs (NSAIDs)

The next step suggests the addition of NSAIDs. Stimulation of the nociceptors, through tissue damage at the site of trauma or surgery, causes inflammation. NSAIDs work to reduce inflammatory pain by inhibition of COX-1 (non-selective) and COX-2 (selective), leading to inhibition of prostaglandin synthesis in inflamed tissues.

In the acute setting for young, fit, and healthy patients, the non-selective NSAIDs are safe and effective: ibuprofen (1200 mg a day or less: in divided doses) or naproxen (1000 mg a day or less: in divided doses) is recommended for prescription at the lowest effective dose and the shortest duration of treatment time necessary to control symptoms. These drugs can be given orally but ibuprofen can also be given transdermally and it is important to know that, whichever route is used to deliver an NSAID, it can still have a systemic effect (NICE 2015a). So, this group of drugs are often best avoided in acutely ill patients because of their adverse pharmacological effects.

Cautions associated with their use include:

1. Symptoms of gastritis which can lead to gastric ulceration by prostaglandin synthesis inhibition in the stomach. This group of patients may be vulnerable particularly if the oral route is unreliable and the patient is under stress. Proton pump inhibitor drugs may help in prevention.

2. Selective COX-2 inhibitor drugs (Coxibs) are associated with a lower incidence of gastritis than the non-selective NSAIDs, but these drugs have been shown to cause an increased risk of myocardial infarction and stroke because they do not inhibit the action of platelets (Neal 2016). However, recently COX-1 drugs too, for example diclofenac and high-dose ibuprofen, have also been shown to increase the risk of cardiovascular events in patients with any cardiac disease (NICE 2015a).
3. Both selective and nonselective NSAIDs can worsen blood pressure control because of sodium retention and decreased kidney perfusion and, because they control blood flow through the renal tubules, they can be nephrotoxic when patients have pre-existing renal impairment, hypovolaemia, and/or hypotension, for example following surgery or trauma (Medicines and Healthcare products Regulatory Agency (MHRA) 2009)
4. Individual NSAIDs can cause bronchospasm in sensitive asthmatics.

Finally, if taken with warfarin, NSAIDs (including topical preparations) have a significant increase of the risk of bleeding and should be avoided.

Opioids

Top of the analgesic ladder are opioids (Figure 9.3). Opioid receptors are found peripherally and throughout the central nervous system (CNS). The analgesic effects are mediated via the μ receptors. Opioids reduce pain transmission at the dorsal horn of the spinal cord by inhibiting excitatory neurotransmitter release, and they act centrally in the brain by enhancing descending inhibition.

Codeine and dihydrocodeine are traditionally known as weak opioids. However, they metabolize to morphine, which has an active metabolite (M6 glucuronide), which is excreted in the urine, and accumulation can occur in patients with renal failure, causing sedation and respiratory depression without careful monitoring, particularly if prescribed regularly. The ability to metabolize codeine can vary between patients: there is a marked increase in morphine toxicity in people who are fast metabolizers and a reduced therapeutic effect in poor metabolizers, so assessment after administration is important (NICE 2015b).

Morphine can be administered intravenously (IV), intramuscularly (IM), or subcutaneously (SC) in acute care. It is usually given IV to manage severe pain but in incremental doses to avoid overdose.

Fentanyl does not have active metabolites and oxycodone does not have clinically significant active metabolites, so these opioids are best used for patients with renal disease (Ashley and Dunleavy 2017). Also, the side effects of oxycodone are often better tolerated than morphine. Fentanyl patches are useful when the oral route is not available to provide pain relief in opioid-tolerant patients, but in hepatic failure transdermal fentanyl can be unpredictably absorbed due to altered skin blood flow.

Tramadol is a centrally acting analgesic that works a little on the μ opioid receptor but also inhibits the reuptake of norepinephrine and serotonin, so unlike pure opioids it is effective for neuropathic pain (ANZCA 2015) but the side effects are similar. It can be administered orally, IV, and IM, and it is often better tolerated as a slow release preparation if given orally.

Common side effects of opioids include euphoria, sedation, and respiratory depression.

Opioid-induced respiratory depression occurs due to high carbon dioxide levels which lead to decreased respiratory rate, increased sedation, and possible upper airway obstruction. Other side effects are nausea and vomiting, hallucinations, and itching.

Opioid-related constipation may be the cause of a paralytic ileus and can also contribute to the retention of urine and add to nausea and vomiting, affecting nutritional status and the healing process. Laxatives should always be prescribed with opioids unless there is a good clinical reason (RCoA 2017).

It is important to note that bradycardia and hypotension are less common side effects but may increase in significance in acutely ill patients. Also, large doses and long-term opioid use can cause the nervous system to become overly sensitive to painful and non-painful stimuli leading to hyperalgesia (see section on acute neuropathic pain).

However, systemic opioids remain the first-line management of severe pain particularly in the Emergency Department (ED) and are usually administered peri- and post-operatively for major surgery.

First pass metabolism

When an opioid is taken orally it is absorbed from the small intestine, travels via the hepatic portal vein to the liver where it is metabolized and enters the systemic circulation, this is called first-pass metabolism (Pond and Tozer 1984). Morphine suffers significant first-pass metabolism so that of a 20 mg dose of oramorph, as little as 10 mg reaches the systemic circulation. Oxycodone suffers less first-pass metabolism so that an approximate equivalent dose to 20 mg of oramorph to immediate release oxycodone is 10 mg. Fentanyl is completely broken down by the liver and is administered transdermally, IV, epidurally, intrathecally, and sub-lingually to avoid first-pass metabolism.

The ratio of the amount of drug entering the circulation to the total dose is the bioavailability: when a patient has liver disease the lack of hepatic blood flow results in increased bioavailability and the necessity to lower the dose. With an acute kidney injury selection of analgesics is crucial because of the potential for the accumulation of active metabolites and/or damage to the kidneys. Changes to mental state in patients on long-term opioid therapy may be the first indication of renal failure (Ashley and Dunleavy 2017).

Patient-controlled analgesia (PCA)

This involves using an electronic device to deliver opioid by patient self-administration usually IV, but can be SC, allowing small and frequent boluses to be given as required by the patient: for example, during mobilization or physiotherapy. The pumps are protocol driven to deliver an opioid in doses and frequency that are most effective and safe for individual patients.

Examples of opioids used include morphine, oxycodone, and fentanyl: patients who are intolerant of the side effects of morphine can often tolerate oxycodone; patients with renal impairment should have fentanyl, because it does not accumulate in renal failure (see earlier).

The indication for PCA, other than for severe pain in the ED or following major surgery, is usually that other routes for the delivery of opioids are unavailable or inappropriate for an individual patient. However, acutely ill patients need to be well enough to be able to control their pain effectively using the machine: when they can, there is often a higher degree of patient satisfaction because patients feel in control (ANZCA 2015).

Monitoring

Monitoring includes a sedation score, respiratory rate, a pain (see section on pain assessment), nausea, and vomiting score, and reports of itching.

Whilst checking respirations: time apnoeic periods which are likely to be due to opioid overdose; be more concerned if respirations are shallow rather than slow, regular, and deep. Remember that oxygen saturation can remain high in the presence of respiratory depression when the patient is receiving oxygen.

Management of opioid-induced respiratory depression

Naloxone is the antagonist for all the opioids. It may be administered to a patient who has stopped breathing following an overdose of opioids in the ED, where it should continue to be administered intravenously until they wake up.

However, if it is being given to a patient who is showing early signs of opioid toxicity postoperatively, 40–100 mcg of naloxone should be given IV and repeated every few minutes until normal respirations resume and the patient is awake. Administration of large doses of naloxone reverses the analgesic effect of all previous opioids given and if a patient has been on long-term opioids for chronic pain then slow titration is essential to prevent pain and withdrawal (NPSA Alert 2014). The side effects of naloxone, including nausea and vomiting, hypertension, and tachycardia, can be avoided by slow administration: arrhythmias and pulmonary oedema are rare.

Naloxone has a shorter half-life than most opioids and so further doses or an infusion may be required to re-establish a normal respiratory pattern whilst keeping the patient's pain under control: the patient needs to be transferred to a Level 2 area for close monitoring of response.

A multimodal approach to managing nausea and vomiting should be used, for example ondansetron, metoclopramide, and cyclizine where appropriate: if severe, an opioid switch may be beneficial. Itching can be treated with chlorphenamine or small doses of naloxone (not reversing the analgesic effect).

Tolerance to opioids means that patients on long-term opioids need an increase in dose over time to have the same effect and can lead to patients receiving huge doses of opioid that have become ineffective. Physical dependence also develops over time, so that patients present with symptoms of withdrawal if long-term opioids are stopped suddenly. Addiction is a personality disorder when an individual continues to take the drug even though they know it is causing them harm: they have tolerance and dependence as well.

Long-term use of opioid prescription medications can cause serious side effects, particularly when taken at doses above an oral morphine equivalent of 120 mg/day (RCoA 2017): this is particularly important for an acutely ill patient with chronic pain or a history of opioid abuse. Opioid-induced immunosuppression allows increased susceptibility to infection and hyperalgesia can mean increased risk of higher reported pain scores (see section on acute neuropathic pain).

Reducing opioid requirements

Opioid-sparing analgesic approaches may be beneficial in patients in whom pain control with opioids is difficult or when it is preferable for opioid consumption to be minimized.

The use of α-2 adrenoreceptor agonists, gabapentinoids (see section on acute neuropathic pain), *N*-methyl-D-aspartate (NMDA) receptor antagonists, and IV lidocaine (see section on local anaesthetics) may reduce opioid-related side effects but they may cause side effects of their own, limiting their use.

Examples of adjuvants to the analgesic ladder

Clonidine

Clonidine is an α-2 adrenoceptor agonist and acts as an analgesic in the dorsal horn of the spinal cord. When it is given during surgery it reduces post-operative pain intensity, opioid consumption, and nausea, however it must be administered and patients monitored with caution because of the side effects, bradycardia and hypotension (Blaudszun *et al.* 2012).

Ketamine

IV morphine is recommended as first line for major trauma patients, with ketamine in analgesic doses as second-line treatment. Ketamine works at NMDA receptors in the dorsal horn of the spinal cord so it is also useful for acute neuropathic pain (preventing hyperexcitability (discussed below), but side effects from overdose include changes to the sense of sight and sound, hallucinations, and a feeling of detachment, so it is prescribed with caution (NICE 2016).

Neuropathic pain

A central mechanism in the spinal cord called 'wind-up', hypersensitivity, or hyperexcitability can occur when noxious stimulation causes the dorsal horn neurons to transmit progressively increasing numbers of pain impulses, which leads to the development of neuropathic pain. Hyperalgesia, which is a heightened pain sensation to a normally painful response, and allodynia, which is a painful response to a non-painful stimulus, can also develop (Cohen and Mao 2014).

Neuropathic pain can be produced by dysfunction of the nervous system itself, physical trauma, repetitive injury, infection, metabolic change, and exposure to toxins or some drugs.

Three types of nerves can be involved:

- Sensory nerves, causing tingling, pain, numbness, or weakness in the feet and hands
- Motor nerves, causing weakness in the lower and upper limbs

- Autonomic nerves, affecting, for example: the gut, bladder; changes heart rate, blood pressure, and sweating.

Patients can develop acute neuropathic pain for example: following acute herpes zoster (shingles); HIV/AIDS; Guillain–Barre syndrome; post stroke pain; diabetic and alcoholic neuropathy, and demyelinating diseases (Macintyre and Schug 2015). Early recognition of neuropathic pain post trauma (e.g. following amputation) is relevant, as early management in the acute phase may help to prevent the development of chronic neuropathic pain following recovery (Clarke *et al.* 2012; Beard and Wood 2015).

The treatment for acute neuropathic pain may include:

1. Gabapentin given orally with a starting dose of 300 mg (or pregabalin 75 mg) titrated with increasing doses against efficacy and side effects. Both drugs modulate calcium channels limiting the influx of calcium ions in hyperexcitable neuronal states, thereby reducing central sensitization (Macintyre and Schug 2015).

   Cautions: gabapentinoids should be administered with caution, particularly in the elderly, as side effects include dizziness, increasing the risk of falls. Also, because of their use as an anticonvulsant, there is a theoretical risk of altering the threshold for seizures, so doses of greater than 900 mg per 24 hours should be reduced slowly after 3 days. Similarly, patients who are acutely ill (e.g. with head injury) and have well-controlled seizure activity with other anticonvulsants should be monitored carefully when managing neuropathic pain with the addition of gabapentinoids. Gabapentin and pregabalin should be dose-limited in patients with renal impairment. For example: patients with an e-GFR of 50–80 mL/minute/1.73 m^2 then gabapentin 0.6–1.8 g daily in 3 divided doses is recommended (NICE 2017a).

2. A serotonin norepinephrine reuptake inhibitor drug (SNRI); for example, duloxetine (NICE 2016). SNRIs increase the concentration of serotonin and noradrenaline in the CNS and are effective by facilitating the descending inhibitory serotonergic and noradrenergic pathways.

   Analgesic drugs with different modes of action target pain at different points along the pain pathway. NSAIDs and local anaesthetics work peripherally, and opioids, antidepressants, anticonvulsants, and paracetamol work centrally. Therefore, 'multimodality' should be applied to the use of analgesia in pain management and by using this approach it may be possible to use lower doses of drugs minimizing unwanted side effects. For example, by using a combination of paracetamol, an NSAID and an opioid, for post-operative pain, the amount of opioid required may be less and opioid-significant related side effects may be reduced.

   Entonox is a 50:50 mixture of nitrous oxide and oxygen. Nitrous oxide is known to act within the brain and in the spinal cord, inhibiting pain impulses by altering pain pathways (British Oxygen Company (BOC) 2015). The analgesic effects are not understood but may be due to the release of endorphins and serotonin.

Indications

Entonox is used for the management of short-term and procedural pain (e.g. acute trauma; dressing changes) and to relieve pain until longer-acting analgesics can be given or have time to take effect. Entonox does not accumulate and it is rapidly eliminated from the lungs during exhalation.

Cautions and side effects

Entonox contains 50% oxygen therefore it must be used with caution in patients with chronic obstructive pulmonary disease (COPD) (BOC 2015).

Nitrous oxide expands in gas-filled spaces so should not be used where the patient has any condition where air is trapped inside the body, particularly if there is a limit to how large the gas-filled space can become or where the increase in size and pressure can compress surrounding structures. For example, Entonox should not be used for patients who have recently had:

- a pneumothorax;
- an air embolism;
- a decompression sickness;
- severe bullous emphysema
- intestinal obstruction/abdominal distension
- maxillofacial injuries: by using the mouthpiece or mask, there is an increased risk of causing further damage and significant risk of blood inhalation
- a head injury; that is, patients with a low GCS because drowsiness could confound neurological observation
- a laryngectomy (due to difficulty in obtaining a seal to enable effective use)
- an episode of vomiting

Non-compliance may be a problem for patients who are unable to self-administer Entonox.

Significant side effects

Bone marrow and neurological complications have been reported in patients exposed to nitrous oxide (BOC 2015). Patients deficient in vitamin B12, including those without associated anaemia, may develop severe myeloneuropathy after even brief exposure to nitrous oxide (MHRA 2009). For this reason, patients must only use Entonox for short-term analgesia.

The use of analgesics in the acutely ill patient requires careful prescribing with consideration of coexisting comorbidities. Patients should be monitored to ensure that changes during an acute illness do not compromise the safety of analgesic choices made or that the analgesics administered do not increase the severity of an acute illness.

Regional analgesia

Regional nerve blocks plus or minus a catheter may provide better pain relief than IV opioids with fewer side effects.

- Indications—the management of trauma (e.g. rib fractures) and surgery (e.g. knee replacement), or when a general anaesthetic (GA) may put the patient at risk (e.g. patients who have COPD).
- Contraindications—coagulopathy, infection, and immune-compromised states or patient refusal.

(Stundner and Memtsoudis 2017)

Spinals

Usually a single shot delivery of local anaesthetic (LA) into the sub-arachnoid space below the level of the spinal cord (usually lumbar vertebrae one to three), which blocks sensory and motor sensation below the level of injection peri-operatively and post-operatively.

Drugs and doses

An LA is used (usually 'heavy' bupivacaine, which contains glucose increasing the specific gravity, thereby ensuring that the drugs do not spread up to the brain), plus or minus an opioid (e.g. fentanyl), which may increase the duration of effectiveness (because of the presence of opioid receptors in the spinal cord). Low LA concentrations (e.g. 0.25%) and volumes (e.g. 1.8 mL) may allow an earlier return to mobility and reduce the likelihood of a significant sympathetic block leading to prolonged hypotension.

Advantages

- Fewer problems with respiratory function and airway management because patients are not ventilated during surgery.
- Reduction in perioperative venous thrombo-embolic disease.
- Reduced incidence of post-operative nausea and vomiting (PONV) with immediate return to normal oral intake (particularly for patients with diabetes) as there is less nausea as fewer opioids are required.
- Cardiovascular stability: even patients with relatively fixed cardiac outputs may remain stable.

(Chou *et al.* 2016)

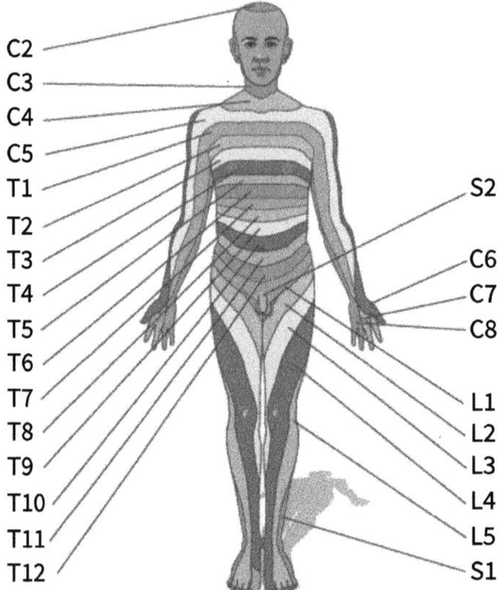

A dermatome is an area of the skin supplied by a single nerve

Levels are:
C = Cervical
T = Thoracic
L = Lumbar
S = Sacral

Figure 9.4 Dermatome map.

Reproduced with permission of Clinical Skills Ltd. Management of continuous epidural infusions, Part 1: insertion, demonstrated by Wendy Caddye, Page 1, pic 2, 'Sensory block (dermatomes)'. © Clinical Skills Ltd. 2014. www.clinicalskills.net.

Nursing management

Observation of vital signs should always be appropriate for the patient's clinical condition. IV access must be maintained to allow management of adverse effects which can include hypotension (which can be treated with sympathomimetic drugs and/or IV fluids) and respiratory depression (which can be treated with naloxone—see p. 267).

Patients, with no sensation and lack of mobility below the dermatome lumbar (L1) (Figure 9.4), are vulnerable to limb damage and pressure sores, so relevant sites need regular assessment of motor power and sensation, based on the 'Bromage' Score (Anaesthesia UK 2004). Also, patients may be at risk of falls if they are unable to stand and/or have hypotension.

Complications

Urinary retention or incontinence of urine is a common complication following spinals and patients may need a urinary catheter until sensation returns: sensory and motor block usually recede within two to six hours.

Severe headache may occur if there is cerebrospinal fluid (CSF) leakage through the dura at the site of injection: diagnosis is suggested when headache occurs as the patient sits up and it is relieved when they lie down again. Lying flat for 48 hours and administering extra fluids may be sufficient to allow the hole to seal but if the headache is not tolerated then a 'blood patch' may be performed. This involves the insertion of 20 mL of the patient's blood into the epidural space at another level to seal the tear: if it is ineffective it may be repeated (Cook *et al.* 2009; Tarkilla 2017).

Finally, there is always a potential risk of local anaesthetic *toxicity* (AAGBI 2010) (see p. 277).

Epidurals

Epidural infusions should selectively block pain messages from the surgical/trauma site, lessen the stress response to surgery (thoracic epidurals), and control pain on movement, providing effective analgesia in the early post-operative period.

Potential benefits include the maintenance of pulmonary function for patients who are unable to tolerate a GA, for example those with COPD; cardiovascular protection as intraoperative blood loss may be reduced with both spinals and epidurals (Kehlet and Holt 2001); and reduction in thromboembolic complications and improved GI function, because fewer opioids are required (Chou *et al.* 2016).

Contraindications

Absolute: bleeding disorders including the use of anticoagulants, patient refusal, local skin sepsis, and inadequate post-operative facilities.

Relative: hypotension/hypovolaemia, septicaemia/bacteraemia, immunocompromised patients (e.g. with HIV/AIDS)

Therefore, use in the acutely ill patient requires a careful risk/benefit assessment by the anaesthetist prior to insertion.

Insertion

Epidural catheters are inserted aseptically, in an anaesthetic room to reduce the risk of infection, and positioned at a level to block sensation at dermatomes (Figure 9.4) appropriate for the surgery performed or the site of trauma; for example, in the lumbar region to block sensory nerves below the level of thoracic (T) dermatome 10 (approx. umbilicus) or higher to block the sensory nerves across the chest and abdomen (RCoA 2010).

Local anaesthetics block the conduction of the sensory, motor, and sympathetic nerve fibres: the action is on nerve roots crossing the epidural space and by diffusion through the dura and subarachnoid membranes. Unlike a spinal, pain relief is usually by continuous administration of LA (plus or minus an opioid) via an indwelling catheter.

Studies have shown that combinations of low concentrations of an LA (e.g. levobupivacaine) and an opioid (e.g. fentanyl) provide better pain relief compared with either of the drugs alone and using lower doses of each reduces the side effects of both drugs (ANZCA 2015). However, an example of surgery where patients could have a plain LA epidural infusion would be following an oesophagectomy, when they can also have an opioid PCA: the latter can manage the pain above which the sensory level is unlikely to be blocked by the LA in the epidural space. Optimization of the analgesic effect of epidural infusions requires individual titration of the infusion rate against the adverse effects, so careful nursing management is essential.

Monitoring

Patients should be monitored hourly in the first 12 hours of the infusion when it is becoming established and should include heart rate, respiratory rate, blood pressure, dynamic pain score (i.e. pain on movement), level of sensory block, and assessment of motor block (RCoA 2010). Additionally, normal clinical considerations should always be applied to determine the frequency of observations in an acutely ill patient.

Measurement of sensory block

A localized area of skin supplying a single nerve from a single nerve root of the spinal cord is called a 'dermatome' (Figure 9.4). Therefore, because the receptors for pain and temperature are the same, sensory block can be measured by testing the levels at which the patient reports a change in sensation from cold to warmth when ice is applied to the skin (Macintyre and Schug 2015).

Motor block usually implies that the local anaesthetic has blocked the motor nerves as well as the sensory nerves (see section on spinals). Prior to mobilizing patients with a lower limb sensory block it is advisable to check that their blood pressure is within their normal range and sit them on the edge of the bed first. Also, lack of power to the legs could cause the patient to collapse on standing and pooling of blood in the legs can make the patient light headed if the blood pressure drops further, due to a sympathetic block. As with spinals, if motor block is present then regularly monitoring of the patient's pressure areas is essential.

Significant clinical signs which require immediate referral to an anaesthetist

- Significant motor block with a thoracic epidural
- Motor block that does not regress when an epidural is stopped
- Unexpectedly dense motor block, including unilateral block
- Markedly increasing motor block during an epidural infusion

(Cook *et al.* 2009)

Temperature should be recorded every four hours (unless otherwise indicated) to ensure that any sign of infection is picked up early. A swinging, high temperature could indicate the presence of an epidural abscess (RCoA 2010; Macintyre and Schug 2015). Also observe the epidural site at least once every shift change and if the patient starts reporting pain, ensure that the epidural catheter is correctly positioned and that there are no signs of infection: if there are signs of leakage at the site this could increase this risk. If a patient reports pain when they were formerly pain free, this may be an indication that the epidural catheter has fallen out. Finally, review the need to continue the infusion, especially after 48 hours, as the risk of infection increases (RCoA 2010).

An epidural bolus of local anaesthetic can cause hypotension within 5 min of administration so monitoring at this time should reflect this. Similarly observations of pain scores, blood pressure, and sensory block should be performed for half an hour following an increase in the infusion rate (RCoA 2010), with continued monitoring depending on patient response.

All patients receiving analgesia via an epidural catheter require careful fluid management because of the increased risk of hypotension. Therefore, intravenous access and a urinary catheter must be continued while the epidural infusion is in place.

Disconnection

If an epidural catheter becomes disconnected from the filter and it was not witnessed then, because of the risk of infection, the catheter must be removed. Before removal always check when the patient last received thromboprophylaxis (Harrop-Griffiths *et al.* 2013) and seek anaesthetic advice if INR > 1.0. If the disconnection is witnessed, use an aseptic non-touch technique to clean the line with 2% chlorhexidine in 70% alcohol, cut a section out of the epidural line with sterile scissors, and reconnect (Macintyre and Schug 2015).

Examples of major risks following insertion of an epidural catheter with percentage risk of related complications

(Cook *et al.* 2009)

- **Neurological damage** (0.016–0.56%) can occur on insertion of an epidural catheter.
- Accidental **dural puncture** (0.3–1.23%) can occur during insertion: leakage of CSF causes a headache (for diagnosis and management: see section on spinals).
- **Epidural haematomas** (0.0004–0.03%) are caused by altered clotting times related to disease or drugs such as warfarin or low-molecular-weight heparins (LMWHs) (Harrop-Griffiths *et al.* 2013).
- **Epidural abscess** (0.01–0.05%) can develop from local or generalized sepsis and/or compromised immunity.

  Motor block may indicate that a haematoma or abscess is pressing on the spinal cord (RCoA 2010), so diagnosis of cauda equina symptoms is made by nurses initially and confirmed by a magnetic resonance imaging (MRI) scan. Early decompression is necessary, as permanent paralysis can occur within four hours.
- **Catheter migration** (0.15–0.18%) into the subarachnoid space can lead to the unexpected development of a high block. A patient may complain of difficulty taking a deep breath if the intercostal muscles are affected, tingling, or numbness in the arms when the block reaches T1 and will stop breathing when the block is at C5 as the diaphragm may be paralysed by lack of phrenic nerve supply. Urgent anaesthetic help is needed.
- **Hypotension** (3–30%) is caused by the blocking of thoracic sympathetic nerves causing vasodilatation of lower limb blood vessels (warm feet, reduced venous return to heart, reduced BP and cardiac output) which may reduce blood flow to vital

organs, including heart, brain, kidneys, and bowel with potential anastomotic-related complications.
However, there are other causes for hypotension, which must be excluded particularly in this group of patients, including bleeding, sepsis, pulmonary embolus, and dehydration, before reducing the rate or stopping the epidural (unless severe).

- **CNS toxicity** (0.01–0.12) can be caused by inadvertent delivery of LA intravenously and is potentially life threatening. For safety, all giving sets, pumps, and equipment related to epidurals should be yellow and all connections should be carefully checked. Specific epidural connectors (non luer lock) are not available at the time of writing (NPSA 2011) so there is the potential risk of attaching the line to an IV cannula.
- **Respiratory depression** (0.13–0.4%) and pruritus (related to fentanyl in the infusion) can be improved with the administration of naloxone.

Removal of the epidural catheter

The patient lies on their side or leans forward with their back slightly curved. Using aseptic non-touch technique (ANTT), the dressing is removed and the catheter gently pulled until the blue curved tip is out. The site is covered with a clear dressing so that it can be observed easily for signs of infection.

There is strict guidance for times of removal of epidural catheters, when patients are taking LMWH or oral anticoagulants to prevent an accidental epidural haematoma (Harrop-Griffiths *et al.* 2013).

Continuous perineural blockade (CPNB)

Local anaesthetics can provide excellent pain relief when administered by a continuous infusion (Macintyre and Schug 2015), either via a catheter sited within a nerve sheath or with the tip sited within a muscle bed. Receptors in the skin and subcutaneous tissue detect pain and this stimulation is transmitted to the spinal cord and the brain (Dickenson 2015). The small diameter C-fibres which carry pain messages are particularly sensitive to LA so sensory nerves can be reversibly blocked. As with epidurals, LA in low doses provide pain relief but still allow the patient to move reducing the risk of pressure sores developing. In addition, the patient can participate in physiotherapy (Neal 2016). The main advantage is that effective analgesia is provided with no effect on the CNS; that is, without the risk of respiratory depression, sedation, or nausea and vomiting associated with the administration of opioids (ANZCA 2015).

Continuous LA infusions may, for example, be used to manage:

- Elderly patients in A&E who have, for example, a fractured neck of femur and are unable to tolerate large doses of opioids and are waiting for surgery (fascia iliac blocks).
- Patients with chest trauma/rib fractures (paravertebral, serratus plane, or interpleural blocks) to improve respiratory effort and the risk of developing pneumonia.
- Patients who need a GA where there are risks of bleeding or haematoma if an epidural is inserted.

Patients with CPNB may also continue to have paracetamol, NSAIDs (if appropriate), and drugs for managing neuropathic pain if prescribed, plus opioids if their pain is not completely controlled using this technique (especially if they are tolerant to opioids, to prevent withdrawal).

The use of dedicated local anaesthetic pumps reduces the risk of inadvertently administering local anaesthetic solutions intravenously with fatal consequences (see Table 9.1).

Other methods of using local anaesthetics for pain management

Intravenous lidocaine (critical care areas only)

When administered IV, lidocaine demonstrates anti-hyperalgesic properties that improve acute post-operative pain management (Eipe *et al.* 2016). Its use in patients following polytrauma (e.g. in Afghanistan) is also recommended for managing acute neuropathic pain in critical care areas because of its opioid-sparing effect (Beard and Wood 2015). Careful use of protocols related to dosing is required as serious adverse effects such as cardiac arrhythmias and haemodynamic instability can occur with large doses (Macintyre and Schug 2015).

Lidocaine plasters

Rib fractures account for 10% of traumatic injuries and have a high incidence of pulmonary complications including chest infections due to the patient's inability to take deep breaths

Table 9.1 Recognition and management of LA toxicity

1. **Recognition**		**Signs of severe toxicity:** • Sudden alteration in mental status, severe agitation or loss of consciousness, with or without tonic-clonic convulsions • Cardiovascular collapse: sinus bradycardia, conduction blocks, asystole, and ventricular tachyarrhythmias
2. **Management**		**Stop LA infusion if appropriate** • Call for help • Maintain the airway • Give 100% oxygen • Confirm or establish intravenous access • Assess cardiovascular status throughout
3. **Treatment**	**In circulatory arrest**	**Without circulatory arrest**
	Follow current resuscitation guidelines,	Treat bradycardia, hypotension, and tachyarrythymias following usual protocols
	administer lipid emulsion	Consider lipid emulsion

Reproduced with the kind permission of the Association of Anaesthetists of Great Britain and Ireland, from Management of Severe Local Anaesthetic Toxicity. AAGBI Safety Guideline. 2010. https://anaesthetists.org/Portals/0/PDFs/Guidelines%20PDFs/Guideline_management_severe_local_anaesthetic_toxicity_v2_2010_final.pdf?ver=2018-07-11-163755-240&ver=2018-07-11-163755-240; accessed 9 December 2019.

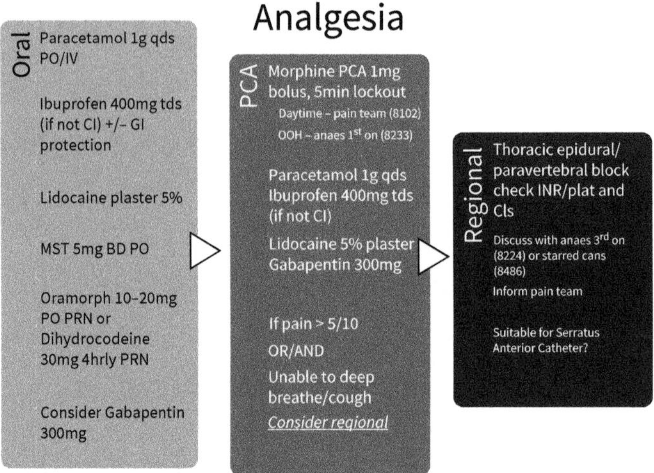

Figure 9.5 Management of rib fractures.

Reproduced from Parras, T. (2015) Case series: Serratus plane block for rib fracture analgesia: Trunk blocks. Available at: https:// academy.esraeurope.org/ esra/ 2015/ 34th/ 105289/ teresa.parras.case.series.serratus. plane. block.for.rib.fracture.analgesia.html?f=m2t1159; accessed 9 December 2019.

because of pain on inhalation. Pulmonary complications are more likely to occur in elderly patients and those with three or more fractures. Despite limited evidence (Ingalls *et al.* 2010; Zink *et al.* 2011) lidocaine plasters have become a useful tool for managing this group of patients. They contain 5% lidocaine and the usual daily dose is between one and three plasters of a size to cover the painful area: they may be cut into smaller pieces to fit. There is limited absorption of the drug so only a small risk of local anaesthetic toxicity, however patients should not use more than 3 plasters at the same time and they should be removed after 12 hours of use, so that there is a 12-hour period with no plaster. They can be applied either during the day or during the night.

The management of pain related to chest trauma clearly needs careful consideration and the use of lidocaine plasters may be insufficient. Blanco, Parras, and colleagues (2013) describe the use of serratus plane blocks for use in rib fractures and, following a case series, Parras (2015) developed a 'traffic light' pain management approach based on severity, shown as an unpublished adapted version (Figure 9.5), which may help to prevent admission to high-dependency areas through early assessment and application.

Non-pharmacological pain management

High pain scores related to prolonged admission may be improved by managing the patient holistically. These could include positioning, pressure area care, comfortable fixation of invasive devices, and reducing noise from alarms. A flexible visiting policy may help decrease pain by allowing more support from family and friends. Physiotherapy maintains range of movement of joints and slows deconditioning, and massage can trigger a relaxation response leading to improved sleep. Listening to music before and during turning a patient may reduce anxiety which may be effective by providing distraction (ANZCA 2015). Trans electrical nerve stimulation (TENS) can be used to modulate acute pain and can relieve pain by stimulating the A-beta nerve fibres, thereby closing the gate on the A-delta and C-fibres (Gate Control theory) and may also be useful.

Psychological factors play a significant role in the aetiology of acute pain, particularly in the transition to chronic pain problems. Assessment and intervention need to reflect the psychological variables mentioned in the 'Biopsychosocial' model discussed earlier, highlighting the need for multidimensional management of the patient.

Clinical link 9.1 (see Appendix for answer)

You are referred a 56-year-old male patient who is having regular haemodialysis who is described as having uncontrolled bilateral foot pain from ischaemia and sepsis. He is awaiting amputation.

- **Pain assessment**—he is in obvious pain and states 8/10 reporting that he has never experienced pain as bad as this. He describes the pain as burning with occasional electric shock pain shooting from his foot up to his knee. He reports being very sleepy with morphine although it did help and the shooting pains improved with gabapentin but his head felt 'awful'.
- **Prescription chart**—he is currently taking: paracetamol 1 gm QDS; oxycodone (IR) 5mg hourly, and pregabalin 75 mg OD.
- **Medical notes**—he has a history of Type 2 diabetes and peripheral vascular disease but has never been seen by a chronic pain consultant in the past.
- **Relevant medical investigations**

Currently – eGFR = 4; CRP = 331 and WCC = 18

Critically discuss his current analgesic regime and any changes you could make.

End of chapter assessment

The following assessment will enable you to evaluate your theoretical knowledge of pain and its management as well as your ability to apply this theory to practice.

Knowledge assessment

With the support of your mentor/supervisor from practice, work through the following prompts to explore your knowledge level.

- Discusses the importance of pain assessment.
- Describes a basic pain pathway/pain physiology.
- Describes the anatomy related to epidural and spinal analgesia.
- Discusses the use of an analgesic ladder and a multimodal approach to pain management.

- Decide which group(s) of analgesic drugs are appropriate for a particular patient group; for example major surgery, chest trauma, chronic kidney disease, etc.
- Lists the drug choices in PCA and the side effects of opioids.
- Understands the difference between tolerance, dependence, and addiction.

Skills assessment

Work with a member of the pain team in clinical practice to find out which skills need further work.

- Demonstrates an appropriate pain assessment using a valid tool.
- Safely assess a patient on a local anaesthetic infusion.
- Safely assess a patient on a continuous epidural infusion.
- Safely assess a patient with a PCA machine.
- Reports concerns to the multidisciplinary team.
- Safely delivers Entonox to a patient during a procedure.

References

Anaesthesia U.K. (2004) *Bromage Scale.* Available at: http://www.frca.co.uk/article.aspx?articleid=100316; accessed 9 December 2019.

Ashley, C., Dunleavy, A. (eds) (2017). *The Renal Drug Handbook.* Available at: https://renaldrugdatabase.com/; accessed 9 December 2019.

Association of Anaesthetists of Great Britain and Ireland (AAGBI) (2010) Management of Severe Local Anaesthetic Toxicity. Available at: https://www.aagbi.org/sites/default/files/la_toxicity_2010_0.pdf; accessed 9 December 2019.

Australian and New Zealand College of Anaesthetists and Faculty of Pain Medicine (ANZCA and FPM), Schug, A., Palmer, G., and Scott D., (eds) (2015) *Acute Pain Management: Scientific Evidence* 4th edn. Melbourne: Australian and New Zealand College of Anaesthetists and Faculty of Pain Medicine. Available at: http://www.fpm.anzca.edu.au/resources/books-and-publications; accessed 9 December 2019.

Barr, J., Fraser, G., Puntillo, K., *et al.* (2013) Clinical practice guidelines for the management of pain, agitation, and delirium in adult patients in the intensive care unit. *Crit Care Med*, 41(1):263–306.

Beard, D.J., Wood, P. (2015) Pain in the complex patient: Lessons from Afghanistan *BJA Education*, 15(4):207–12.

Blanco, R., Parras, T., MacDonnell, J.G., *et al.* (2013) Serratus plane block: A novel ultrasound-guided thoracic wall nerve block. *Anaesthesia*, 68(11):1107–13.

Blaudszun, G., Lysakowski, C., Elia, N., *et al.* (2012) Effect of perioperative systemic alpha 2 agonists on postoperative morphine consumption and pain intensity: Systemic review and meta-analysis of randomised controlled trials. *Anesthesiology*, 116(6):1312–22.

British Oxygen Company (BOC) (2015) Entonox: The Essential Guide. Available at: http://www.bochealthcare.co.uk/internet.lh.lh.gbr/en/images/entonox_essential_guide_hlc401955_Sep10409_64836.pdf; accessed 9 December 2019.

Bosilkovska, M., Walder, B., Besson, M., *et al.* (2012) Analgesics in patients with hepatic impairment: Pharmacology and clinical implications. *Drugs*, 72(12):1645–69.

Chou, R., Gordon, D., de Leon-Casasola, O. (2016) Management of postoperative pain: A clinical practice guideline from the American Pain Society, the American Society of Regional Anesthesia and Pain Medicine, and the American Society of Anesthesiologists' Committee on Regional Anesthesia, Executive Committee, and Administrative Council. *J Pain*, 17(2):131–57.

Clarke, H., Bonin, R.P., Orser, B.A., *et al.* (2012) The prevention *of* chronic postsurgical pain using gabapentin and pregabalin: A combined systematic review and meta-analysis. *Anesth Analg*, 115(2):428–42.

Clinical Skills (2014) Management of continuous epidural infusions, Part 1: Insertion. Available at: http://www.clinicalskills.net; accessed 9 December 2019.

Cohen, S., Mao, J. (2014) Neuropathic pain mechanisms and their clinical implications *Br Med J*, 348:7656.

Cook, T., Counsell, D., Wildsmith., J. (2009) on behalf of the Royal College of Anaesthetists (RCoA). Major complications of central neuraxial block: Report on the Third National Audit Project of the Royal College of Anaesthetists. *Br J Anaesth*, 102(2):179–90.

Descartes, R. Clerselier C., La Forge L., *et al.* (1664) *L'homme et un Traitté de la formation du Foetus du Mesme Autheur*. Paris: Charles Angot (cited in Moayedi M., and Davis K., 2013).

Dickenson, A. (2015) Update on pain Mechanisms (Online) Available at: http://www.paincommunitycentre.org/article/update-pain-mechanisms-tony-dickenson; accessed 10 December 2019.

Eipe, N., Gupta, S., Penning, J. (2016) Intravenous lidocaine for acute pain: An evidence-based clinical update. *BJA Education*, 16(9):292–8.

Erb W., (1874) *Handbuch der Krankheiten des Nervensystems II* (F.C.W. Vogel, Leipzig) (cited in: Perl E., (2011) Pain Mechanisms: A Commentary on Concepts & Issues) *Prog Neurobiol*, 94(1):20–38.

Gregory, J., Richardson, C. (2014) The use of pain assessment tools in clinical practice: A pilot survey. *Journal of Pain and Relief*, 3(2):140–6.

Gregory, J., Vernon, C., Onwudike, F., *et al.* (2014) The Bolton Pain assessment tool: Devising and implementing a pain assessment tool for patients unable to communicate. *Age Ageing*, 43 (Suppl 2):ii1.

Grisell, V.S. (2010) Is the WHO analgesic ladder still valid? Twenty-four years of experience. *Can Fam Physician*, 56(6):514–17.

Harrop-Griffiths, W., Cook, T., Gill, H., *et al.* (2013) Regional anaesthesia and patients with abnormalities of anticoagulation. *Anaesthesia*, 68(9):966–72.

Hardy, J., Wolff, H.G., and Goodell, H., (1940) Studies on Pain. A new method for measuring pain threshold: observations on spatial summation of pain. *J Clin Invest*, 19(4):649–57.

Ingalls, N.K., Horton, Z.A., Bettendorf, M., *et al.* (2010) Randomised, double-blind, placebo-controlled trial using lidocaine patch 5% in traumatic rib fractures. *J Am Col Surg*, 210(2):205–9.

International Association for the Study of Pain (IASP) (2012) Definition of Pain. Available at: http://www.iasp-pain.org/Taxonomy; accessed 9 December 2019.

Kehlet, H., Holte, K. (2001) Effect of postoperative analgesia on surgical outcome. *Br J Anaesth*, 87(1):62–72.

Macintyre, P.E., Schug, S.A. (2015) *Acute Pain Management: A Practical Guide* 4th edn. Boca Raton, FL: CRC Press

Medicines and Healthcare products Regulatory Agency (MHRA) Guidance (2009) Non-steroidal anti-inflammatory drugs (NSAIDs): Reminder on renal failure and impairment. Available at: https://www.gov.uk/drug-safety-update/non-steroidal-anti-inflammatory-drugs-nsaids-reminder-on-renal-failure-and-impairment; accessed 9 December 2019.

Melzack, R., and Wall, P., (1965) Pain Mechanisms: A new theory. *Science*, 150(3699):971–9.

Moayedi, M., and Davis, K. (2013) Theories of pain: From specificity to gate control. *J Neurophysiol*, 109:5–12.

Muller J. (1840) *Handbuch der Physiologie des Menschen für Vorlesungen*. Coblenz: Verlag von J. Hölscher, (cited in Moayedi M., and Davis K., 2013).

Neal, M.J. (2016) *Medical Pharmacology at a Glance* 8th edn. Chichester: Wiley Blackwell.

NICE (2015a) Non-Steroidal Anti-inflammatory Drugs. Available at: https://www.nice.org.uk/guidance/ktt13/resources/nonsteroidal-antiinflammatory-drugs-58757951055301; accessed 9 December 2019.

NICE (2015b) Scenario: Weak Opioids. Available at: https://cks.nice.org.uk/analgesia-mild-to-moderate-pain#!scenario:4; accessed 9 December 2019.

NICE (2016) Major Trauma: Assessment and Initial Management. Available at: http://www.nice.org.uk/guidance/ng39; accessed 9 December 2019.

NICE (2017a) Guidance for Gabapentin in Renal Disease. Available at: https://www.evidence.nhs.uk/formulary/bnf/current/4-central-nervous-system/48-antiepileptic-drugs/481-control-of-the-epilepsies/gabapentin-and-pregabalin/gabapentin; accessed 9 December 2019.

NICE (2017a) Neuropathic Pain: Pharmacological Management (Online). Available at: https://www.nice.org.uk/guidance/cg173/evidence/full-guideline-pdf-191621341; accessed 9 December 2019.

NPSA Alert (2011) Safer spinal (intrathecal), epidural and regional devices. Available at: http://www.nrls.npsa.nhs.uk/resources/?entryid45=94529; accessed 9 December 2019.

NPSA Alert (2014) Risk of distress and death from inappropriate doses of naloxone in patients on long-term opioid/opiate treatment. Available at: https://www.england.nhs.uk/wp-content/uploads/2014/11/psa-inappropriate-doses-naloxone.pdf; accessed 9 December 2019.

Parras, T. (2015) Case series: Serratus plane block for rib fracture analgesia: Trunk blocks. Available at: https://academy.esraeurope.org/esra/2015/34th/105289/teresa.parras.case.series.serratus.plane.block.for.rib.fracture.analgesia.html?f=m2t1159; accessed 9 December 2019.

Pond, S., Tozer, T. (1984) First-pass elimination: Basic concepts and clinical consequences. *Clin Pharmacokinet*, 9(1):1–25.

Royal College of Anaesthetists (2010) Best Practice in the Management of Epidural Analgesia in the hospital setting. Available at: https://www.britishpainsociety.org/static/uploads/resources/files/pub_prof_EpiduralAnalgesia2010.pdf; accessed January 2020.

Royal College of Anaesthetists (2017) Opioids Aware: A resource for patients and healthcare professionals to support prescribing of opioid medicines for pain. Available at: http://www.fpm.ac.uk/faculty-of-pain-medicine/opioids-aware; accessed 9 December 2019.

Strong, C.A. (1895) The psychology of pain. *Psychol Rev*, 2(4):329–47.

Stundner, O., Memtsoudis, S.G. (2017) Regional anesthesia and analgesia in critically ill patients: A systematic review. *Rev Esp Anestesiol Reanim*, 64(3):144–56.

Sullivan, M., Feuerstein, M., Gatchel, R., *et al.* (2006) Integrating psychosocial and behavioural interventions to achieve optimal rehabilitation outcomes. *J Occup Rehabil*, 15:475.

Tarkkila, P., (2017) Spinal Anesthesia: Safe Practice and Management of Adverse Events in B. Finucane and B. Tsui (eds). New York, NY: Springer, pp. 245–58.

Varndell, W., Fry, M., Elliott, D. (2017) A systematic review of observational pain assessment instruments for use with nonverbal intubated critically ill adult patients in the emergency department: An assessment of their suitability and psychometric properties. *J Clin Nurs*, 26(1–2):7–32.

Von Frey, M. (1895) Beiträge zur physiologie des schmerzsinns. *Königl. Sächs. Ges. Wiss., Math. Phys. Classe* 46:185–96 (cited in Melzack R. and Wall P. 1965).

World Health Organization (WHO) ladder (1996) Cancer Pain Relief. Available at: http://apps.who.int/iris/bitstream/10665/37896/1/9241544821.pdf; accessed 9 December 2019.

Zink, K.A., Mayberry, J.C., Peck, E.G., *et al.* (2011) Lidocaine patches reduce pain in trauma patients with rib fractures. *American Surgeon*, 77(4):238–442.

10
Systematic assessment, early warning scores, and patient escalation

Fiona Creed

Chapter contents

The need for rapid and accurate assessment, treatment, and escalation of the patient whose condition is deteriorating is beyond refute. Several initiatives have been developed to facilitate this and most focus upon an ABCDE-type (Airway, Breathing, Circulation, Disability, and Exposure) assessment tool (Resuscitation Council 2015) and use of an Early Warning Score (RCP 2012/ 2017).

Understanding the importance of assessment, interpretation of findings, and escalation are important determinants of patient outcome (RCP 2012). Therefore, this chapter will focus on:

- systematic assessment using an ABCDE approach
- understanding of alterations in observations and their significance to the patient's condition
- the use of track-and-trigger tools to facilitate the assessment and escalation of patients whose condition is deteriorating
- the use of electronic early warning scores
- appropriate escalation of the patient whose condition is deteriorating
- the use of communication tools to communicate concern
- the role of critical care outreach/patient at risk teams
- the deteriorating patient in the community setting

Learning outcomes

This chapter will enable you to:

- apply systematic assessment principles to your patient
- explore signs of deterioration and how they may be identified during patient assessment
- explore the need for robust escalation systems
- understand the need for an updated track-and-trigger system (NEWS2)
- review the need for effective communication and escalation protocols

- explore the role of critical care outreach and medical emergency teams
- consider how these tools may be utilized in the community setting

Systematic assessment: A stepwise approach to assessment

The Acute Life-Threatening Events Recognition and Treatment tool (ALERT©) was first introduced by Smith in 2003. This teaching programme focused upon an A–E assessment encouraging practitioners initially to identify potentially life-threatening problems using a look and listen approach. Since the implementation of the programme, this systematic assessment tool has been widely implemented to acute and, more recently, community settings (Salim 2014). Several adaptions of this tool have been introduced into clinical practice including the A–G assessment (Benson 2017). For the purpose of simplicity and standardization, the book will focus upon the A–E assessment advocated by the Resuscitation Council (2015). Variations will be discussed, and limitations of the system identified.

The ABCDE tool

The Resuscitation Council (2015) emphasizes the need to complete all stages of the tool if the patient's condition permits. Simple alterations to patient treatment should be implemented as assessment progresses in an endeavour to rectify the abnormality and practitioners are advised to follow the assessment and initial treatment recommendations for each step. However, if a life-threatening alteration is detected help should be summoned immediately and appropriate protocols followed (see Chapter 11). Practitioners are reminded that this tool should be used in conjunction with clinical expertise and professional judgement.

Step 1: Assessment of patient airway

Airway obstruction is a medical emergency and requires immediate medical attention. If there are concerns about the patient's ability to maintain their airway emergency help should be summoned. Most patients' airway patency can be assessed by means of asking a question. If the patient can clearly speak it is unlikely that there will be airway patency issues. However, if there is concern further assessment may be required. This should include visual, auditory, and tactile assessment.

Visual signs of airway obstruction include: changes in patient colour such as pallor or central cyanosis, paradoxical chest movement, or no chest movement. If the patient is awake and has aspirated food or a foreign object, the patient may also look panicked.

Auditory signs of airway obstruction vary depending upon the severity of obstruction. For partial obstruction noises such as snoring, gurgling, wheezing, coughing, and stridor may be evident. These may be rectified by the use of suction, airway adjuncts, and changes to patient position. If patients do not respond to these interventions immediate help should be summoned. If there is absence of sound, total airway obstruction should be suspected and practitioners can feel for the presence of air movement by simply placing their hand over the patient's mouth and noting whether respiration is taking place. If this is absent and there is no respiratory effort this situation requires advanced airway management skills; immediate help should be summoned because untreated airway obstruction can quickly lead to cardiac arrest and patient death (Resuscitation Council, 2015).

Step 2: Assessment of breathing

Assessment of respiratory effort is an important and often overlooked aspect of patient assessment. A full description of respiratory assessment is included in Chapter 2, however; an abridged version is included here to facilitate a timely respiratory assessment.

The Resuscitation Council (2015) advocates that visual inspection is a critical aspect of assessment and should include observation of respiratory rate and the pattern and depth of respiration. The patient's colour and visual signs of respiratory failure such as pallor, central cyanosis, and diaphoresis should be observed. If equipment is available then recording of oxygen saturations is helpful and these should be interpreted in the light of the oxygen requirement of the patient. It is important to remember that release of the vasopressor catecholamines in response to acute illness may cause peripheral vasoconstriction: in this event centrally recorded saturations are more reliable.

The nature of chest movement (bilateral or unilateral) and shape of the thorax should be observed for signs of kyphosis, scoliosis, or anything else that might impede breathing (such as obvious thoracic injury). The increased use of accessory muscles should also be noted as this indicates worsening respiration function and may be related to changes in ventilation and gaseous exchange. This may be best observed from the foot of the bed (Bickley *et al.* 2017).

Advanced visual inspection may also include observation of tracheal deviation (as this indicates mediastinal shift and may be indicative of tension pneumothorax). Raised jugular venous distension (JVD) should also be noted; this may indicate tension pneumothorax or worsening air trapping in severe asthma. It is important also to inspect the abdomen as diaphragmatic splinting may occur in patients with obesity, abdominal distension, and pregnancy. In this case a semi-recumbent position may be favoured to reduce splinting and thus improve ventilation and gaseous exchange.

Initial auditory assessment can be performed without the use of equipment and practitioners are advised to assess for obvious audible sounds such as coughing, wheezing, and stridor that may indicate patient deterioration such as worsening infection, asthma, and partial airway obstruction.

Chest auscultation is an important tool in the assessment of an acutely breathless patient. From 2020 all pre-registration nurse education will include training in chest auscultation (NMC 2017). Practitioners are advised to auscultate the chest in a systematic manner noting for any concerns. Of particular importance are reduced or absent sounds and adventitious sounds (see Chapter 2).

In certain groups of patients such as trauma and post-surgical patients it may be useful to palpate the chest for signs of surgical emphysema or crepitus.

The assessment of respiratory status should also consider the patient's perception of the difficulty associated with breathing. This is referred to as dyspnoea and is a particularly useful measure in patients with chronic lung disease who may present with signs of respiratory failure, but this is 'normal' for that patient. Understanding how this presentation compares to their 'normal' is useful in this group of patients and will indicate when concern is warranted.

Assessment of the inspired oxygen concentration is useful and should include observation of an increasing need for oxygen as this requires urgent escalation (Resuscitation Council 2015; Vaughan and Parry 2016).

Initial treatment may include simple steps such as alteration in position if the patient's condition permits. In the majority of patients an upright position facilitates ventilation and gaseous exchange, but professional judgement should be used and consideration given to other injuries or conditions that may prohibit position change. Oxygen should be administered in accordance with the British Thoracic Society guidance (2017). Psychological support and reassurance is paramount for the patient as acute breathlessness is a frightening experience. Frequent reassessment is required in patients with deteriorating respiratory function and if there is concern then the patient should not be left unattended and should be supervised by a registered practitioner.

Step 3: Assessment of cardiovascular status

The assessment of circulatory status should include general observation of the patient, alongside recording of cardiovascular measurements (Vaughan and Parry 2016).

Initial assessment of patient colour may identify circulatory problems therefore patients should be observed for pallor, flushing, or cyanosis. Peripheral vasoconstriction and diaphoresis are indicators of deterioration and should be noted. The Resuscitation Council (2015) suggests noting for presence of intravenous cannulae as venous access may be required for more advanced treatment.

Following initial assessment, the patient's radial pulse should be recorded manually. The pulse should be felt for one minute noting for rate, regularity, and strength/magnitude. Patients presenting with excessively fast heart rates may require early anti-arrhythmic medication and urgent medical attention should be sought. Patients with bradycardia should also trigger a review.

The patient's skin temperature should be felt as this may indicate vasoconstriction or vasodilation. If vasoconstriction is noted, it may be useful to note the level (e.g. cold peripheries to ankle/knee level) as this may indicate severity of deterioration. Capillary refill may be a useful indicator (normal is less than 2 s). This may not be a helpful measure in patients with hypothermia, peripheral vascular disease, and the elderly.

Blood pressure must be recorded. In acute deterioration an electronic device may not function and it may be necessary to revert to manual recordings of blood pressure. The practitioner should note the systolic, diastolic pressures and also consider the pulse pressure and mean arterial pressure. Note however that in early stages of deterioration the systolic blood pressure may appear to be within normal parameters.

Additional cardiovascular assessment should include assessment of fluid status. This is often problematic in clinical practice and the NICE (2013) fluid guidance highlights the importance of practitioners understanding other signs of fluid depletion/fluid overload (see Chapter 8) as fluid balance charts may not be available or may be poorly recorded and inaccurate. Measurement of urine output may be advisable and, in some patients, urinary catheter insertion may be required to facilitate accurate fluid balance assessment.

Sepsis is an increasingly common issue in clinical practice (Sepsis Trust 2017). Vaughan and Parry (2016) highlight the need to record the temperature during the systematic assessment. Within the literature there is conflicting evidence about where, in the systematic ABCDE process, to record the temperature. This is arbitrary as temperature changes may significantly impact upon cardiovascular stability it would appear fitting to include it with cardiovascular assessment, however RCP (2017) guidance includes temperature assessment with exposure and therefore assessment occurs later in the NEWS2 assessment process. If a clinically significant pyrexia is noted the sepsis guidance from NICE (2016) should be rapidly implemented (see Chapter 8).

More advanced assessment may be required such as recording and accurate interpretation of cardiac rhythm, 12-lead ECGs (electrocardiograms), and cardiac auscultation (see Chapter 3). It is also advisable to check for the presence of chest pain, which may be indicative of cardiac disease, and to review the patient's medication prescription as polypharmacy in the elderly may impact upon cardiovascular findings (Cowan 2015).

Initial treatment should include repositioning of the patient. For most patients presenting with hypotension an upright position is detrimental due to the impact of gravity on circulation. It is generally advisable to lower the bedhead of the patient to recumbent or semi-recumbent position. Conflicting evidence exists exploring the usefulness of elevating the patient's feet. In some patients with cardiac conditions, this position is not advisable and professional judgement should be used and Nurse Specialist/medical advice should be sought if unsure.

The practitioner should increase the frequency of observations and may consider the need for advanced cardiovascular monitoring tools such as a 3- or 5-lead ECG. It may be necessary to begin automated blood pressure recordings. In both incidences appropriate alarm parameters should be set to notify the practitioner of changes in the patient's condition.

It is advisable to seek advice for cannula insertion as this may be required for medication or fluids in the acutely ill patient. Fluid resuscitation may be utilized and this should be in consultation with the medical staff unless you are working in a level 2/3 area where goal-directed fluids are prescribed. Fluid resuscitation should be in accordance to the NICE (2013) guidance noting that attention is required when caring for elderly patients and patients with a history of cardiac or renal disease. In patients presenting with right- or left-sided heart failure, fluid resuscitation is not generally recommended and medication may be required to improve blood pressure.

Frequent reassessment is required in patients with deteriorating cardiovascular function and if there is concern the patient should not be left unattended and should be supervised by a registered practitioner.

Step 4: Assessment of neurological status (disability assessment)

For the majority of patients, a simplistic ACVPU tool can be used to assess consciousness levels (see Chapter 4 to review when a formal neurological assessment encompassing the Glasgow Coma Scale may be required). The patient should be assessed to determine whether they are:

- Awake/Alert
- **Confused**/New confusion noted
- Awoken to **Voice**
- Awoken to **Pain**
- Are **Unarousable/Unconscious**

The patient's pain levels should also be assessed as this may be a physiological sign of deterioration. Pain should be assessed using a systematic pain assessment tool (see Chapter 9). It is also important to note that pain may be indicative of deterioration; for example, abdominal pain may indicate haemorrhage. Therefore, it is vital to understand the cause of the pain prior to its treatment. Analgesia may worsen hypotension and therefore should be used with caution in patients presenting with cardiovascular instability.

Changes in neurological function may impact upon the patient's ability to maintain their airway and to maintain a safe environment. Frequent reassessment is required in patients with deteriorating neurological function and if there is concern the patient should not be left unattended and should be supervised by a registered practitioner.

Step 5a: Exposure

Having completed an A–D assessment it is vital to examine the patient for potential causes of deterioration if these have not already been identified. During exposure it will be necessary to expose the patient's body fully to observe for indicators of the cause of deterioration. If this is required it is essential to respect the patient's dignity and maintain a compassionate approach whilst minimizing heat loss. It is important to examine the patient from head to toe and back to front, clearly explaining each step to the patient and gaining consent where possible (Barker 2015).

It is important to look for any obvious signs of injury (traumatic or otherwise) and signs that may indicate reasons for respiratory failure or shock.

Respiratory distress: check legs for swelling pain and redness that may indicate the presence of a venous thromboembolism (VTE). In patients with centrally inserted cannulae it is possible to have a thrombus in the arms. If signs of VTE are present, urgent medical attention is required.

Hypovolemic shock: observe for signs of external haemorrhage or fluid loss. Review wounds and wound drains if they are present. Remember in some instances blood loss may be underneath the patient and it is important to roll the patient over to observe for this. Observe for signs of internal haemorrhage such as swelling/distension and increased pain. Remember a significant amount of blood can be lost into the peritoneal cavity before abdominal distension occurs, and the first sign may be patient discomfort and worsening pain.

Sepsis: observe for signs of infection in wound sites, line sites, drains, and other invasive devices. Observe patient color and general presentation. In the early stages patients may be flushed and vasodilated; in later stages they may present with mottling and feel cool to touch. Some patients with sepsis may present with peripheral oedema due to fluid shifts (see Chapter 8).

Anaphylaxis: patients may present with extreme breathlessness, wheezing, stridor, angioedema, urticarial rashes, and marked flushing due to vasodilation as a result of the non-specific immune response. If intravenous medication or blood is in progress it should be immediately stopped and the lines disconnected from the patient to avoid further infusion (see Chapters 7 and 8).

Where possible the patient's recent blood results, recent investigation results, medication charts, and nursing/medical notes should be reviewed and available to the attending medical team.

Step 5b: Escalation

The need for prompt escalation is noted throughout the literature (NICE 2016; Waldie *et al.* 2016). It is important when escalating care that the patient is referred to the appropriate medical practitioner and communication is effective. These will be discussed later in the chapter in the section on track-and-trigger and communication tools.

Alterations to ABCDE assessment tools

Some Trusts and publications (e.g. Benson 2017) may advocate the use of a different tool and there is discussion within the literature for an A–G tool, the last two elements referring to:

F = **Fluids:** assessment of input/output and assessment of fluid status
G = **Glucose:** assessment and management of blood glucose status

However, the difference is negligible as the assessment contains all the same elements but in a slightly different order. For sake of ease, the Resuscitation Council (2015) guidance has been used in this chapter. Perhaps the most significant thing to consider is not variations in tools but interpretation of clinical signs and symptoms, the need for timely escalation and intervention, and the vital need for accurate documentation of all events.

Interpretation of clinical signs of deterioration

Registered professionals are expected to be able to assess the patient accurately and, more importantly, comprehend the significance of the changes in physiological signs so that they can appropriately manage the care of patients whose condition is deteriorating (NICE 2012).

Alterations in respiratory rate

Respiratory rate changes are arguably the most sensitive indicator of deterioration (Elliot 2016). Increases in respiratory rate can occur due to many causes and further detailed information is given in Chapter 2. However simplistically, chemoreceptors will detect changes in blood carbon dioxide levels, oxygen levels, and pH, and this will trigger an increase in respiratory rate. The respiratory system may indicate metabolic and/or respiratory disturbances and is therefore an important indicator of patient deterioration. It is therefore the initial cardinal sign of patient deterioration. It is argued that an increase in the respiratory rate by just three to five breaths may be clinically significant and should certainly prompt closer observation unless there is an obvious cause (Elliot 2016).

A study by Gerogake and colleagues (2012) identified that respiratory rate is the most frequently omitted vital sign and this study also suggested that there is an over reliance on other variables, such as the oxygen saturation. Mok and colleagues (2015) identified that a quarter of nurses erroneously felt that oxygen saturation can effectively replace respiratory observation. It is important to acknowledge that compensatory mechanisms will normalize saturation recordings in the early stages of deterioration and therefore it should never be used as a replacement for accurate respiratory assessment. Mok and colleagues (2015) argue that staff should be more aware of signs that may indicate deterioration such as:

- an increasing respiratory rate, when resting;
- staccato speech;
- increased workload of breathing (increased use of accessory muscles, nasal flaring, increased depth and effort);
- reports of dyspnoea; and
- patient's colour and appearance.

A reduction in respiratory rate is also another potential sign of deterioration. Low respiratory rates may indicate central nervous system (CNS) depression or narcosis and prompt intervention is required if the respiratory rate is low (RCP 2012).

Changes in oxygen saturation

There is limited evidence that this is an effective early sign of deterioration as increased respiratory rate in the early stages of deterioration may ensure normal oxygen saturation levels (Mok *et al.* 2015). Whilst it is included in the National Early Warning Score (NEWS) calculation (RCP 2012), it is important to note that:

- saturation provides no indication of the adequacy of ventilation (Mok *et al.* 2012; Elliot 2016).
- a variety of factors will affect the accuracy of saturation recording such as poor perfusion, anaemia, arrhythmia, bright lighting, skin colouration, and reduced temperature. Nurses should be aware of factors that limit the reliability of saturation measurements (NICE 2012).
- it may be inaccurate in the acutely ill patient due to peripheral circulation compromise.
- it should always be viewed in the light of the patient's oxygen demand. Therefore, a patient with an increasing oxygen demand and decreasing saturation is of particular concern.
- a patient's comorbidities should be taken into account, in particular in patients with suspected hypercapnic respiratory failure.

Changes in heart rate

Variations in the heart rate are important to acknowledge and these should be assessed in conjunction with the strength of the pulse. Bradycardia and tachycardia may both be signs of patient deterioration.

Tachycardia may be a result of a cardiac condition and patients with cardiac conditions may require additional monitoring and serial ECGs to assess for cardiac abnormality.

Tachycardia will also occur in most shock states and is caused by the release of catecholamines as part of the compensatory mechanism.

It is important to note here that most of ventricular and coronary artery filling occurs during diastole. When heart rate increases, diastolic time reduces and so, if the heart rate increase is excessive, reductions in cardiac output and coronary perfusion may result. This will be reflected in changes to the blood pressure and possibly the onset of ischaemic chest pain and is more likely to occur in the elderly and in patients with pre-existing cardiac conditions.

Additionally, it is important to consider the heart rate in relation to the systolic pressure (the Portsmouth sign) as this may be a useful indicator of patient deterioration. Concern should be raised if the patient's heart rate is higher than the systolic pressure. This may indicate that the patient's cardiovascular status is significantly compromised. The NEWS2 chart prohibits the plotting of these two variables in the same section and Christofidus and colleagues (2014) argue that there is no evidence to suggest that plotting blood pressure (BP) and heart rate together increases identification of deterioration. However, it is important to acknowledge that this a late sign of patient deterioration and therefore requires rapid escalation.

Elderly patients and patients on β-blockade may not exhibit normal tachycardia responses and it is important that the patient's observations are reviewed in an holistic manner and medication history reviewed, especially if other clinical signs of deterioration are present.

Bradycardia may be caused by certain drugs, cardiac conditions, and diseased cardiac conduction pathways or raised intracranial pressure. Severe bradycardia will have a direct effect on blood pressure and this may drop dramatically. Patients with bradycardia may benefit from continuous ECG measurement and this should be instigated immediately if there is concern about the patient's heart rate or rhythm. It may be beneficial, if the patient is sufficiently stable, to record a 12-lead ECG whilst waiting for review from the medical staff (see Chapter 3).

Changes in blood pressure

It is important to state that the blood pressure will remain stable during the initial stages of deterioration because of the effects of compensatory catecholamines and other stress hormones (Felton 2012). The release of adrenalin, noradrenalin, and arginine vasopressin causes vasoconstriction and increased rate and contractility of the heart muscle. These responses divert the blood away from the peripheries, increase cardiac output, and thus increase blood pressure. The patient therefore may appear to be stable until compensatory mechanisms fail. Generally, the systolic blood pressure will not reduce until approximately one-third of the circulating volume has been depleted or the heart begins to fail. It is also worth noting that the advent of track-and-trigger systems has caused an emphasis on the recording and interpretation of the systolic pressure and this is unfortunate as in the early stages all elements of the blood pressure should be considered.

Perhaps the most significance measurement is the diastolic pressure. During compensatory mechanisms the diastolic pressure will begin to increase as the patient develops vasoconstriction. The importance of this is often overlooked and it is vital to look out for an increasing diastolic pressure with a normal or slightly elevated systolic pressure. This may reflect the presence of compensatory mechanisms and can be an early warning of impending deterioration.

The pulse pressure is another important and often overlooked indicator of deterioration. The pulse pressure is a simple calculated value:

$$\text{Pulse pressure} = \text{Systolic Pressure} - \text{Diastolic Pressure}$$

A decreasing or narrowing pulse pressure may indicate vasoconstriction and may be suggestive of hypovolaemic or cardiogenic shock. An increasing or widening pulse pressure may be indicative of vasodilatation and may suggest sepsis or the early stages of anaphylaxis.

The mean arterial pressure (MAP) is another important indicator as this reflects perfusion of major organs. Most electronic sphygmomanometers will display the MAP, but this is generally not documented in most clinical settings. A MAP of 60 is generally required to maintain adequate organ perfusion; below this level, blood flow to the organs is compromised. Elderly patients or those with persistent or untreated hypertension may require a higher MAP to perfuse organs.

It is essential to compare current readings with normal blood pressure readings. A drop of pressure from normal may indicate patient deterioration but if the patient is normally hypertensive this may not trigger on NEWS2 scores. Therefore, it is important to investigate the cause of a drop from the patient's norm as this may also signify deterioration.

Hypertension is given less weighting in the context of acute-illness assessment. There are a number of causes of hypertension and typically hypertension may be seen in the context of pain or increased anxiety in acute care settings (RCP 2017). However systolic blood pressure increases should be noted and escalated if there are any causes of concern. Persistent hypertension will require medical assessment and potential intervention with antihypertensive medication.

Changes in temperature

It is important to note for changes to temperature that may indicate patient deterioration. There are, of course several reasons for a raised temperature but it is important to treat any raise in temperature (above 38.1°C) as potential sepsis, especially if accompanied by other indicators (see Box 10.1) which indicates that infection may be present and medical attention sought.

Presence of a red flag (see Box 10.2) indicator indicates the need for an immediate medical response and instigation of an appropriate sepsis bundle.

Box 10.1 Signs of sepsis

Are any of the following two features present?

- Temperature > 38.1°C or < 36°C
- Respiratory rate > 20 per minute
- Heart rate > 90 per minute
- Acute confusion/ reduced conscious level
- Glucose > 7.7 mmol/l (unless diabetes mellitus)

Source data from NICE 2016 Sepsis: recognition, diagnosis and early management NG51. London: TSO.

Further discussion on the assessment and management of the septic patient is included in Chapter 8.

Hypothermia is defined as a temperature below 35°C. Potential causes of hypothermia should be evaluated and include:

- environmental factors
- exposure
- large fluid replacement
- massive blood transfusion
- post-operative complications
- extra corporeal blood circulation (e.g. dialysis)

The practitioner should monitor for side effects of hypothermia (cardiac arrhythmias, blood coagulopathies, hypotension, etc.) and attempt to increase core body temperature slowly.

Box 10.2 Red flag criteria

- Systolic BP < 90 mmHg or MAP < 65 mmHg
- Lactate > 2 mmol/l
- Heart rate > 130 per minute
- Respiratory rate > 25 per minute
- Oxygen saturations < 91%
- Responds only to voice or pain/unresponsive
- Purpuric rash

Source data from NICE 2016 Sepsis: recognition, diagnosis and early management NG51. London: TSO.

Changes in consciousness levels

The Resuscitation Council (2015) identifies that causes of reduced consciousness may include hypoxia, hypercapnia, cerebral hypoperfusion, or the recent administration of sedatives or analgesic drugs. Where possible these should be reviewed to investigate whether they are impacting on the patient's consciousness.

Additionally, it is important to remember that one of the most common causes of deterioration/alteration in consciousness is changes in blood glucose levels. A blood glucose level should be recorded. The practitioner should note that hypoglycaemia may be accompanied by increasing confusion, agitation, or lack of patient cooperation. Patients with hypoglycaemia are prone to rapid deterioration because of the detrimental effects of hypoglycaemia on the central nervous system. It is therefore essential that hypoglycaemia is quickly identified and managed following guidance from the Joint British Diabetes Society guidelines (2013).

Hyperglycaemia may also affect consciousness levels; again, this is normally accompanied by other signs such as Kussmaul's respirations, extreme thirst, excessive urine output, and signs of dehydration. This should also be managed in accordance the British Joint Diabetes Society guidelines (2013).

New confusion or worsening confusion is a common sign of deterioration in patients (especially elderly patients). The RCP (2017) highlight that deteriorating mental status may represent sepsis, hypoxia, hypotension, or metabolic disturbance, all of which should be considered within the assessment process.

Changes in other physiological variables

It is important for the practising nurse to identify other variables that may be impacted by deteriorating conditions. These variables for many complex reasons do not add to the numerical rating of the aggregated NEW score (RCP 2017), however; they may allow the nurse to identify other important clinical signs of deterioration. These include:

- urine output
- pain
- age and comorbidities
- changes in blood analysis

Urine output

In shocked states the body will normally attempt to conserve water by releasing anti-diuretic hormone and aldosterone. Anti-diuretic hormone causes adaptations to the renal tubule, increasing the amount of fluid reabsorbed. Aldosterone increases renal reabsorption of sodium and thus increases retention of fluid. Both these mechanisms will see a decreased urine output that is often concentrated in nature with a high osmolality.

In the later stages of deterioration, the urine output may be affected by decreased perfusion to the kidneys. In health the kidneys require a constant perfusion pressure in order to function effectively. If the MAP drops below 60 mmHg for any sustained period of time renal function will deteriorate. NICE (2013) identify the importance in assessing urine output. Any signs of oliguria (a urine output less than 0.5 mL/kg /hr.) may indicate development of acute kidney injury (AKI). They identify that other associated factors such as sepsis, hypovolaemia, and increasing early warning scores may increase the likelihood of AKI. Any episodes of oliguria should be escalated to the medical staff and immediate treatment required (see Chapter 5).

There are fewer incidences of increased urine output signifying patient deterioration. Nurses caring for patients with acquired brain injury (head injury/stroke/subarachnoid haemorrhage) should be alert to excessive urine output as these may indicate the presence of either cerebral salt wasting or diabetes insipidus. Most cases of diabetes insipidus are caused by damage to the pituitary gland, inhibiting the release of anti-diuretic hormone, and are normally related to head injury and increasing intracerebral pressure. Cerebral salt wasting is caused by excessive sodium excretion by the kidney which in turn causes excessive water removal (due to the effect of the osmotic gradient caused by sodium). Both these conditions require immediate medical escalation as prompt medical intervention is necessary to prevent dehydration, sodium imbalance, and associated impact on the cardiovascular and central nervous systems.

Pain

Assessment of pain is important in acutely ill patients for a number of reasons:

- Practitioners have a professional and ethical duty to ensure that adequate analgesia is provided to all patients.
- The presence of pain may adversely affect some of the core variables. Heart rate and respiratory rate may be increased in the presence of pain and it is useful to exclude pain as the cause for any changes documented.
- Analgesia may directly affect the core variables; in particular, opiate-based analgesia may cause hypotension, bradycardia, or tachycardia, and may cause respiratory depression. Side effects of analgesia require careful monitoring in the acute patient.
- Increases in pain levels may be signs of the patient's condition worsening; for example, increased levels of pain in a patient who has undergone abdominal surgery, may indicate haemorrhage.
- Although pain assessment is clearly relevant in assessment of the acutely ill adult the Royal College of Physicians (2017) has decided to exclude the pain score from the aggregate value that triggers escalation. However, a pain score is documented on the chart as the RCP identifies the importance of assessing pain in acutely ill adults and feel the presence of a pain score will encourage assessment of levels of pain. There appears to be little guidance on type of score to use and therefore local policy should be followed, and concerns escalated if pain is increasing or failing to respond to analgesia.

Age and comorbidities

The RCP (2017) highlights that deterioration is more likely in older patients and those patients who present with comorbidities or immunosuppression. However, the RCP (2017) argues that chronological age is not always a good indicator of biological age. Patients with complex comorbidities may require assessment using a range of different tools and these should be discussed with the medical team. The need to include NEWS2 in a patient's generic assessment is emphasized.

Changes in blood analysis

Blood results may enable the medical staff to make a differential diagnosis. A large number of blood results may be requested when caring for an acutely ill adult. However, the complexity and range of blood results available prohibit their use on a track-and-trigger scoring system. Commonly requested blood tests in acute situations include:

- suspected bleeding: full blood count, clotting studies
- suspected infection: full blood count (white cell count and neutrophils), C-reactive protein, blood lactate
- suspected respiratory problems: full blood count, arterial blood gas analysis
- fluid overload: full blood count (haematocrit), urea, and electrolytes
- suspected pulmonary embolism: full blood count, clotting studies, D-dimers

This list is not extensive and other blood tests and investigations may be requested by the medical team. It is useful to locate recent blood results for the patient wherever possible as the medical team may require these to make a differential diagnosis.

Early warning scores

A variety of early warning systems are utilized throughout the world and these may be single parameter (usually respiration rate or nurses concern) or aggregate scores (each abnormal variable measurement receives a value and the score is added together to form an aggregate score).

In 2012 in the United Kingdom, the Royal College of Physicians initially launched the National Early Warning Score (NEWS) in an attempt to standardize assessment of acutely ill patients across the country. Other countries such as Ireland have also implemented National Early Warning Scores (National Clinical Effectiveness Committee 2013). Both these tools provide national aggregate scores which standardize assessment and associated scoring and have several benefits which include:

- standardization of a format to facilitate recognition of the deteriorating patient;
- potential to standardize training and education packages for staff who deliver acute hospital care;

- standard response to deterioration across the United Kingdom;
- potential to standardize assessment pre-hospital with a growing move to utilize NEWS systems in community and primary care settings;
- an opportunity to allow standardized data collection and analysis in relation to acute deterioration;
- an ability to develop severity of illness protocols that could impact upon resourcing the delivery of care to this group of patients.

Evaluation of the National Early Warning Score tools is ongoing. The York and Humber Academic Health Science Network (2014) identifies that aggregate scores appear to be more beneficial than single parameter scores and this would therefore support the development of the NEWS system. They also identified that Early Warning Scores (EWS) appear to work better in surgical patient populations where deterioration patterns are perhaps more predictable. They also identified several issues arising from use of EWS. These included some doubts about the accuracy of the recorded information on the systems which at times was compounded by inaccuracies in the calculation of an aggregate score when manual EWS systems are utilized.

Other studies have highlighted the potential advantages of the NEWS system. An early review of the NEWS tool by Smith and colleagues (2013) found that the NEWS score enabled more accurate discrimination of patients at risk of cardiac arrest and unanticipated admission to critical care than 33 previous EWS reviewed in their study. Subsequent work by Abbott and colleagues (2015) echoes the view that the NEWS provides an increased sensitivity for identifying patients at risk of deterioration and cardiac arrest.

More recent discussions have highlighted the use of NEWS in certain subgroups of patients including those with chronic obstructive pulmonary disease (COPD) and community-acquired pneumonia (CAP). Sbiti-Rohr and colleagues (2016) identified that the NEWS was a good prognostic tool for assessing likely critical care admissions and deterioration in patients admitted to the Emergency Department with CAP. However, O'Driscoll and co-workers (2014) have begun to explore subgroup limitations of the NEWS, highlighting that it is less reliable when used with patients with COPD, particularly those with long-term hypoxia as difficulties occurred with scoring in relation to adjusted target values of peripheral capillary oxygen saturation (SpO_2) in this subgroup. They suggested that modification may be required in this group.

Other issues related to the NEWS concern inaccuracies related to human factors. Rather worryingly, error in calculations and inability to follow escalation procedures were identified by Kolic and colleagues (2015). Their study identified an 18% error rate in manual calculations of NEWS scores and a 26% error in following correct escalation processes. Whilst this can easily be rectified by implementation of electronic scoring systems it must be acknowledged that these are not available widely across all healthcare system for all patients. Care is still therefore required to avoid these human errors and the need for accurate recordings, calculations, and understanding of assessment results must be emphasized in all education programmes for nurses and medical staff.

Response to evaluation: The development of NEWS2

The Royal College of Physicians (2017) recently released a new version of the UK early warning score, NEWS2, in response to a report from the NEWS review group. Whilst the group highlights that the core principles of NEWS remain unchanged, a number of modifications have been made that respond to previous criticisms of NEWS. It is anticipated that these modifications will enable earlier escalation of the acutely ill patient. The key changes include:

- reconfiguring the chart to match resuscitation guidance to enable assessment to follow an ABCDE approach (see earlier section on patient assessment).
- additional assessment area for patients with hypercapnic respiratory failure (including patients with COPD, but also other groups who may have a hypercapnic drive such as the morbidly obese, patients with chest wall deformities, and those with neuromuscular problems). The decision to use the amended scale should be made by a competent decision-maker and this decision should be recorded in the patient's records. To avoid any doubt, the section not being used should be clearly crossed out by the clinician who has decided to utilize the hypercapnic respiratory failure section.
- the need to include precise recording of oxygen delivery systems as this was often poorly documented on the previous chart. Documentation should follow the standard British Thoracic Society (BTS) guidance on delivery devices; for example, A = breathing air N = nasal cannula.
- the clinical response to NEWS has been modified to enable early escalation of patients whose condition is deteriorating.
- addition of Confusion within the AVPU section which is now recorded as ACVPU and helps facilitate early identification of deteriorating patients and encourage urgent escalation of this group of patients.
- an emphasis on signs and symptoms that may indicate early sepsis. Several tools have been endorsed by the International Sepsis Consensus group (2016) to facilitate early identification of sepsis however this is clearly a complex area and several parameters need to be considered as temperature changes are not always a reliable tool. To simplify identification of sepsis NEWS2 guidance prompts clinicians to consider sepsis in any patients whose NEWS is 5 and emergency escalation if the NEWS is 7 or above.

Electronic scoring systems

Several commercially available electronic scoring systems are linked to the National early warning score. NICE (2016) identified the use of systems across the NHS and these included VitalPAC©, Patientrack©, Nervecentre©, Wardware©, Visensia©, and IntelliVue©. Other currently noncommercial systems such as SEND© have also been developed.

These electronic tools clearly have some simplistic advantages over paper charts in that they require all data to be inputted and calculate score automatically. The devices can be linked to automated escalation devices and allow instant recognition of the patients scoring highly in individual ward areas and across a hospital system which may be advantageous to medical emergency and critical care outreach teams.

Alongside this ward managers can draw data from these systems to facilitate audit and improve patient care. Most systems will permit the real-time audit of data to see whether observations are recorded in a timely manner or omitted. This may be utilized alongside other patient-related activity data to assess the need for higher staffing levels and in monitoring patient safety.

One of the most interesting potential benefits of the electronic scoring systems is the ability to utilize data for retrospective research purposes. Wong and colleagues (2015) argue that there is currently little evidence that supports the benefits of electronic scoring devices in identifying at-risk patients over paper scoring systems. His team is utilizing a bespoke electronic tool (SEND©) to explore whether an electronic system can be used to improve recognition of deterioration in a tertiary healthcare setting. Another research use of these systems is that data collected from these may be used to inform future early warning scores to enhance their reliability in detecting earlier signs of clinical deterioration.

The RCP (2017) have acknowledged that several NHS Trusts now utilize mature electronic patient databases and agree that these tools reduce the likelihood of human error in the calculation of the NEWS2 score. However, they stress the importance of utilizing the standardized NEWS2 assessment criteria to ensure accurate recognition of signs and symptoms of deterioration and facilitate comparative research studies.

Clinical trigger questions

Carberry and colleagues (2014) suggests the adjunct of trigger questions to be used alongside traditional track-and-trigger systems. This small-scale study explored the use of trigger questions to help ward staff identify patients of concern. They focused upon clear signs of deterioration and prompts related to:

- high track-and-trigger scores;
- use of high concentration oxygen via non re-breath masks;
- patients requiring rapid fluid resuscitation;
- need for medical review.

Whilst this was a very small study, staff found the trigger questions a useful adjunct that increased staff's perceptions of key factors that represent a deteriorating patient. The authors argued that trigger questions can help to identify and facilitate rapid escalation of deteriorating patients.

Escalation tools

The RCP (2012) identifies a clear need for the NEWS system (paper or electronic) to be linked to a robust escalation system that triggers the nurse to escalate concern about patient deterioration. An escalation tool developed by the RCP (2017) can be found at: https://www.rcplondon.ac.uk/projects/outputs/national-early-warning-score-news-2

The nurse is reminded of the importance of correct calculation of the NEWS, the advice from the escalation protocol, and the need to use professional judgement at all times. For example, the NEWS may be low and clinical judgement and concern for the patient's well-being can of course allow the nurse to override the escalation tool if required.

Communication tools

The need for effective communication of the patient's condition cannot be over-emphasized and the nurse clearly has a duty of care to their patients (NMC 2015). Almost universally, communication in healthcare poses a concern and in 2007 the World Health Organization (WHO) first recommended the universal adoption of a systematic escalation tool. It identified that acute patient deterioration often necessitated involvement of several nursing, medical, and allied health professional teams and therefore the scope to miss important information during rapid patient handover was significant. This could lead to breakdown in continuity of care, missed treatment, misunderstandings, and potential patient harm.

In standardizing communication, the WHO (2007) recommended:

- implementation of the SBAR (Situation, Background, Assessment, and Recommendation) tool;
- allocating sufficient time to communicating and ensuring that the message is understood. Repetition of main points should allow the communicator to check understanding;
- clear provision of information relating to treatment plans, response to treatment, and the patient's resuscitation status or advanced directives (see Chapter 13);
- ensuring that communication is limited to that which is essential to providing safe and effective patient care.

Alongside recommendations from the WHO, the RCP (2012) also advocates the use of a systematic tool such as SBAR that is standardized across the United Kingdom.

It argues that utilization of a standardized approach such as SBAR:

- reduces the barriers to effective communication across all disciplines.
- creates a shared model that relates to critical exchange of information.
- serves as a memory prompt and therefore encourages staff to prepare to communicate.
- reduces the likelihood of missed communications.

The SBAR tool consists of four standardized prompts that encourage the communicator to explain the:

Situation

- Identify yourself and ward area
- State patient's name and rationale for calling
- State concern

Background

- Provide background information including:
    - patient's history, reason for admission, a brief summary of treatment to date (e.g. medications, blood results, diagnostic test results), resuscitation status.

Assessment

- Provide assessment information including:
    - Any observations you are concerned about, the patient's NEWS and GCS, a recent fluid balance if available, mental state.
    - Any suspicions about diagnosis may also be provided. Do not be afraid to state you do not know what is wrong but you are concerned or that the patient's condition appears to be deteriorating.

Recommendation

- Explain what you require the person you are communicating with to do and clarify your expectations, for example state 'I would like the patient reviewed within 10 minutes'.

Some NHS Trusts have added a final R stage of repetition or read back. This allows the person communicating to check that the message they have conveyed has been understood and avoids misunderstandings due to human factors.

Clinical link 10.1

Mrs Johnston is a 55-year-old lady admitted to your ward following abdominal surgery two days ago. She was stable during the initial recovery had been progressing well. You have been asked to review Mrs Johnston by the healthcare assistant as she is worried that Mrs Johnston reports feeling generally unwell and says her joints ache and she feels like she has the flu.

Her observations are as follows:

- RR 28
- Saturations 98
- On-room air
- HR 132
- BP 110/40
- CRT 1 second
- Temperature 39.2°C

On examination her airway is intact and she is talking to you, she is visibly shivering and asking for more blankets, repeatedly telling you she is cold and her joints ache. She is breathing without use of accessory muscles, but her breathing is shallow. Her pulse is bounding, and she feels very warm to the touch. She is alert and orientated but tells you she does feel quite tired. On exposure her wound is red and inflamed. Arterial blood gas: pH 7.34; PaO_2 14.1; PCO_2 4.1; HCO_3 21; Lactate 3 mmol/l

- Identify the significant findings in this patient
- Discuss any changes you would make to her care during the assessment
- Calculate the NEWS2 score
- Discuss how you would escalate this patient

Critical care outreach

The development of critical care outreach teams was recommended in the Department of Health (2000) report, Comprehensive Critical Care: A Review of Adult Critical Care Services. Since this publication was released, many NHS Trusts have instigated a variety of outreach services to meet the report's requirements.

NICE (2007) highlighted that the primary role of Critical Care Outreach teams (CCOT) was to ensure that all patients at risk of deterioration or patients who are deteriorating have timely treatment in the most suitable area. Initially role development was idiosyncratic, and a variety of teams were developed with significantly different functions with little standardization of roles and no clear operational guidance for the development of services.

However, in 2012 the UK National Outreach Forum published the operational standards framework for outreach teams. The paper redefined outreach as a 'multidisciplinary organisational approach to ensure safe, equitable and quality care for all acutely unwell, critically ill and recovering patients irrespective of location or pathway'.

The core operational elements of outreach roles were identified, and the acronym PREPARE was used to highlight the key roles of outreach. PREPARE includes seven core operational elements:

- Patient track and trigger
- Rapid response
- Education, training, and support
- Patient safety and clinical governance
- Audit and evaluation; monitoring of patient outcome and continuing quality care
- Rehabilitation after critical illness
- Enhancing service delivery

The PREPARE tool has been devised to provide organizations with an operational framework of standards and competencies. Organizations with CCOT are encouraged to measure their own performance and use a red, amber, green (RAG) rating tool to identify areas of strength and areas where further improvement is needed. This work is ongoing and data from studies will prove useful in evaluating the role of a standardized CCOT.

Evaluation of the effectiveness of outreach teams has been undertaken over the past decade and unfortunately this has proved inconclusive, perhaps because of the lack of a unified approach to the teams and research.

Seminal work by Rowan and colleagues (2009) highlighted the overwhelming variations in the provision of outreach services, identifying considerable differences in the composition and availability of outreach teams and the types of roles undertaken by the teams. It identified that the recommendations for continuous 24-hour outreach provision were not met and several areas failed to meet minimum staffing requirements.

One of the positive aspects of outreach was that the presence of an outreach team was associated with a significant decrease in resuscitation rates, out-of-hours admissions to intensive therapy unit (ITU), and the level of acuity of patients when admitted to ITU.

Sadly, the study was unable to either prove or disprove the relative benefits of outreach services and stressed the need for further evaluation, especially in relation to the financial implications of outreach services. It concluded that ultimately management of the acutely ill patient should be the responsibility of appropriately trained professionals who possess in-depth knowledge and skills.

Subsequent studies have echoed similar findings about the impact of outreach on patient outcome. Jeddian and colleagues (2016) review of outreach intervention in Birmingham identified no significant impact of outreach on either patient outcome or mortality rates. Kovac's (2016) meta-analysis of previous studies again found no conclusive evidence for CCOT related to patient outcome, however she did acknowledge that internationally clinicians perceived that CCOT was of benefit. These benefits related to:

- empowerment of the ward nurse
- effective communication
- prompt escalation of patients

Other benefits that have been found in the literature include the positive effect that CCOTs have on junior and inexperienced ward staff, providing them with support and prompt response during episodes of acute deterioration (Rowan *et al.* 2009). The presence of CCOTs does appear to improve connectivity of patient care and enhance communication across organizational and specialty settings which clearly enhances quality of the patient journey (Moody and Griffiths 2011).

A NICE (2017) meta-analysis again concluded an overall effect on patient outcome however they did identify an overall increase in the number of do not attempt resuscitation (DNAR) orders where CCOT teams were present, perhaps reflecting the significant role the teams play in preventing unnecessary resuscitation attempts and enhancing the quality of end of life care for acutely ill patients. This is clearly another significant role of CCOT.

An almost universal agreement within the literature is that more contemporary evidence and robust research is needed to explore the role of CCOT and the impact and potential benefits of CCOT on the patient journey in acute care hospitals (Rowan *et al.* 2009; Moody and Griffiths 2011; Kovac 2016; NICE 2017). Much of the current evidence is dated and does not reflect the potential impact of the National Outreach Forum standards.

Acute care in the community

The focus on acute illness is increasingly becoming a priority in primary care as patients are being discharged home earlier or having their care managed in ambulatory settings and then transferred home. In 2009 the Department of Health highlighted the need to adequately recognize, assess, and diagnose patients who may become acutely unwell in the community setting. Over the last decade an increasing awareness to ensure early detection of acutely ill patients in the community has been increasingly recognized (Salim 2014; Silcock *et al.* 2015).

To this end, several developments have occurred within community settings as there is an increased drive for acute care skills. The ALERT course has been taught in some NHS Trusts and the aims as highlighted by Salim (2014) are:

- improvement of recognition of acute illness;
- earlier recognition of deterioration;
- reduction in avoidable admissions to secondary and tertiary care;
- facilitation of early hospital discharges;
- facilitation of communication across all healthcare providers;
- reduction in avoidable deaths.

The implementation of a modified ALERT course for community staff has demonstrated positive benefits and staff feel more confident to identify patient deterioration and escalate patients to secondary care where required.

Alongside this innovation, Silcock and colleagues (2015) undertook a study exploring the relevance of the NEWS score in primary healthcare settings which highlighted that use of the NEWS tool enable paramedics to recognize those patients appropriately who required urgent medical intervention and a rapid transfer to a hospital setting.

This stance is echoed by the Royal College of Physicians (2017) who emphasize the need for all early responders to utilize NEWS 2 assessment in primary care settings.

The future

Significant research continues into patient assessment tools, track-and-trigger scoring systems, communication tools, and critical care outreach and other support services. This, combined with increasing technology, highlights the dynamic nature of acute care delivery and the need for all acute care staff to update their knowledge in these areas frequently.

End of chapter test

Reflect upon your own practice area and test your knowledge in relation to the following.

- Discuss why systematic assessment of the patient is beneficial.
- Identify the key components of each step of the ABCDE model.
- Identify key changes that may indicate patient deterioration.

- Consider what other factors should be considered when assessing a patient.
- Discuss why track-and-trigger systems were introduced.
- Analyse which changes in track-and-trigger parameters may cause concern, providing rationale for your answer.
- Explain why aggregate scoring systems are the most appropriate tool and explore why these are recommended by NICE.
- Analyse advantages and disadvantages of using track-and-trigger systems to enhance patient assessment.
- Identify the advantages of using an electronic track-and-trigger system.
- Discuss limitations of the National Early Warning.
- Identify the model of outreach used within own hospital area.
- Describe main objectives of outreach services.
- Discuss situations in which outreach intervention would be appropriate.
- Discuss situations that should trigger emergency call to medical/outreach staff.
- Discuss potential problems with communication of concern about a patient.
- Describe use of SBAR tool to improve escalation of concern.

References

Abbott, T.E., Vaid., N. Cron, N. *et al.* (2015) A single-centre observational cohort study of admission National Early Warning Score (NEWS). *Resuscitation*, 92:89–93.

Barker, M. (2015) How to assess deteriorating patients *Nursing Standard*, 30:34–36.

Benson (2017) The A–G assessment tool (Airway, Breathing, Circulation, Disability, Exposure, Further information and Goals). Clinical Skills. Net Clinical Skills Limited.

Bickley, L.S., Szilagyl, P.G., Hoffman, R.M. (2017). *Bates' Guide to Physical Examination and History Taking* 12th edn. Philadelphia, PA: Wolters Kluwer.

British Thoracic Society (2017) *BTS Guideline for Oxygen Use in Healthcare and Emergency Settings.* London: British Thoracic Society.

Carberry, M., Clements, P., Headley, E. (2014) Ward nurses perceptions of clinical trigger questions. *Nursing Times*, 110:1–3.

Christofidis M.J., Hill A., Horswill M.S., *et al.* (2014) Observation charts with overlapping blood pressure and heart rate graphs do not yield the performance advantage that health professionals assume: An experimental study. *J Adv Nurs*, 70:610–24.

Cowan, H. (2015) Polypharmacy in the cardiac patient and chronocardiology. *Br J Card Nurs*, 10:268–9.

Department of Health (2000) *Comprehensive Critical Care, a Review of Adult Critical Care Services.* London: TSO.

Elliot, M. (2016) Why is respiratory rate the neglected vital sign? A narrative review. *Int Arch Nurs Health Care*, 2(3):1–4.

Felton, M. (2012) Recognising signs and symptoms of patient deterioration. *Emergency Nurse*, 20: 23–9.

Georgaka, D., Mparmparousi, M. Vitos, M. (2012) Early warning systems. *Hospital Chronicles*, 7:37–43.

Jeddian, A., Hemmings, K., Lindermayer, A. *et al.* (2016) Clinical Research—Clinical Trials And Studies; New findings from University of Birmingham in clinical trials and studies provides new insights (Evaluation of a critical care outreach service in a middle-income country: A stepped wedge cluster randomized trial and nested qualitative study). *J Crit Care*, 36:212–17.

Joint British Diabetes Societies Inpatient Care Group (2013) The management of diabetic ketoacidosis in adults British Joint Diabetes Society. Available at: https://www.diabetes.org.uk/resources-s3/2017-09/Management-of-DKA-241013.pdf?_ga=2.158769599.468428599.1505127410-1295258485.1505127410; accessed 9 December 2019.

Kolic, I., Crane, S., McCartney, S. *et al.* (2015) Factors affecting response to National Early Warning Score (NEWS). *Resuscitation*, 90:85–90.

Kovac, C. (2016) Outreach and early warning systems for the prevention of intensive care admission and death of critically ill adult patients on general hospital wards *Int J Nurs Practice*, 22:523–5.

Kovac, C. Jarvis, S., Prytherch, D.R., *et al.* (2016) Comparison of the National Early Warning Score in non-elective medical and surgical patients. *Br J Surgery*, 103:1385–93.

Mok, W., Wang. W., Cooper, S. *et al* (2015) Attitudes towards vital signs monitoring in the detection of clinical deterioration: Scale development and survey of ward nurses. *Int J Qual Health Care* 27: 207–13.

Moody, S., Griffiths, P. (2011) Effectiveness of Critical Care Outreach Services Working Papers in Health Science. Available at: https://www.southampton.ac.uk/assets/centresresearch/documents/wphs/Effectiveness%20of%20Critical%20Care%20Outreach%20Services.pdf; accessed 9 December 2019.

National Clinical Effectiveness Committee (2013) *National Early Warning Score: National clinical guidance number 1.* Available at: http://health.gov.ie/wp-content/uploads/2015/01/NEWSFull-ReportAugust2014.pdf; accessed 9 December 2019.

National Outreach Forum (2012) *Operational Standards and Competencies for Critical Care Outreach Services.* Available at: https://www.norf.org.uk/Resources/Documents/NOrF%20CCCO%20and%20standards/National%20Outreach%20Forum%20report%202014.pdf; accessed 9 December 2019.

NMC (2015) *The Code: Professional Standards of Practice and Behavior for Nurses and Midwives.* London: Nursing and Midwifery Council.

NMC (2017) *Standards of Proficiency for Registered Nurses* (Draft). London: Nursing and Midwifery Council.

O'Driscoll, B.R. (2014). The national early warning score gives misleading scores for oxygen saturation in patients at risk of hypercapnia. *Clin Med*, 14:695–6.

Resuscitation Council (2015) The ABCDE approach. Available at: https://www.resus.org.uk/resuscitation-guidelines/abcde-approach/; accessed 9 December 2019.

Rowan, K., Adam, S., Ball, C., *et al.* (2009) *Evaluation of Outreach Services in Critical Care.* London: Intensive Care National Audit and Research Committee.

RCP (2012) *National Early Warning Scores: Standardising the Assessment of Acute Illness Severity in the NHS.* London: Royal College of Physicians.

RCP (2017) *National Early Warning Scores 2: Standardising the Assessment of Acute Illness Severity in the NHS.* London: Royal College of Physicians.

Salim, S. (2014) Recognition and treatment of life-threatening events in the community setting Part 1: Tthe journey. *Br J Community Nurs*, 19:453–6.

Sbiti-Rohr, D., Kutz, A., Christ-Crain, M., *et al.* (2016) The National Early Warning Score (NEWS) for outcome prediction in emergency department patients with community-acquired pneumonia: Results from a 6-year prospective cohort study. *BMJ Open*, 2016. Available at: http://bmjopen.bmj.com/content/6/9/e011021; accessed 9 December 2019.

Sepsis UK (2017) *The Sepsis manual.* Available at: https://sepsistrust.org/wp-content/uploads/2018/06/Sepsis_Manual_2017_web_download.pdf, accessed 13 January 2020.

Singer, M., Clifford, S., Duetchsman, M.D., *et al.* (2016) The Third International Consensus Definitions for Sepsis and Septic Shock (Sepsis-3). Available at: https://www.ncbi.nlm.nih.gov/entrez/eutils/elink.fcgi?dbfrom=pubmed&retmode=ref&cmd=prlinks&id=26903338; accessed 9 December 2019.

Silcock, D., Corfield, A., Gowens, P. (2015) Validation of the National Early Warning Score in the pre-hospital setting. *Resuscitation*, 89:31–5.

Smith, G. (2003) *ALERT: Acute Life Threatening Events, Treatment and Recognition.* 2nd edn. Portsmouth: University of Portsmouth.

Smith, G., Prytherch, D.R., Meredith, P., *et al.* (2013) The ability of the National Early Warning Score (NEWS) to discriminate patients at risk of early cardiac arrest, unanticipated intensive care unit admission, and death. *Resuscitation*, 84:465–70.

Vaughan, J., Parry, A. (2016) Assessment and management of the septic patient: Part 1. *Br J Nurs*, 25:958–64.

Waldie, J., Tee, S., Day, T. (2016) Reducing avoidable deaths from failure to rescue: A discussion paper. *Br J Nurs*, 25:1–7

Wong, D., Bonnici, T., Knight, J., *et al.* (2015) SEND: A system for electronic notification and documentation of vital signs. *BMC Medical Informatics and Decision Making*, 15:1–12.

World Health Organization (2007) *Communication During Patient Hand-Overs*. Available at: http://www.who.int/patientsafety/solutions/patientsafety/PS-Solution3.pdf; accessed 9 December 2019.

York and Humber Academic Health Science Network (2014) Effectiveness matters, the impact of early warning scores on patient outcomes. Centre for Reviews and Dissemination, University of York. Available at: http://www.improvementacademy.org/documents/resources/effectiveness_matters/Effectiveness%20Matters%20Early%20Warning%20Systems%20(September%202014).pdf; accessed 9 December 2019.

11
Acute emergency situations

Lorna East, Fiona Creed, and Christine Spiers

Chapter contents

Maximizing survival from cardiac arrest in hospital requires a coordinated and rapid response, skilled practitioners performing resuscitation procedures correctly and utilizing evidence-based guidelines. This chapter will therefore examine:

- causes and prevention of acute emergency situations
- initial assessment of the patient in acute emergency situations
- management of the patient in cardiac arrest
- management of the patient with anaphylaxis
- management of the patient in peri-arrest arrhythmias
- post-resuscitation care

Learning outcomes

This chapter will enable you to:

- be able to define cardiac arrest and CPR
- explore a structured approach to assessing an acutely sick patient
- identify early recognition and cardiac arrest prevention in acute care patients
- identify causes of cardiac arrest
- identify all the known cardiac arrest rhythms and differentiate the management for shockable versus non-shockable arrests
- consider the assessment, diagnosis, and management of the patient in cardiac arrest
- understand the importance of chest compressions and early defibrillation
- be familiar with management of peri-arrest arrhythmias, including pacing and synchronized cardioversion
- evaluate the nursing management of a patient with anaphylaxis

An essential part of nursing in an acute care area is to be fully prepared to deal promptly and effectively with any acute emergency situation. More acutely ill patients are being cared for within ward environments, which place an ever-increasing need for staff to be competent and confident in the care and management of those at risk of cardiac arrest. Approximately 80% of cardiac arrests are predictable, with patients displaying adverse clinical signs in the few hours preceding the event. Strategies to prevent cardiac arrest are therefore paramount. The assessment of simple vital signs helps to predict cardiorespiratory arrest (Resuscitation Council (UK) 2016a, 2016b). Recognition of adverse signs from the deteriorating patient, calling for early expert assistance and intervention of key therapies such as airway management, oxygen, and fluid resuscitation, must therefore aim to prevent cardiac arrest occurring in the first instance. It is clear that the current and future focus on resuscitation must be to ensure that all healthcare professionals are able to recognize the deteriorating patient and to be able to respond appropriately to signs of clinical deterioration, using NEWS2 (RCP 2017), within our acute hospitals (further information can be obtained from Chapter 10 on systematic patient assessment).

It is crucially important that deterioration is quickly identified and responded to in a timely manner so that survival from cardiac arrests within our hospitals can significantly improve.

Recognition and prevention of cardiac arrest

Evidence suggests that patients who become acutely unwell in hospital may still receive suboptimal care (Waldie *et al.* 2016). Communication and documentation are often poor, experience might be lacking, and provision of critical care expertise, including admission to critical care areas, could be delayed. In 2007 the National Patient Safety Agency found that when patients had died, staff demonstrated the inability to seek advice and even appreciate any sense of clinical urgency.

Following this, NICE (2007) emphasized the importance of evidence-based practice emphasizing the necessity for effective communication and collaboration between nursing and medical teams. The need for robust assessment systems, medical emergency teams, and a system approach to the deteriorating patient is again highlighted by McNeill and Bryden (2013) and the Royal College of Physicians (2017). It is argued that early recognition of deterioration may prevent:

- cardiac arrests and deaths
- inappropriate resuscitation attempts
- admissions to intensive therapy unit (ITU) (Resuscitation Council UK 2016a, 2016b)

In the United Kingdom, a system of pre-emptive ward care called critical care outreach has developed and aims to reduce ward deaths and post-operative adverse events. Critical care outreach teams also play a role in educating and improving acute care skills of ward personnel.

Over the last few decades, early recognition and cardiac arrest prevention has been a heavily weighted component of hospital resuscitation training programmes (ALERT™ 2003, Advanced Life Support 2016, Immediate Life Support 2016). Greater emphasis is now placed on earlier recognition of the deteriorating patient (National Patient Safety Agency 2007; NICE 2007; RCP 2017). Using a framework ensures the identification of the life-threatening needs and care to be prioritized in a structured ABCDE (airway, breathing, circulation, disability, and exposure) approach (Smith 2000; NICE 2007; RCP 2017). The aim of initial treatment is to keep the patient alive and achieve some clinical improvement to buy time for further treatment (Resuscitation Council (UK) 2016b).

ABCDE approach

In general, the clinical signs of critical illness are similar whatever the underlying pathology, before there is failure of the respiratory, cardiovascular, and neurological systems; the ABCDE problems (Resuscitation Council (UK) 2016a/b).

This rapid assessment is performed in a structured order so that life-threatening symptoms can be dealt with along the way. If at any stage life-threatening signs are evident, the emergency team, depending on your local Trust policy, must be called; you must recognize when you need extra help and call for this help early (Resuscitation Council (UK) 2016a, 2016b).

Situations that are likely to result in serious harm should be dealt with first. For instance, a blocked airway should be prioritized before breathing or circulation difficulties and these areas must be assessed and supported in order of priority. Guidelines on the ABCDE approach are now embedded in current resuscitation documentation (Resuscitation Council (UK) 2016a, 2016b) adapted originally from the ALERT™ course (Smith 2003):

- Airway
- Breathing
- Circulation
- Disability
- Exposure

Airway

It is vital to look, listen, and feel in the assessment of the airway (Box 11.1). Detail on airway assessment can be found in Chapter 11. Simple measures will almost always open an obstructed airway.

Box 11.1 Airway assessment in the acutely ill patient

- Is the airway patent? Is the patient talking or mumbling?
- Are there any added noises/sounds?
- Is suction required?
- What is the patient's colour?
- Are airway opening manoeuvres required? Consider c-spine.
- Apply O_2 high flow.
- Check oropharyngeal/nasopharyngeal airways.

Box 11.2 Breathing assessment in the acutely ill patient

- Rate.
- Effort.
- Depth.
- Bilateral chest movement and equal air entry.
- Breath sounds/added sounds.
- O_2 saturations (Note: this does not detect raised CO_2)/ABGs.
- Colour.
- Sweating/clammy.
- Use of accessory muscles.
- Position of patient.

Breathing

Evidence of respiratory distress or inadequate ventilation can also be determined using a simple 'look, listen, feel' approach (Smith 2003).

Along with the assessments identified in Box 11.2 it is essential that the patient is ventilating adequately. If the patient's ventilations are inadequate, then the heart rate will increase, the skin colour will deteriorate, become grey/pale, and even cyanosed. This is a peri-arrest sign. The patient may also become anxious, restless, or even drowsy if ventilation is inadequate because oxygen to the brain is significantly reduced.

Again, simple measures can be applied, for example sitting your patient upright if possible to optimize oxygenation and ventilation. All acutely ill patients should receive oxygen to maintain adequate oxygen saturation and it is important to treat all underlying causes of respiratory problems. The emergency team must be called immediately if acute life-threatening conditions occur, such as acute asthma or pulmonary oedema. (See Chapter 2 for a detailed discussion of respiratory assessment and care.)

Circulation

It is important to assess the patient's circulatory status using the same look, listen, and feel approach (Box 11.3). In almost all medical and surgical emergencies, hypovolaemia should be considered the primary cause of shock until proven otherwise (Smith 2003; Resuscitation Council (UK) 2016a, 2016b). If the patient has a normal blood pressure it does not exclude shock, severe blood loss, or critical illness. (For further information see Chapters 3 and 7.)

Disability (neurological)

A rapid assessment of the patient's neurological function should follow a quick reassessment of ABC. See Box 11.4 for neurological assessment. (See Chapter 4 on neurological assessment and care.)

Box 11.3 Circulation assessment in the acutely ill patient

- Reassess airway and breathing.
- Pulses: peripheral/central? Rate? Rhythm? Volume?
- Peripheral circulation: Cool? Clammy? Warm/hot?
- Capillary refill time.
- Blood pressure.
- Any blood/fluid loss? Wounds? Drains? Dressings? Arterial lines? Haemorrhage control.
- CVP.
- Urine output.
- 12-lead ECG interpretation.
- Need intravenous access? Take bloods.
- Fluid challenge.

Exposure

Finally, 'a top to toe' look at the patient should be conducted, to check that no other cause of their acute episode has been missed (see Box 11.5).

The aim of treating the acutely ill patient is the early anticipation and detection of abnormal physiology at a stage before organ failure is established and to initiate simple preventative therapies and interventions (RCP 2017).

Cardiac arrest: Causes, rhythms

Cardiac arrest can be defined as the cessation of circulation along with absent signs of life such as normal respirations or movement. The patient will have loss of consciousness and become unresponsive and lifeless. Respiratory effort will be absent or gasping, along with an

Box 11.4 Disability (neurological) assessment in the acutely ill patient

- Reassess ABC. Is it still hypoxic or hypotensive?
- ACVPU (Alert, Confusion, responds to Voice, responds to Pain, Unresponsive).
- Blood sugar.
- Pupil(s) reaction.
- Posture.
- Anxious? Restless? Aggressive? Fidgety?
- Airway secure? Left lateral position (if C-spine ok).
- Look at drug chart/blood results.

Box 11.5 Exposure in the acutely ill patient

- Rashes? Wounds? Lines?
- Top to toe look.
- Signs of deep vein thrombosis?
- Central temperature.
- Maintain dignity.
- Reassess ABCDE.

absent pulse in a major artery (carotid or femoral). UK ambulance data indicates out of hospital arrest occurs at a rate of 52 per 100,000 inhabitants with a survival to discharge of 8%. UK National Cardiac Arrest Audit (NCAA) data indicate in-hospital cardiac arrest occurs in 1.6 per 1,000 hospital admissions with the rate of survival to discharge of 18.4%. Recent international data suggest that survival rates after both in- and out-of-hospital cardiac arrest are slowly improving (Resuscitation Council UK 2015). Sudden cardiac arrest is responsible for more than 60% of adult deaths from coronary heart disease. Other causes can be viewed in Box 11.6.

Those who survive to discharge tend to sustain cardiac arrest from a primary ventricular fibrillation (VF) or pulseless ventricular tachycardia (VT) rhythm. Treatment for these arrest rhythms is prompt defibrillation. Defibrillation is the only treatment for sustained ventricular arrhythmias.

Box 11.7 identifies all four cardiac arrest rhythms.

Box 11.6 Causes of cardiorespiratory arrest in acute care

- Airway obstruction.
- Hypoxia.
- Anaphylaxis.
- Pulmonary embolism.
- Hypovolaemia (sepsis and/or haemorrhage).
- Acute coronary syndrome.
- Metabolic and electrolyte disturbances.
- Cardiac arrhythmias.
- Drugs (i.e. anti-arrhythmic drugs; opiates).
- Neurological insult (i.e. CVA; head injury).
- Tension pneumothorax.

Box 11.7 The four cardiac arrest rhythms

These two rhythms together are known as the shockable cardiac arrest rhythms:

- ventricular fibrillation
- ventricular tachycardia (pulseless)

These two rhythms are known as the *non-shockable* cardiac arrest rhythms:

- pulseless electrical activity (PEA)
- asystole (including *p*-wave asystole)

Clinical link 11.1 (see Appendix for answers)

Part A

A 43-year-old patient has been admitted to hospital with anaemia, cause unknown. She returns to the ward after having an endoscopy procedure. She is supine in the bed. Your initial assessment reveals respirations 10/min, heart rate 115 and regular, blood pressure 130/80, central temperature 36.3°C, and O_2 saturations 86%. She is pale and clammy. She is responding to voice.

- What would your immediate actions be and why?
- What other assessments would you consider?

Part B

After your initial intervention and treatment her condition appeared to improve. However, on your return with more help to change her position and to recheck further observations, you notice she is cyanosed around her lips and a noise is coming from her airway.

- What are your priorities for this patient?
- What interventions/actions will you take?
- Can you list all the signs of complete and partial airway obstruction?

The concept of the 'chain of survival' (Cummins *et al.* 1991) still remains true to current recommendations, with emphasis on swift implementation of good-quality chest compressions and early defibrillation (Figure 11.1). Effectiveness of defibrillation falls rapidly with even small delays to treatment. The chain is only as strong as its weakest link. To optimize the chances of a successful outcome, each link in the chain needs to be strong.

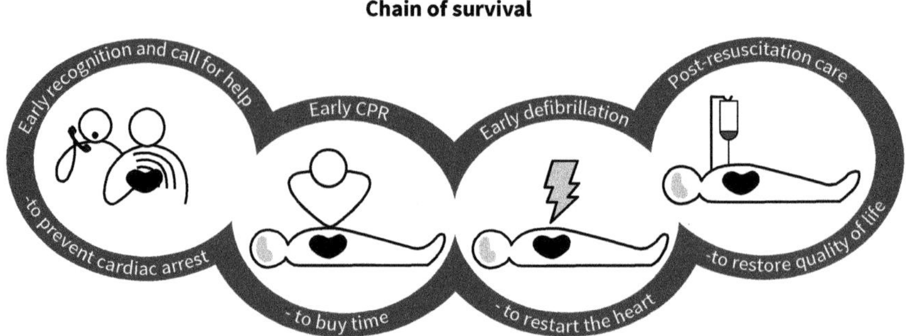

Figure 11.1 Chain of survival.

Reproduced with the kind permission of the Resuscitation Council (UK). Adult basic life support and automated external defibrillation. © Resuscitation Council (UK). 2015. [https://www.resus.org.uk/resuscitation-guidelines/adult-basic-life-support-and-automated-external-defibrillation/] accessed 07/06/19.

Cardiopulmonary resuscitation

Cardiopulmonary resuscitation (CPR) is an emergency procedure required for someone in cardiac arrest. It combines techniques of providing external chest compressions creating artificial blood circulation and delivering artificial respirations to create lung inflation and oxygen delivery. A combination of these more modern techniques have been used over the past 50 years but have been fine-tuned according to current evidence-based medicine. CPR may have been known in theory, if not in practice, for hundreds or even thousands of years. The first ever written account of a resuscitation attempt was of Elijah, the prophet, who warmed a dead boy's body and placed his mouth over the boy's mouth.

CPR is unlikely to restart the heart but is a holding measure delaying cell death. Irreversible tissue death occurs within 4–5 min if resuscitation attempts are not commenced. Good-quality CPR will extend this very brief window in order for advanced life support (ALS) techniques to be implemented. The brain and the heart will be oxygenated, albeit to only approximately 30% of normal cardiac output. The aim therefore is for a successful resuscitation attempt to occur without permanent brain damage.

Resuscitation equipment

In every emergency situation a speedy response is crucial. It is vital that all essential equipment is ready, accessible, functional, and is in date. A designated trolley must be set up and should only be used in an emergency and checked on a daily basis. It must be restocked and checked again after use. Your hospital's own resuscitation department should advise a checklist; it is important that an agreed system is in place and monitored. The defibrillator must also be checked according to the manufacturer's guidelines. Any faults must be reported to your maintenance team. To avoid the machine's battery failing it is important to ensure that the machine is always plugged into the mains, ready for use. Most manufacturers recommend that electrocardiogram (ECG) and defibrillator electrodes should not be opened until required for use.

Most acute care bed areas are equipped with individual suction and bedside piped oxygen facility, however an emergency mobile suction unit, and spare oxygen cylinder (which must be over half full) must be readily available as a backup. In theory, any patient, relative, or member of staff could collapse beyond a bed space area. The suction units must be tested to ensure that they are working (that they can create suction up to 300 mmHg) and that enough tubing is available to reach a patient, with ample room. A recent NHS Improvement alert (2018) has highlighted the failure of healthcare practitioners to use portable O_2 cylinders correctly and NHS Trusts must ensure that appropriate training is offered to all healthcare personnel. A wide-bore suction catheter should also be attached ready for use (after the suction has been tested). There must also be a non-rebreathe oxygen mask and reservoir device available and access to a bag valve mask (BVM) unit with its own oxygen tubing. All bed spaces must be kept tidy and free from clutter so that the resuscitation team can easily and swiftly access the patient safely from all sides of the bed if required.

In-hospital resuscitation

The public expect that clinical staff can undertake CPR (Resuscitation Council (UK) 2016a). All healthcare professionals should be able to recognize cardiorespiratory arrest, call for help, and start CPR (see Box 11.8).

All staff who attend a cardiac arrest may have different competencies in managing the airway, breathing, or circulation and should use skills in which they have been trained. Communication skills and other non-technical skills are just as important for successful resuscitation outcomes. There is also a current trend for pre-allocation of roles and responsibilities for dealing with an emergency to ward staff, at the start of each shift.

Safety

Your personal safety and that of the resuscitation team members is the first priority during any resuscitation attempt (Resuscitation Council (UK) 2016a, 2016b). It is therefore essential to check the patient's surroundings are safe and there are no hazards. It is important that protective equipment is used, with gloves and aprons as standard. A sharps box must be readily available on the emergency trolley and staff must be fastidious in their use and disposal. Local infection control policies must be followed to minimize risks.

Box 11.8 Sequence of events in hospital cardiac arrest

In hospital, all healthcare professionals should:

- immediately recognize cardiorespiratory arrest
- ensure that emergency team has been dispatched using standard number (e.g. 2222)
- commence CPR immediately; using airway adjuncts once arrived: pocket mask or two-person technique BVM
- defibrillate, if indicated, and attempt this within 3 min.

Data from Resuscitation Council (UK) (2016) Immediate Life Support. 4th edn. Resuscitation Council (UK), London; and Resuscitation Council (UK) (2016) Advanced Life Support. 7th edn. Resuscitation Council (UK), London.

Call for help early

It is vital to shout 'Help!' whilst approaching the patient, having assessed it is safe to do so. Your colleagues are therefore alerted to assist you and more importantly your experienced senior nurses will also be there to help. The single rescuer must always ensure that help is coming (Resuscitation Council (UK) 2016a, 2016b) and therefore emergency buzzers should also be deployed.

Responsive patient

Check the patient's responsiveness with a gentle shake and ask loudly, 'Are you alright?' (Resuscitation Council (UK) 2016a, 2016b). If there is a response, assess the patient using the ABCDE approach (Resuscitation Council (UK) 2016a, 2016b) and call either the medical emergency team (MET) or outreach team depending what policy is in place in your Trust. (See Chapter 11 on track-and-trigger systems). Ensure that the patient has high-flow oxygen, sit them upright if tolerated, insert a cannula to obtain venous access and take bloods, and start blood pressure, ECG, and O_2 saturation monitoring. Ensure vital signs are recorded and a NEWS2 score obtained. Be prepared to hand over to the team when they arrive using an SBAR (situation, background, assessment, recommendation) technique. Always ensure that medical notes are available and observation and fluid charts visible.

Unresponsive patient

If the patient does not respond, the nurse must perform a quick and timely ABC assessment to confirm cardiac arrest. Ideally, the patient should be flat on their back. As recommended by the Resuscitation Council (UK) (2016a, 2016b), keeping the airway open with either head tilt, chin lift, or jaw thrust (in cervical spine injury patients) ensures that it is clear from any obstruction. The rescuer needs to determine if the patient is breathing normally or has any other signs of life (i.e. coughing, moving) for no longer than 10 seconds. Gasping or very slow irregular breathing (agonal breathing) is abnormal and not adequate. This is commonly seen in the early stages of an arrest and is a sign of cardiac arrest and not to be mistaken as a sign of life Resuscitation Council UK (2016a, 2016b). It is essential to look for normal rise and fall of the chest wall, listen for breath sounds, and feel for air on your cheek.

The cardiac arrest call of 2222 or designated number in your NHS Trust has to be made immediately and practical resuscitative measures commenced. Box 11.9 demonstrates the key personnel involved in a cardiac arrest procedure and their position and roles.

Fortunately, within acute care areas, staff members are usually within closer working distances and many actions can be performed at the same time. One nurse can make the call, one can bring the resuscitation trolley with the defibrillator, and one can start immediate chest compressions. Whilst the defibrillator is being brought to the resuscitation attempt, chest compressions must be ongoing. Only if there are adequate personnel with the correct equipment should the compressions be halted, to allow pocket mask or BVM ventilation to occur. Without effective head tilt, chin lift, and a good effective tight seal, ventilations will not be successful, and the patient's chest will not rise and fall. If this is the case, chest

Box 11.9 Cardiac arrest team members, roles, and positions

F1, foundation year 1 doctor; F2, foundation year 2 doctor; IV, intravenous; ODP, operating department practitioner; BLS, basic life support.

Anaesthetist ± ODP

Airway protection & ventilation/oxygenation

F1/2 Doctor

IV access & drugs

Trained nurse

Defibrillation

2 BLS providers

Good-quality chest compressions

Senior Nurse

Documentation & audit form (may also be required for family presence)

(back-up defibrillator)

Team Leader

On-call medical doctor/ALS provider

compressions *must not* stop in order for any more ventilatory attempts until the next group of uninterrupted 30 compressions. The only time immediate interruption should occur is when the rescuer is ready to assess the heart rhythm to determine whether it is shockable or non-shockable or if there are signs of life from the patient. If the patient is in VF or pulseless VT, then immediate safe defibrillation must occur. For non-VF/non-VT arrest rhythms, compressions and ventilations at 30:2 must resume.

Remember if there is no evidence of normal breathing, coughing, and/or any movement, then there are no signs of life: this is a cardiac arrest. If there are any doubts you must ensure that help and equipment, including a defibrillator and pocket mask, is coming and commence immediate CPR, starting with 30 chest compressions then 2 ventilations.

If there is any doubt the nurse must commence CPR, as delays in chest compressions will affect a positive outcome. It must be noted that starting CPR on a very sick patient with a low cardiac output is unlikely to be harmful and may even be beneficial (Resuscitation Council (UK 2016b).

It is important to remember that if you have taken your patient to the magnetic resonance imaging (MRI) or computerized tomography (CT) scanning areas or are transferring your patient to another area within the hospital, you may have to call the resuscitation team yourself. This must be done prior to commencing resuscitation measures if you are the single responder. It is also the nurse who is responsible when chaperoning patients to these areas, therefore take adequate equipment in the event of their patient's condition deteriorating (see Chapter 14 on safe transfer of the acutely ill). These patients should, on any transfer, have a defibrillator/monitor, suction equipment, and a pocket mask, with a full oxygen cylinder, in the event of a cardiac arrest occurring outside the acute care area. Within some NHS Trusts the portering staff may be trained in chest compression-only CPR, in which case they could commence this immediately whilst the single rescuer (the acute care nurse) makes the call.

Within NHS Trusts, basic life support skills are mandatory for all healthcare professionals. This arguably makes it a little less stressful for the nurse, if anything sudden should occur outside of their acute care area.

Chest compressions

These have been called external cardiac massage or cardiac massage in the past but this can be extremely misleading as a great amount of effort is required to perform them correctly and to be as effective as possible for the patient. Chest compressions need to be at the correct rate, depth, position, and recoil with the patient lying on their back, face up, ideally on a solid surface. They must be performed using a vertical force directed in the middle of the patient's sternum. Two hands should be on the centre of the chest (sternum) with straight arms, elbows locked, and shoulders directly over the patient. If the patient is on the floor, the nurse must ensure that their knees are as close to the patient as possible; this will allow the optimum position. Remember to lower any hospital beds or trolleys as low as possible to optimize good-quality compressions. It is also important to deflate low air loss mattresses using the CPR handle or button. The sternum must be compressed hard and fast. The depth should be 5–6 cm (2 inches) and the rate of 100–120 a minute (almost 2 compressions every second!). Ideally, try not to allow your fingers to press on the chest wall over the ribs. The heels of your hands are much stronger. With the wrists bent and fingers up, it allows better force to be applied. After each compression the pressure must be released to allow full recoil of the chest, but without taking away the hand position. This allows for better cardiac filling and blood flow to the myocardium. Compression and release (recoil) should take the same time and this should avoid any jerky compressions. *Use 30 compressions to 2 ventilations.*

The only times the ratio of compressions changes are:

- when first commencing CPR and waiting for the resuscitation trolley and defibrillator to arrive, continuous compressions should prevail unless there are signs of life.
- when the patient is already intubated or has a secure airway with a supraglottic device, compressions should be continuous. The patient will be ventilated independently of the compressions, so the ratio becomes asynchronous.
- for basic life support purposes *if you are not in the hospital setting*: if you are not able or are unwilling to give rescue breaths, give chest compressions only (Resuscitation Council (UK) 2015).

Chest compressions provide critical but limited blood flow to the brain and heart. They also increase the likelihood that a defibrillatory shock will terminate VF (Resuscitation Council (UK) 2015). This is achieved by increasing intrathoracic pressure within the chest cavity and also by directly pushing down on the heart itself. Almost a third of cardiac output can be created with good-quality chest compressions; therefore, minimizing chest compression interruptions cannot be over emphasized. To reduce fatigue, it is important to change the individual undertaking compressions every 2 min (Resuscitation Council (UK) 2016a, 2016b).

Advanced life support

The current guidelines published in 2016 (Resuscitation Council (UK) 2016) were introduced to simplify the teaching process and to encourage retention of skills. Emphasis is aimed at improved care and implementation of the ALS Guidelines in order to improve patient outcomes. The main changes of minimally interrupted high-quality chest compressions during CPR are based on studies showing circulating blood increases during chest compressions. Even delays of 10–20 s can reduce the chances of successful defibrillation, therefore new changes recommend pauses (hands off) of less than five seconds (Figure 11.2).

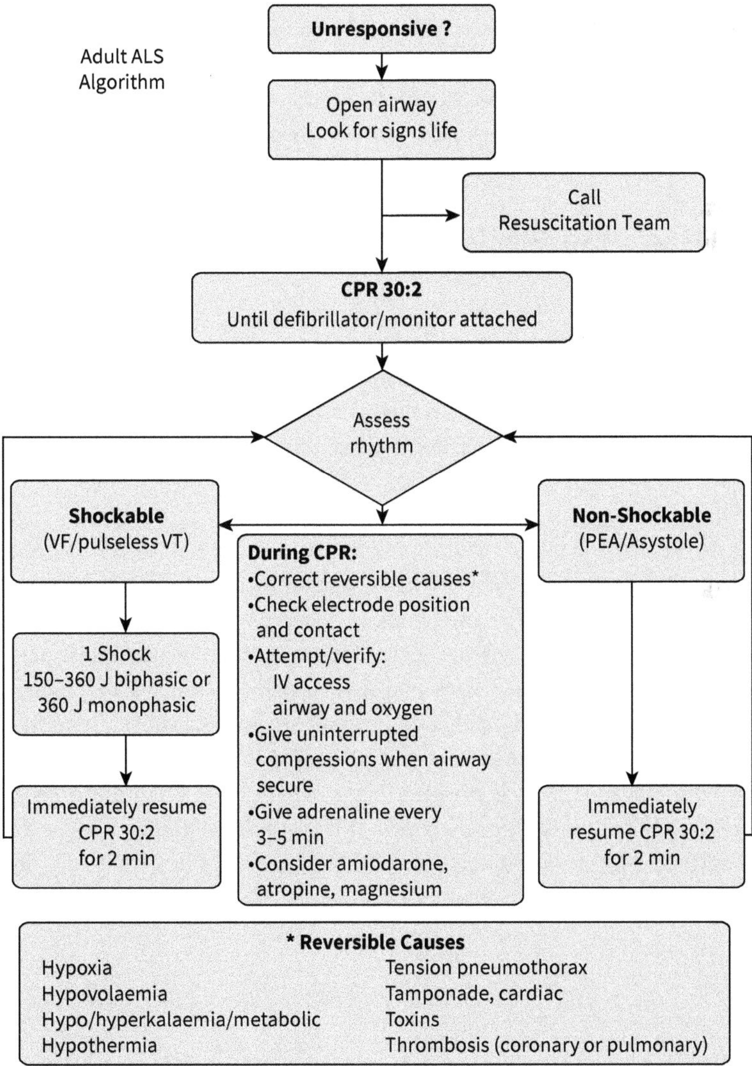

Figure 11.2 ALS algorithm.

Reproduced with the kind permission of the Resuscitation Council (UK). Adult basic life support and automated external defibrillation. © Resuscitation Council (UK). 2015. [https://www.resus.org.uk/resuscitation-guidelines/adult-basic-life-support-and-automated-external-defibrillation/] accessed 07/06/19.

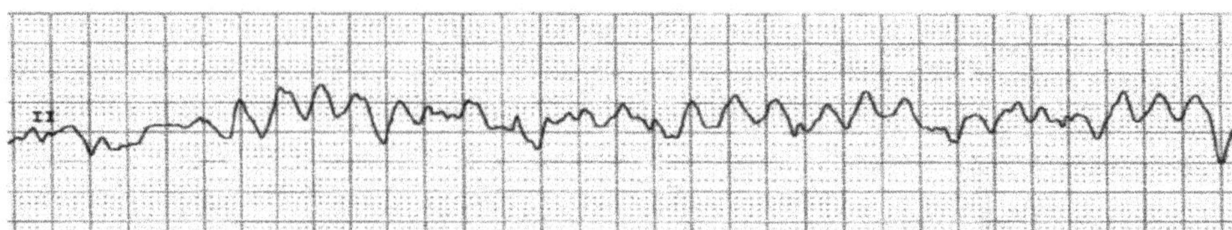

Figure 11.3 Fine ventricular fibrillation.

Management of shockable arrest rhythms

Ventricular fibrillation

- A chaotic bizarre disorganized waveform. No recognizable QRS complex.
- The ventricles are fibrillating like a plate of jelly. There is absence of any ventricular contraction, hence immediate loss of output and sudden cardiac arrest occurs.
- VF may present in a 'fine' or 'coarse' form as highlighted in Figures 11.3 and 11.4.

Ventricular tachycardia (pulseless VT)

- Fast, broad, regular complexes.
- Treat as ventricular fibrillation until proven otherwise.
- Most patients cannot tolerate this rhythm for very long, if at all. The ventricles are contracting so fast that venous return is impeded and the patient will be in cardiac arrest.
- VT will often deteriorate into VF if not managed effectively.
- VT with a pulse is a peri-arrest situation, which will be discussed later.

As soon as the defibrillator arrives, the rhythm needs to be assessed once the pads have been applied. If VF or VT (Figure 11.5) has been confirmed, then charge immediately and give *one shock*. Immediately after the shock is delivered chest compressions are resumed without checking for a pulse or rhythm. Even if the defibrillation attempt is successful in restoring a perfusing rhythm, it is rare for a pulse to be palpable immediately after a shock and the delay in trying to palpate will further compromise the myocardium if a perfusing rhythm has not been restored (Resuscitation Council 2016a, 2016b)

After two minutes of CPR, it is prudent to glance quickly at the monitor to do a rhythm check. Do *NOT* take more than five seconds. If it is still VF/VT then a second shock must be given and then two more uninterrupted minutes of CPR *unless* there are obvious signs

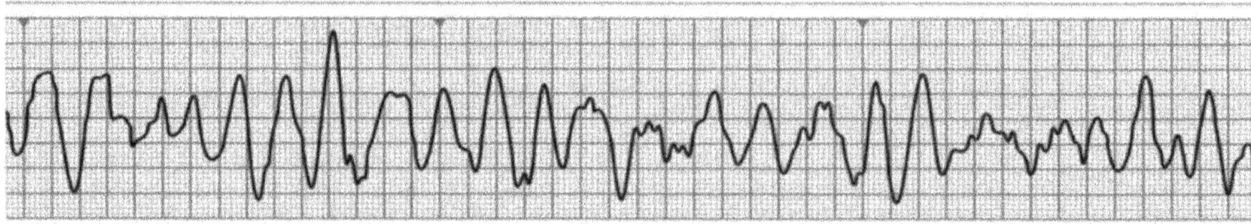

Figure 11.4 Coarse ventricular fibrillation.

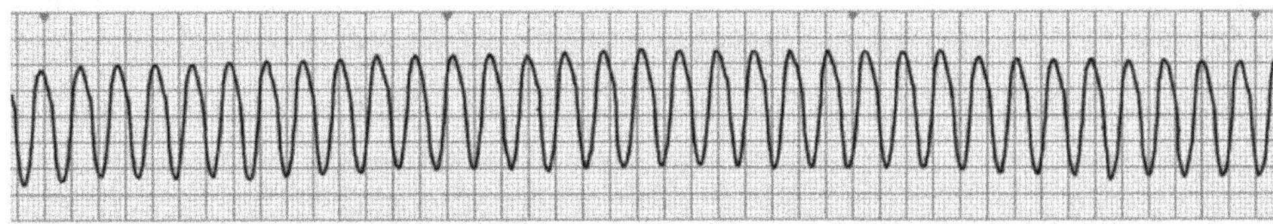

Figure 11.5 Ventricular tachycardia.

of life. After two more minutes of CPR pause for a third rhythm check and if it is still VF/VT, deliver a third shock. Adrenaline 1 mg and amiodarone 300 mg are given after the third shock once CPR has been recommenced. Adrenaline 1 mg is given every other loop (every three to five minutes) regardless of the arrest rhythm until return of spontaneous circulation (ROSC) is achieved. Check the monitor if there are obvious signs of life from the patient, for example movement, coughing, groaning, and normal breathing or any other evidence such as end-tidal CO_2 if available. If a recognized and organized rhythm is evident then an ABC assessment must be made, but for no longer than five seconds (Resuscitation Council (UK) 2015). If normal breathing and pulse is absent and without signs of life, recommence chest compressions and follow the non-shockable arm of the algorithm (asystole/PEA). If a pulse is present and there are signs of life, reassess ABCDE optimizing patient care and start post-resuscitation care (see Table 11.1).

Defibrillation

Defibrillation is the application of a direct current (DC) electric shock through large sticky electrode pads to the heart via the chest wall. It is a quick shock with extremely high energy aiming to terminate life-threatening tachy-arrhythmias. The energy, which is measured in joules, creates mass depolarization of the myocardium. It halters the chaotic arrhythmia by prolonging refractoriness and therefore fibrillation wave fronts. This allows the natural pacemaker, the sino-atrial node, to take over the normal electrical function of the heart and therefore maintain mechanical stability.

In 1947, the first human was defibrillated successfully directly on the heart itself, which is called internal defibrillation. Dr Paul Zoll in 1956 was the first to be successful in closed-chest defibrillation. Initially, the defibrillators were used with alternating current (AC) and changing to DC shocks meant that they could be battery operated, portable, and also proved to have fewer side effects. 1980 witnessed the first implanted internal defibrillator in Baltimore, Maryland. Over the past 10 years further information has become available from the defibrillators themselves in predicting the success of defibrillation using ECG analysis. Evidence suggests that higher VF amplitude and frequency correlates to success, along with minimizing interruption of chest compressions and the number of shocks delivered.

Early defibrillation has been demonstrated to be the key factor in the treatment of cardiac arrest (Resuscitation Council (UK) 2016b). There are several types of defibrillators and all healthcare professionals should be trained in the safe use of their particular model.

Manual defibrillators

It is beneficial to have manual-type defibrillators in acute care areas as they can also be used as a transfer monitor, have added facilities for synchronized cardioversion, and provide

Table 11.1 Post-resuscitation care: patient assessment and treatment after return of spontaneous circulation

Problem area	Assessment	Nursing care/intervention
Airway and breathing Aim: a patent airway, good oxygenation and ventilation	Look, listen, and feel Rate and effort of breathing Added sounds/noises Equal chest movement Pulse oximetry/ABGs Colour Chest X-ray: overall picture also for lines, fractures, and tubes Mental state Sweating/clammy	Head tilt/chin lift Oro/nasopharyngeal airway Suction as required using a wide bore suction catheter High-flow O_2 via non-rebreathe. Aim for sats 90% BVM ventilation (two-person technique) if in ratio 15 compressions to 2 breaths Prepare equipment for intubation and escalation of care/ITU Nasogastric tube if intubated Document observations and NEWS2 scores
Circulation Aim: maintain adequate cardiac output/organ perfusion and arrhythmia control	Monitor heart rate and rhythm Central/peripheral pulses and temperature/capillary refill time Observe colour Blood pressure Adequate intravenous access Assess recent blood results CVP/arterial lines and monitor Assess drains/wounds Urine output	Attach to heart monitor Cannulate into two large veins and send bloods Aim blood pressure systolic 100 mmHg Evaluate 12-lead recording/contact cardiology physicians/?PCI Urinary catheter insertion and hourly measurements Take blood cultures Administer fluids as prescribed Replace electrolytes as prescribed Documentation and care bundles Blood group and save/note location of O-negative blood if required
Disability Aim: maintain brain perfusion and optimise neurological recovery	ACVPU/GCS Pupils Posture/limb movements Blood sugar	Blood sugar control and monitoring (aim for normoglycaemic); may require sliding scale Regular neurological observations If GCS 8, prepare equipment to secure airway Seizure control/sedation as prescribed if required Ensure communication is maintained to patient with reduced conscious level

Table 11.1 *Continued*

Problem area	Assessment	Nursing care/intervention
Exposure Aim: to ensure any other underlying causes are excluded	Temperature Skin Lesions/wounds/holes/rashes Any bleeding areas/points Assess for DVT	Full observation of patient top to toe maintaining dignity at all times Control any bleeding points Send any infective-looking sources for microscopy, culture, and sensitivity from wound swabs, lesions, pus from any source. Administer analgesia as prescribed and monitor effect Maintain privacy and dignity

ABGs, arterial blood gases; BVM, bag valve mask; ITU, intensive therapy unit; MEWS, modified early warning score; CVP, central venous pressure; PCI, percutaneous coronary intervention; ACVPU, Alert, Confused, responds to Voice, responds to Pain, Unresponsive; GCS, Glasgow Coma Score; DVT, deep vein thrombosis.

external pacing, which may be required in the peri-arrest management (see section on peri-arrest). The user needs to interpret the rhythm and make the decision to defibrillate. The joules must also be set by the user (according to manufacturer), the charge button deployed, and, in turn, the shock button when it is safe to do so.

Automated external defibrillators

Automated external defibrillators (AEDs) analyse the rhythm and decide if a shock is required. If a shock is required, the AED will charge up the machine and then indicate to the user when the shock is ready to be delivered. The user then pushes the shock button when it is safe to do so. AEDs are used in the community setting. With widespread increase in public access defibrillation programmes, many more lives will undoubtedly be saved (Box 11.10).

Implantable cardiac defibrillators

Implantable cardiac defibrillators (ICD) look very similar to pacemakers. They are implanted in a subcutaneous pocket and will detect a life-threatening arrhythmia and either attempt to overdrive pace or deliver a shock. This can be very distressing and painful for patients if shocks are discharged unnecessarily, which can sometimes happen. The healthcare team can

Box 11.10 Hands-free pad position for defibrillation

- Top pad/adhesive electrode below the right clavicle to the right of the sternum, thus avoiding large bone mass.
- Lower electrode/apical pad because it lies closer to the apex of the heart. It should be placed just below the left nipple, avoiding breast tissue in mid-axillary line (in line to V6).

care for and touch the patient in a normal manner as they are at no risk of feeling or getting a shock themselves. For the patient's well-being and comfort the critical care unit or cardiac departments within your Trust should have large magnets available which, when placed over the ICD, will deactivate it. This should only be performed in an emergency situation and it is essential that the trust's electrophysiologist or cardiac consultant review the patient as soon as possible.

There are also a number of important safety issues with which you should be familiar in relation to defibrillation—these are identified in Table 11.2.

Precordial thump

This is a sharp blow from a tightly clenched fist with immediate release, on the middle of the sternum. Only those who have been trained in this technique should perform this (Resuscitation Council (UK) 2016a, 2016b). It should be performed when cardiac arrest is witnessed *and* monitored in a shockable rhythm (VF/pulseless VT). If the defibrillator is situated next to the patient then the defibrillator must be used and the precordial thump is no longer recommended. Immediately after the precordial thump, if there are no obvious signs of life or you are unsure then chest compressions must be commenced and await the defibrillator.

Table 11.2 Defibrillation safety

Defibrillation preparation and safety	Intervention
Team and self	The person using the defibrillator must take responsibility for ensuring the area is safe. Visual checks all around the bedspace must be performed in addition to warning all to 'stand clear' before the machine is charged Ensure that neither you nor anyone else are not touching the patient or bed and beware of any stray clothing such as ties, coats, or dangling stethoscopes
Oxygen	Remove any O_2 mask and place at least 1 metre away Leave connected to closed circuit unless ventilator unable to achieve adequate tidal volumes due to chest compressions
Hands-free pads/hand-held paddles	Use of large adhesive electrodes (hands-free) rather than held paddles may reduce risk of sparks Only charge defibrillator when paddles/pads are on the patient's chest
Chest hair	Can reduce chance of successful defibrillation as impedance can be reduced with a lot of chest hair The patient will need to be shaved very rapidly using razor from trolley, this should be performed only where the pads/paddles need to be placed Remember to minimize interruptions on chest compressions therefore the second rescuer will need to quickly shave the chest areas
Drug patches	Remove any transdermal drug patches as they may create unnecessary impedance to defibrillation They may also cause burns to the patient
Fluids	Ensure no-one is left holding attached bags of fluids, as there is an indirect risk to that person Be aware of wet surroundings; make sure patient's chest is dry and ensure team are not standing in puddles of fluid

Consider reversible causes

After ensuring good quality chest compressions between shocks and checking that electrodes are positioned and adhered correctly, a search for other reversible causes should commence. These are known as the 4Hs and 4Ts and are identified in Table 11.3 (Resuscitation Guidelines (UK) 2015). Consider changing electrodes or defibrillator if VF/VT persists after all Hs and Ts have been corrected.

Airway and ventilation

Once the anaesthetist has arrived the airway can be secured and intubation still remains the gold standard. Avoid interruptions to chest compressions during laryngoscopy and intubation, however a brief pause in compressions may be required as the tube is passed through the vocal cords, but this pause should not be for more than five seconds (Resuscitation Council (UK) 2016b). If skilled clinicians are not present then the use of a supraglottic airway is recommended.

It is important for the team leader, when working through the Hs and Ts, to confirm high-flow oxygen is still attached, turned on, and that the patient's chest is rising and falling with each ventilation breath. Some hospitals do not always have anaesthetists available and alternative policies must be put in place. Once the airway is secure, ventilations will be 10/min and asynchronous to compressions; at 100–120/min.

Management of non-shockable arrest rhythms

Pulseless electrical activity (PEA)

- Cardiac electrical activity on the monitor *without* any palpable pulse/signs of life (Figures 11.6 and 11.7).
- Patients can have very weak mechanical function but will be too weak to produce signs of life/pulse.
- Often caused by reversible causes.

Asystole

- The heart has absent electrical or mechanical activity.
- Wandering baseline (Figure 11.8). (Exact straight line could indicate the pads/leads have fallen off the patient therefore check this.)

Asystole with p-waves (ventricular standstill)

- Sino-atrial node firing and atrial contraction only (p-waves) therefore no cardiac output (Figure 11.9).
- Attempt pacing once sticky pads applied.

The use of chest compressions, intubation and ventilation, reversible causes, intravenous access, and adrenaline are common to both shockable and non-shockable arrest rhythms. In PEA or asystole as soon as chest compressions are underway administer 1 mg adrenaline. Ensure that the leads are attached in asystole to confirm the rhythm. If only p-waves are visible, attempt to externally pace (see section on peri-arrest management).

Table 11.3 Potentially reversible causes during cardiac arrest (4Hs and 4Ts)

H or T	Causes	Intervention
Hypoxia	Airway obstruction Respiratory failure Sepsis	Clear, open, suction High O_2 attached BVM, ETT gold standard Check bilateral air entry/chest movement
Hypovolamia	Haemorrhage Trauma Sepsis Gastrointestinal bleed Ruptured aortic aneurysm	2 large-bore cannulae Aggressive IV fluids Blood, O-negative supplies Urgent surgical referral
Hypothermia (< 35°C, severe < 30°C)	Exposure—collapse outside Immersion in water Ingestion of drugs/alcohol	Remove wet clothes and dry ↑ABC assessment time IV fluids at 40°C/warmed air through ventilator/hugger/bypass if available/dialysis DC shock may not work < 30°
Hyper/hypokalaemia and metabolic disorders	Renal disease Calcium channel blocker overdose Documented electrolyte imbalance	Look at current results ABG to see electrolytes Replace electrolytes if low Ca chloride 10 mL 10% IV for hyperkalaemia and OD channel blockers
Tamponade	Penetrating chest trauma Myocardial infarction Cardiac surgery	Needle pericardiocentesis—long cardiac needle (and large syringe) at base of sternum towards left shoulder at 45% angle pulling back whilst inserting Ideally, under echocardiogram if on unit at time of arrest In cardiothoracic centres prepare for urgent chest opening procedure
Tension pneumothorax	History of chest trauma Asthma CVP line insertion Missed pneumothorax plus positive pressure ventilation	Absent breath sounds and chest wall rise and fall Tracheal shift—often late sign Large-bore cannula mid-clavicular line second intercostal space→chest drain
Toxic/therapeutic disorders	Drug overdose A good history Industrial exposure	Protection of team National poisons unit/toxbase Rapid administration of known antidotes
Thrombo-embolic	Pulmonary embolism (surgery/pregnancy/DVT/long-haul travel)	Immediate thrombolysis IV: for known or high suspicion pulmonary embolism: full resuscitation commitment of ALS up to 1 hour. Although routine use is not yet recommended, mechanical devices for continuous chest compressions are available in most acute hospital trusts and can be considered for use in prolonged resuscitations.

BVM, bag valve mask; ETT, endo-tracheal tube; ABC, airway, breathing, circulation; DC, direct current; OD, overdose; DVT, deep vein thrombosis; ALS, advanced life support.

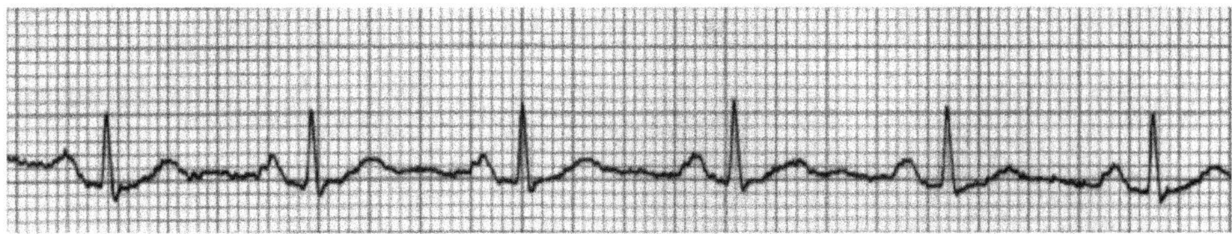

Figure 11.6 Pulseless electrical activity 1 (PEA).

If the cardiac arrest rhythm changes to a VF/VT shockable rhythm, change sides on the algorithm and prepare to shock the patient.

Fine VF or asystole?

If it is unclear whether the patient is in asystole or fine VF, compressions must recommence. Defibrillation at this point is no longer recommended by the Resuscitation Guidelines (UK) 2015. In fact, by compressing the chest uninterrupted, the fibrillating heart should become much more responsive to defibrillation. It is important to remember even if the patient is already being monitored, confirmation of cardiac arrest must be a clinical observation. Always treat the patient and not the monitor.

> **Clinical link 11.2 (see Appendix for answers)**
>
> You walk into the ward bathroom and find Mrs Patel aged 65 collapsed on the floor. She is for CPR. She has no signs of life and you begin immediate CPR and call the cardiac arrest team. Once Mrs Patel is connected to the defibrillator and ECG the cardiac arrest team diagnose PEA arrest. It is suspected that she has had a pulmonary embolism.
>
> - At what rate and depth should you be performing CPR?
> - Explain the reversible causes of cardiac arrest.
> - What treatment might Mrs Patel require?

Drugs used in advanced life support

In past years a great deal of emphasis was given to the administration of drugs in resuscitation. Currently, there is much debate over the use of so many drugs and whether the evidence

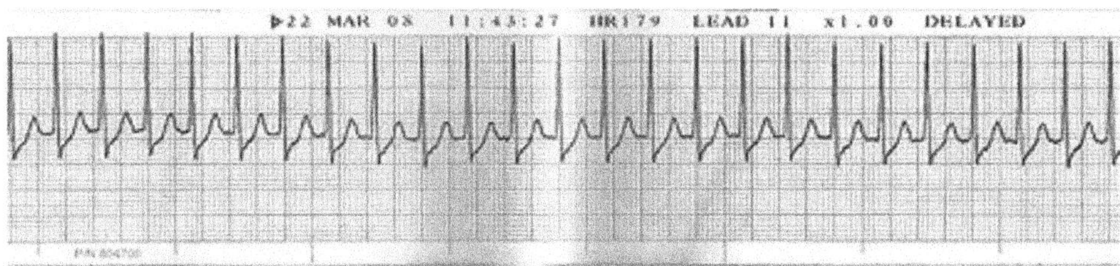

Figure 11.7 Pulseless electrical activity 2 (PEA).

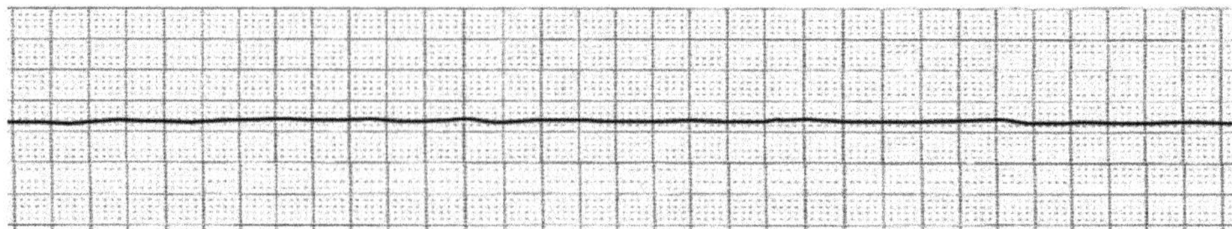

Figure 11.8 Asystole.

supports long-term survival from cardiac arrest. Drugs now play their part much further down the ALS algorithm so other crucial components are emphasized first. Provision of drug therapy must not delay defibrillation and continuous chest compressions, but it is important to secure intravenous or intraosseous access as soon as possible, if this has not already been done.

Routes

Intravenous access (*IV*) remains the best route for delivery of drugs during ALS. The peripheral route is easier and safer to insert than central access in an emergency and has far fewer complications. The *intraosseous* (*IO*) route has been advocated in paediatric guidelines and is now the second-choice route in adult guidelines. Further information can be obtained through hospital resuscitation departments and advance life support courses. After each drug, it is important to give a 10 mL bolus of 0.9% saline or 5% dextrose after amiodarone. The *endotracheal* (*ET*) route for the administration of drugs is no longer recommended.

Below is a list of drugs and their actions recommended by the current European Resuscitation Council (2015) and UK Resuscitation Guidelines (2015).

Adrenaline

Indication during cardiac arrest

- First drug to be given during cardiac arrest.
- Given to increase cerebral and coronary perfusion.

Dose

- 1 mg IV/IO.
- Half-life 3 min.

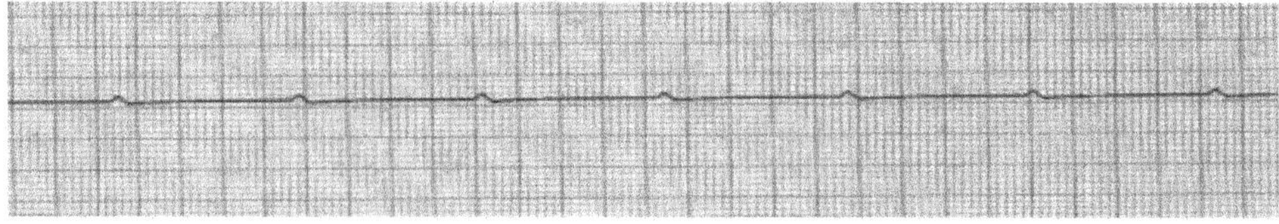

Figure 11.9 Asystole with p-waves (ventricular standstill).

Frequency

- Note: If VF/VT persists after three shocks then give adrenaline. Then give adrenaline every 3–5 min (every other loop).
- For asystole/PEA give with chest compressions and every 3–5 min thereafter.

Desired effects

- Stimulates alpha 1 and alpha 2 receptors to produce vasoconstriction.
- Increases systemic vascular resistance during CPR, producing an increase in coronary and cerebral perfusion.

Undesired effects

- Post arrest: increase in heart rate and force of contraction, therefore increasing the work of the heart.
- Subsequently increasing myocardial oxygen demand and consumption may increase ischaemia and or infarct size.
- Pro-arrhythmogenic due to an increase in myocardial excitability.

Amiodarone

Indication during cardiac arrest

- Shock resistant VF/pulseless VT: give only *AFTER* first three defibrillation attempts

Dose

- 300 mg IV preloaded syringe or diluted in 20 mL 5% dextrose.

Frequency

- 300 mg dose recommended for use.
- 150 mg dose can be given if VF/pulseless VT persists/reoccurs after total of five defibrillation attempts.

Desired effects

- Increases the entire action potential duration, therefore reducing the rate of repolarization.
- Reduces the excitability of all cardiac tissues by increasing the refractory period.
- Reduces the automaticity of the sino-atrial and atrio-ventricular nodes.
- Facilitation of electrical or DC cardioversion.

Undesired effects

- Prolongation of the Q-T interval and may therefore induce polymorphic VT, called torsades des points.

- Pro-arrhythmic.
- Extravasation may cause necrotic tissue damage, therefore ideally given via a central line. If this is not possible a large-bore cannula in a large peripheral vein should be used, such as the ante cubital fossa region.
- Post arrest: bradycardia and hypotension.

Magnesium

Indications during cardiac arrest

- Hypokalaemia/hypomagnesaemia.
- Shock resistant/refractory VF/VT.
- Torsades des pointes.
- Digoxin toxicity.

Dose

- 8 mmols (2 g) as bolus in cardiac arrest over 1–2 min.

Frequency

- May be repeated during resuscitation attempt.

Desired effects

- Improves contraction of a stunned myocardium.
- Neurochemical transmission properties.

Undesired effects

- Post arrest: acute overdosage may cause bradycardias due to inhibition of the sino-atrial node.
- Post arrest: magnesium and calcium work against each other at the cell membrane of vascular smooth muscle, therefore an excess of magnesium or if it has been given too rapidly may cause vasodilation therefore hypotension.

Calcium

Indication during cardiac arrest

- Hyperkalaemia.
- Hypocalcaemia.
- Overdose of calcium channel blockers.

Dose

- 10 mL of 10% calcium chloride IV.

Frequency

- Usually one single dose but may need to be repeated.

Desired effects

- Protects the heart from the toxic effects of potassium in hyperkalaemia.
- An increase of serum calcium. Will need serum levels checking post arrest.

Undesired effects

- Does not lower serum potassium in hyperkalaemia. Dextrose and insulin pre and post arrest most effective.
- Extravasation may cause soft tissue damage.
- Post arrest: bradycardia and arrhythmias.

Sodium bicarbonate

Indication during cardiac arrest

- Hyperkalaemia.
- Tricyclic overdose.
- Consider in severe metabolic acidosis.

Dose

- 50 mmol (50 mL of 8.4% sodium bicarbonate) IV bolus.

Frequency

- Titrated to acid/base values (venous or arterial blood).

Desired effects

- Acts as the buffer in a severe acidotic state. Only consider use if pH is < 7.1 or base excess ≤ 10 mmols/L.
- Some evidence to show benefit in cardiac arrest due to tricyclic anti-depressants.
- An increased sodium load pushes potassium back into the cells.

Undesired effects

- It causes production of carbon dioxide (CO_2), which diffuses into the cells causing a rebound intracellular acidosis.
- Negative inotropic effect on the myocardium.
- Produces a shift to the left on the oxygen (O_2) dissociation curve, which inhibits further oxygen delivery to the tissues (see Chapter 2).

Post-resuscitation management

ROSC is the first step in the continuum of resuscitation (Resuscitation Council (UK) 2016b). Some patients who survive cardiac arrest are resuscitated easily and quickly. They rapidly regain consciousness and resume breathing. Treatment then concentrates on preventing a recurrence. These patients may well stay on the high dependency unit for close monitoring and continuing care. However, some patients who have ROSC will remain unconscious and may or may not be able to breathe satisfactorily for themselves. They may also have poor cardiac output and will therefore be hypotensive. Treatment for these patients is aimed at restoring cardiovascular and respiratory function so that cerebral and systemic tissue perfusion is maintained. As soon as ROSC occurs, post-resuscitation care will begin and it is the final link in the chain of survival. Table 11.1 identifies patient assessment and nursing care/treatment after ROSC. This care must be altered and adapted to meet the patient's own individual needs to provide the best possible chance of leaving hospital. Most patients will be moved to an area for ongoing care and support, whether it is the intensive care unit, the cardiac catheter laboratory, or the coronary care unit.

Percutaneous coronary intervention

Patients who show signs of acute myocardial infarction on a post-cardiac arrest 12-lead ECG will require an immediate review by the on-call cardiologist. Patients who have sustained a VT/VF arrest during or after their acute myocardial infarction are extremely high risk and may require immediate transfer to the cardiac catheter laboratory for percutaneous coronary intervention (PCI) to ensure the best possible outcome for the patient (Thygesen *et al.* 2018). The term percutaneous coronary intervention (sometimes called PTCA, angioplasty, or stenting) describes a range of procedures that treat narrowing or blockages in coronary arteries, supplying blood to the heart (see Chapter 3).

Peri-arrest arrhythmias

These rhythms are life-threatening to patients if left untreated. Peri-arrest rhythms can either be narrow complex arrhythmias, originating from the atrium, or broad complex arrhythmias, which usually (but not always) originate from the ventricles.

This section will pay close attention to the recognition and treatment of an unstable patient with a bradyarrhythmia and/or tachyarrhythmia (see Chapter 3 for a general overview of rhythms and stable arrhythmia management). If the patient is unstable the acute care nurse must focus on initiating early treatment and calling for the appropriate help, instead of becoming too engrossed in interpreting the exact rhythm. Peri-arrest arrhythmias are life-threatening emergency situations, therefore it is crucial that the patient is assessed first. The acute care nurse must be aware of the presence of any *adverse signs*, which will indicate the need for immediate treatment (Box 11.11) Patients who are not acutely ill can often be seen by a member of the cardiology team for advice on appropriate treatment.

Peri-arrest: Bradycardia

This is defined as a heart rate of below 60 beats a minute. For many patients this can be entirely normal and is not dangerous. Athletes especially have very low resting heart rates and

Box 11.11 Immediate treatment in peri-arrest

In the peri-arrest situation many treatment principles are common to all the tachycardias (Resuscitation Council UK 2016b)

- call for help
- high-flow oxygen
- IV access
- blood pressure, oxygen saturations, respirations, and pulse
- 12-lead ECG
- correct any electrolyte imbalances.

can often be around 40 beats a minute. Patients who are prescribed β-blockers also have lower heart rates. Severe or extreme bradycardia of below 40 beats a minute is rarely physiological and usually needs urgent treatment (Resuscitation Council (UK) 2016b).

As the heart rate falls cardiac output is increased by an increase in stroke volume (see Chapter 3), but when this compensation fails cardiac output and blood pressure fall. Coronary filling is also reduced, which will reduce blood supply to the myocardium. The patient may show signs of pallor, be sweaty or clammy, and have an altered level of consciousness.

Bradyarrythmias include extreme sinus bradycardia (Figure 11.10) and first-, second-, and third-degree atrioventricular block (Figure 11.11).

The causes of bradyarrythmias include:

- myocardial infarction (especially inferior wall)
- hypothyroidism
- raised intracranial pressure
- hypothermia
- electrolyte imbalances, such as hyponatraemia
- drug effects, particularly β-blockers and digoxin
- severe hypoxia
- severe hypovolaemia

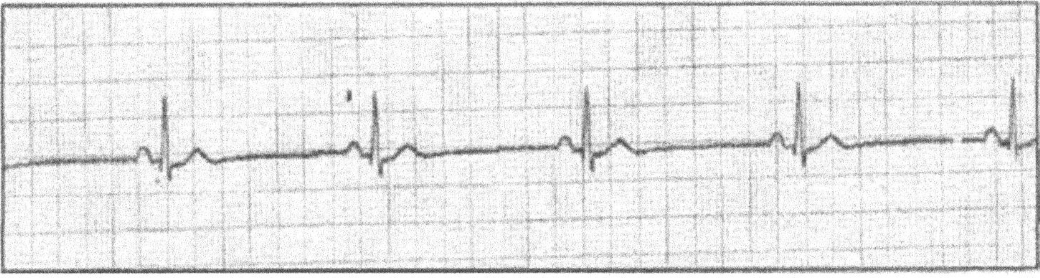

Figure 11.10 Sinus bradycardia.

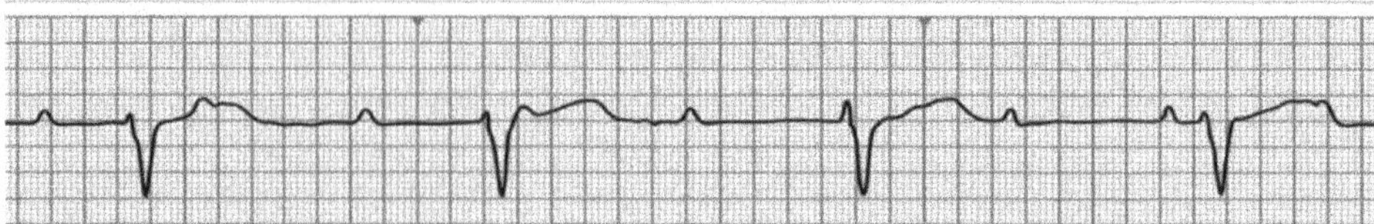

Figure 11.11 Third-degree AV block.

If the patient is at risk of asystole and/or there are any adverse signs proceed to:

- calling 2222 medical emergency
- atropine 500 µg IV increments according to response (max 3 mg)
- adrenaline infusion (2–10 µg/min) if required
- pacing

Pacing

There are four types of pacing: permanent pacing, temporary transvenous pacing, emergency external or transcutaneous pacing, and emergency percussion pacing (fist pacing). Inserting a permanent system and even a temporary transvenous wire is *invasive* and takes time, requiring skilled personnel and specialist radiological equipment. In an acute situation therefore, a quick life-saving interim measure that is *non-invasive* is required that can be started within a minute by trained nursing staff within the acute setting.

Transcutaneous pacing

Non-invasive pacing is achieved easily and is an immediate treatment for bradyarrhythmia, which is a potential risk to the patient who is not responding to drug therapy (Resuscitation Council (UK) 2016b).

Large adhesive electrodes should be placed in the same place as for defibrillation or alternatively in an anterior posterior (A/P) position. A 10–200 milliamp pulse several milliseconds long can be delivered by turning on the pacing facility on the defibrillator. The aim is to achieve cardiac capture, as long as the myocardium still has some evidence of spontaneous electrical activity, by increasing the amount of milliamps until electrical capture is seen on the monitor. Most modern defibrillators placed in an acute area will have a pacing facility capable of demand pacing, whereby the patients' intrinsic QRS complexes are sensed and pacing stimuli will be delivered only if needed. To make it much easier and quicker, modern hands-free defibrillation electrodes (sticky pads) are multifunctional and are capable of monitoring the ECG, defibrillation/cardioversion, and pacing as required.

Due to the stimulation to the nerve endings and skeletal muscle it can be very uncomfortable and can cause distress and pain to conscious patients. The patient's upper body can also jerk along with each stimulus, therefore it is very important to explain what will happen in order to pre-warn the patient. Strong analgesia, for example morphine, should be prescribed by the doctor to ensure comfort.

An appropriate demand rate should be set, which is usually around 60–80 a minute. In some situations a much lower rate should be set, especially if the patient has third-degree AV block with wide QRS, extreme bradycardia, or at risk of ventricular standstill (p-wave asystole), for example patients in Mobitz type 2 second-degree AV block (refer to Chapter 3).

External transcutaneous pacing must only be used in an acute medical emergency to gain time before more definitive treatment can be organized. Once electrical capture has been achieved it is vital to immediately check a central pulse to ensure that mechanical capture has also occurred. This will confirm that the stimulus has created a myocardial contraction. As soon as this is confirmed expert help will arrange for urgent insertion of a temporary transvenous pacing wire. The acute care nurse must be vigilant, organized, and prepare for safe transfer to the cardiac catheter lab/suite (see Chapter 14 on transfer of the acutely ill patient).

Remember it is quite safe to touch the patient during external pacing as less than 1 J is delivered through extremely well-insulated electrodes/pads.

Percussion pacing

This is also an emergency type of pacing. It is not as reliable as electrical pacing. It can be used if there is a delay in activating or preparing the defibrillator ready for external transcutaneous pacing. Deliver firm repeated blows over the precordium to the side of the lower left sternal edge at about 10 cm above the chest. They should be gentle enough so that the conscious patient tolerates them. If capture does not occur, attempt to move the blows around to change the point of contact and also make them more gentle (Resuscitation Council (UK) 2016b).

Peri-arrest: Tachycardia

This is defined as a heart rate of above 100 beats a minute. Sinus tachycardia, however, is not an arrhythmia. Whether the patient is stable or unstable affects the treatment options during peri-arrest arrhythmias. If the patient is *stable* they should be given drug therapy to cardiovert the arrhythmia chemically (see Chapter 3). If the patient is *unstable* and compromised (see Box 11.12; Resuscitation Council (UK) 2016b) then electricity is used to cardiovert the arrhythmia (urgent synchronized cardioversion).

Tachyarrhythmias include narrow complex tachycardias, atrial flutter (Figure 11.12), atrial fibrillation (Figure 11.13), and supraventricular tachycardia (Figure 11.14). These tachycardias are usually less life-threatening than broad complex tachycardias.

Causes of narrow complex tachycardia include:

- electrolyte abnormalities
- alcohol/caffeine

Box 11.12 Adverse signs in peri-arrest

- Systolic blood pressure < 90 mmHg.
- Heart failure.
- Chest pain.
- Heart rate < 40 or ≥ 150.
- Drowsiness/confusion.

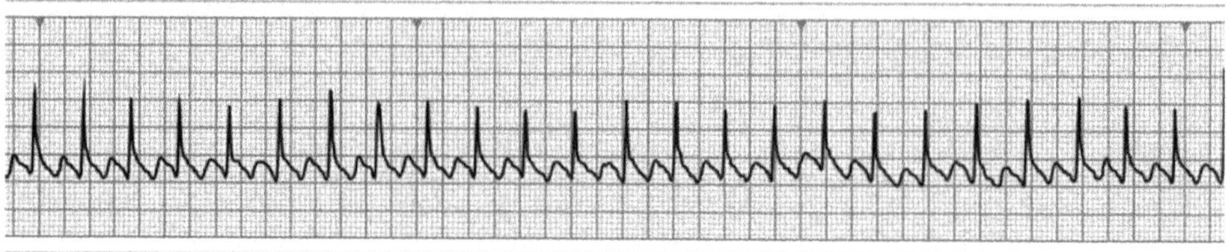

Figure 11.12 Atrial flutter.

- myocardial infarction
- antiarrhythmic drugs
- Wolff–Parkinson–White syndrome
- thyrotoxicosis
- coronary heart disease
- heart failure

VT is a broad complex tachycardia (Figure 11.15), the causes of which include:

- myocardial infarction
- cardiomyopathy
- long QT syndrome
- Brugada syndrome
- antiarrythmic drugs
- heart failure
- R on T phenomenon
- electrolyte imbalances
- tricyclic antidepressant overdose

If the patient with broad complex tachycardia has any adverse signs proceed to:

- calling 2222 medical emergency
- support ABCs
- giving O_2, cannulating, and correcting electrolytes
- if possible perform 12-lead ECG
- synchronized DC shock three attempts (range of 80–360 J depending on trust policy and type of defibrillator used)
- amiodarone 300 mg IV over 10–20 min
- repeat DC synchronized shock

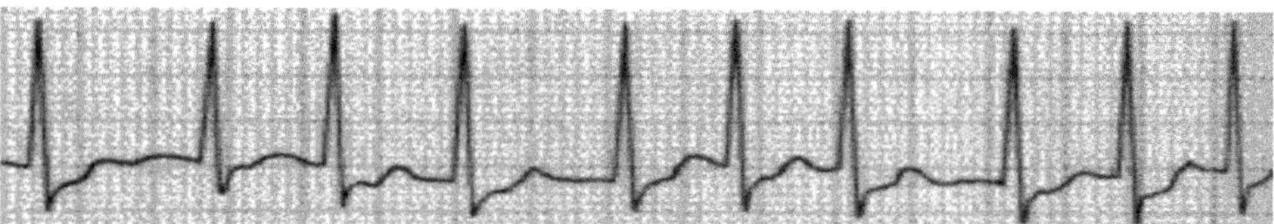

Figure 11.13 Atrial fibrillation.

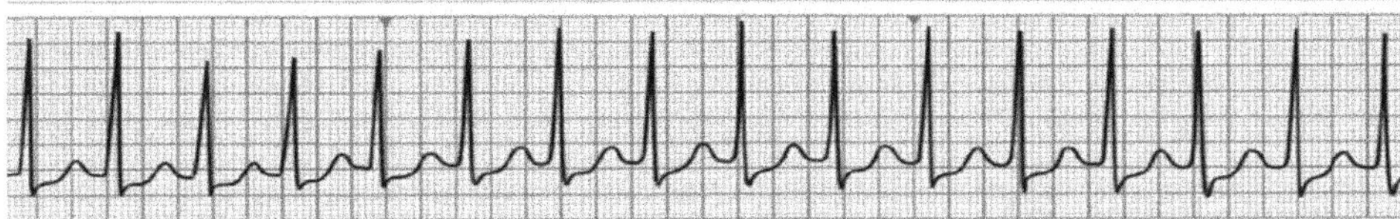

Figure 11.14 Atrial tachycardia.

Synchronized cardioversion for unstable tachyarrhythmias

The patient needs to be prepared for urgent synchronized cardioversion whilst the nurse waits for medical support. Full explanation and reassurance to the patient is essential. The anaesthetist will need to sedate heavily or even anaesthetize before cardioversion because it is an extremely painful procedure. In readiness for synchronized shock, the large adhesive electrodes (defib pads) will be placed on the patient's chest). Energy levels may differ according to trust policy but usually start at less than for VF/VT cardiac arrest. Once the energy is selected on the defibrillator the synchronized button needs to be turned on. The shock delivered needs to be synchronized onto the patient's own R-wave, to avoid the DC shock affecting the unstable part of the cardiac cycle. If this occurred the patient's rhythm could deteriorate into pulseless VT or VF. All safety aspects apply as for defibrillation during cardiac arrest. The person responsible for defibrillating must ensure that all the safety checks are performed and must only deliver the shock when they are sure the rhythm is being synchronized and it is safe to do so. Once the synchronized shock is delivered the patient's central pulse must be checked in case the patient's condition has deteriorated. A cardiac monitor along with non-invasive saturation, respirations, and blood pressure monitoring must be recorded throughout and also post procedure. A repeat 12-lead ECG should be recorded to rule out myocardial infarction or other cardiac causes for the arrhythmia after the procedure. Electrolytes will also need to be checked as shocks can cause loss of available potassium and/or magnesium within the circulation to the myocardium. The patient may need to be transferred to the coronary care unit for escalation of care.

Anaphylaxis

Anaphylaxis is an acute, severe, and life-threatening allergic reaction. The term comes from the Greek words *ana* meaning 'against' and *phylaxis* meaning 'protection'. It is undoubtedly an acute emergency and unfortunately its occurrence appears to be on the increase. Twenty deaths in the United Kingdom every year are due to anaphylaxis, but this number is

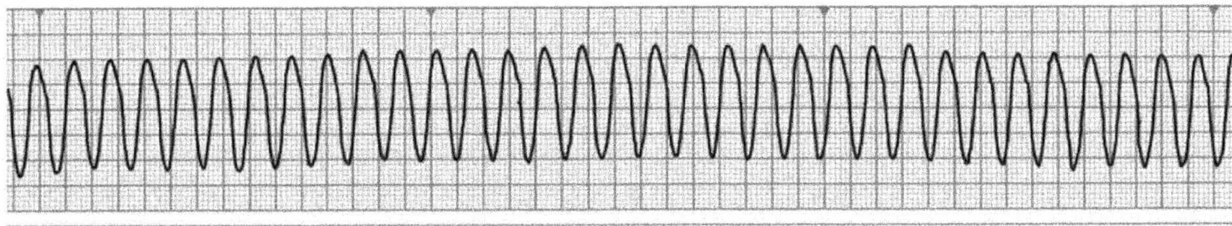

Figure 11.15 Broad complex tachycardia (ventricular tachycardia).

probably an underestimation as many will probably be unrecognized (Resuscitation Council (UK) 2011).

Common triggers

- Insect stings/bites: wasps, bees, and others.
- Foods: nuts, fish and seafood, strawberries, milk, chickpeas, bananas.
- Drugs: antibiotics, non-steroidal anti-inflammatory drugs, muscle relaxants, contrast medium, colloids, angiotensin-converting enzyme inhibitors.
- Blood transfusions.
- Others: hair dye, latex.
- Idiopathic.

Anaphylaxis is triggered by something (the antigen) that sensitizes the immunoglobulin antibodies (IgE mediated). In many cases no cause can be identified and these are generally idiopathic and non-IgE mediated.

An allergic response triggers a quick release of many immunological mediators from mast cells. Mast cells can be found in connective tissue and are required as part of the body's normal inflammatory process within the immune system. Large quantities of released histamines, prostaglandins, and leukotrienes cause blood vessels to dilate and capillaries to leak out plasma into tissues.

Life-threatening signs and symptoms of anaphylaxis

- Gross oedema, especially around the face (angioedema) and upper airway, causing airway obstruction.
- Severe bronchoconstriction/bronchospasm and lung oedema (non-cardiac), causing extreme breathing difficulties, hypoxaemia, and respiratory failure.
- Profound vasodilatation, causing severe hypotension, circulatory collapse, unconsciousness, and cardiac arrest.
- Looks and feels unwell.

Other symptoms may include:

- wheezing
- urticaria (hives/rash)
- itching
- anxiety, 'impending doom'
- abdominal cramps and diarrhoea
- flushed appearance or pallor
- runny eyes

These other symptoms alone do *not* indicate an anaphylactic reaction but may occur alongside the life-threatening symptoms.

The Resuscitation Council (UK) updated the guidelines on anaphylaxis in 2011. Criteria for anaphylaxis (Resuscitation Council (UK) 2011) include:

- the sudden onset and rapid progression of symptoms.
- life-threatening airway and/or breathing and/or circulation problems.
- skin and/or mucosal changes such as flushing, urticaria, and angioedema.

Symptoms can occur immediately, after a few minutes (usually within 5–35 min). or can be delayed up to hours after exposure. Some cases have been reported anything up to 72 h after the triggering event. Episodes may also occur whereby symptoms improve, only to worsen again, each time in a more severe fashion until they are severe enough to threaten life. Death caused by intravenous medications occurs most commonly within 5 min, but rarely over 6 h from contact with the trigger (Resuscitation Council (UK) 2011). There is also a strong link of severity of reaction and risk of death associated with patients with asthma (Pumphrey and Gowland 2007).

Using the ABCDE approach (Resuscitation Council (UK) 2016a, 2016b) in an acute emergency is important as anaphylaxis can be very difficult to diagnose. In any critical illness the clinical signs will always be similar, therefore adopting a structured approach will ensure life-threatening symptoms will be recognized and treated quickly and appropriately.

It is essential that the patient has a full investigation by their medical team after the reaction has occurred, so that they are followed up as soon as possible by an allergy specialist. To help confirm diagnosis blood samples should be obtained. Mast cells degranulate in anaphylaxis, which increases levels of blood tryptase levels. Peak time is 1–2 h after start of symptoms and is back to normal at 6–8 h (Schwartz 2006), therefore it is important to take samples at the correct times. A 24-h sample or at follow up should be analysed to show baseline levels of tryptase.

Treatment

Please refer to Figure 11.16 (with kind permission from the Resuscitation Council (UK)).

It is vitally important to firstly remove the suspected trigger. As IV injections usually cause a rapid reaction, if suspicions are raised then the IV drug must be stopped immediately. With suspected food-induced anaphylaxis, attempts to make the patient vomit are not recommended by the Resuscitation Council (UK) (2008). During your ABCDE assessment it is important to remember that you are treating life-threatening problems as you find each one. Calling for support from your nurse colleagues early is essential and if the three criteria are met then a medical emergency call (or cardiac arrest call if your hospital does not have a separate MET) must be deployed.

Intramuscular (IM) adrenaline 0.5 mg (1/2 mL 1:1,000 adrenaline) should be given immediately (refer to algorithm for child doses) and can be repeated after 5 min if there is no improvement (1:10,000 IV adrenaline can be given by an intensivist/anaesthetist because they will be experienced in using IV adrenaline). The IM route is safer, easier to administer, and does not require IV access. There are no randomized controlled trials to support the use of adrenaline; however, there is good anecdotal evidence of adrenaline as a known vasoconstrictor thereby restoring cardiac output and reducing angioedema. Adrenaline also acts as a bronchodilator. Its β-adrenergic receptor activity helps to cause bronchodilation of the bronchial airways and also increasing the force of myocardial contraction and suppressing the

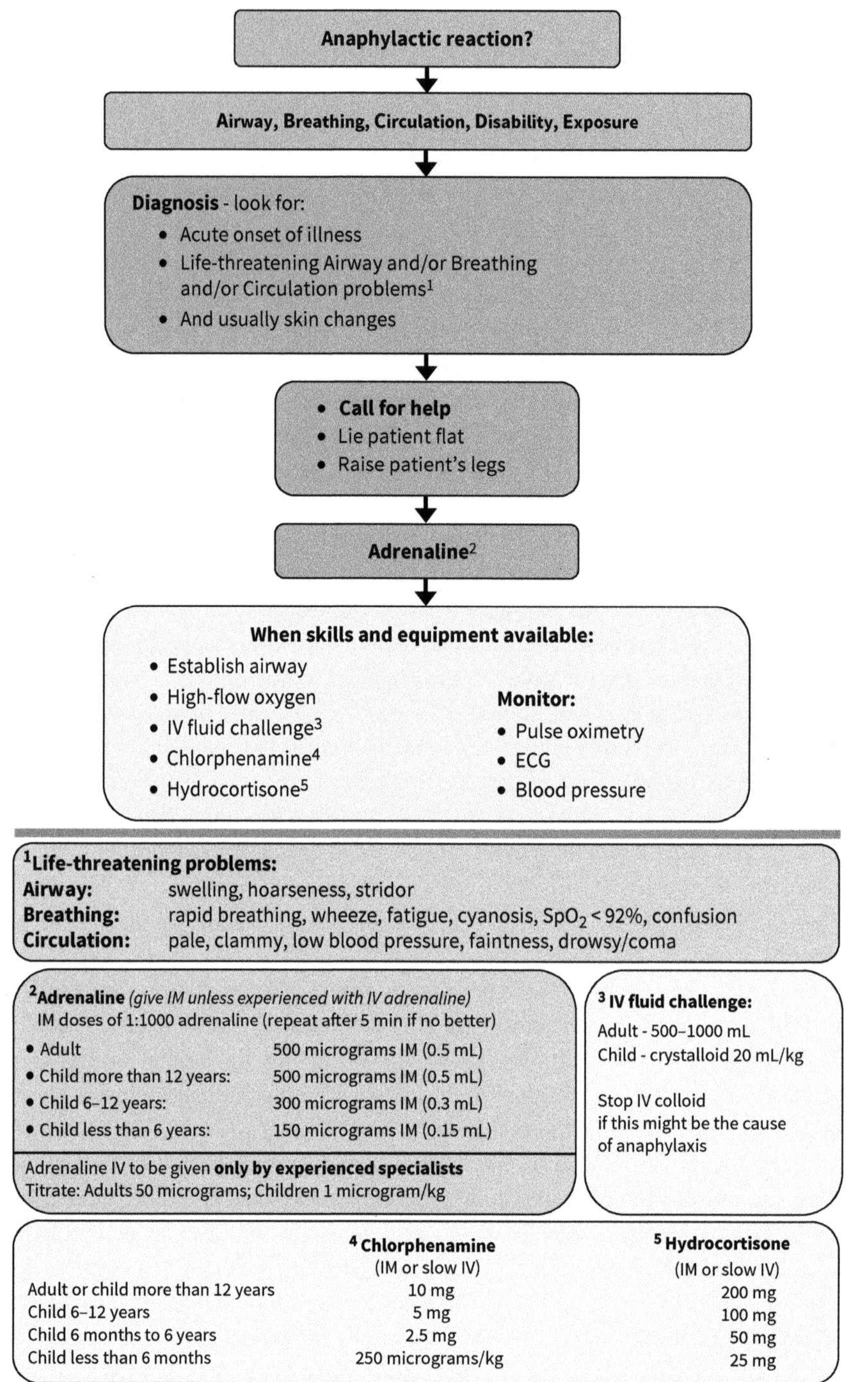

Figure 11.16 Anaphylaxis algorithm.

Reproduced with the kind permission of the Resuscitation Council (UK). Emergency Treatment of Anaphylactic Reactions: Guidelines for Healthcare Providers. In *Anaphylaxis*. Copyright ©208, Resuscitation Council (UK). https://www.resus.org.uk/anaphylaxis/emergency-treatment-of-anaphylactic-reactions/.

negative effects of histamine and leukotriene release. It is essential the patient is given high-concentration oxygen via a non-rebreathe mask with reservoir. Ensure that the resuscitation trolley is nearby, with airway protecting and intubation equipment ready for the anaesthetist to use if required. Ensure all monitoring is available including pulse oximetry, ECG, and blood pressure. If you are trained in cannulation skills, attempt to secure a cannula in a large vein and prepare for IV crystalloid fluid challenge.

Other medications

Antihistamines and steroids are only for second-line treatment and can be given after the acute emergency and initial resuscitation. There is no evidence to support their usage in the initial stages and they should not be given before adrenaline, oxygen, or fluids.

Cardiac arrest following anaphylaxis

If the patient has sustained a cardiac arrest, start immediate CPR and instigate in-hospital resuscitation, as already discussed earlier in this chapter. ALS remains unchanged and adrenaline doses and routes are stated in the ALS guidelines (2015) (see Figure 11.8). The IM route is not recommended once the patient has sustained a cardiac arrest from anaphylaxis.

Conclusion

Reversibility of cardiac arrest has only in recent times been made a practical reality. If patients in peri- and/or cardiac arrest are to receive high-quality care and treatment to have a chance to survive, it is essential that management and treatment are based on sound evidence supported by clear concise guidelines. These guidelines need to be available to all involved in patient care and this, along with further staff education, training and audit of practice, will help to ensure patients receive the optimum care they deserve.

Early recognition and treatment of critically ill patients will prevent some cardiac arrests (Resuscitation Council (UK) 2016a, 20016b). The most important factor in the survival from a cardiac arrest is the presence of a trained rescuer who is equipped to intervene. As identified, the most effective tools of the trained rescuer are CPR and defibrillation.

The nurse working in the acute care arena will undoubtedly gain knowledge, experience, and an increased level of skill and confidence by reflecting on each acute emergency situation they face. The opportunity to regularly undertake practical updates and practice scenarios in the classroom is also essential for the retention of these skills. This will reduce stress, improve performance, and enhance understanding. To this end, acute care nurses will become a crucial component of any resuscitation team.

Patients with acute emergencies present the nurse with a wide range of problems and challenges that test knowledge, abilities, and skills. The systems of patient assessment can be easily applied to any clinical area. Using this prior knowledge, experience, and reflection in assessment and treatment will undoubtedly assist the acute care nurse with the next acutely sick patient presented. Above all it is vital to have the understanding that an emergency situation actually exists. Hopefully this chapter has given you this understanding and an increased confidence to ensure that happens.

References

Cummins, R.O., Ornato, J.P., Thies, W.K., *et al.* (1991) Improving the survival from sudden cardiac arrest: The 'chain of survival' concept. *Circulation*, 83:1832–47.

McNeill, G., Bryden, D. (2013) Do either early warning systems or emergency response teams improve hospital patient survival? A systematic review. *Resuscitation*, 84:1652–67.

National Confidential Enquiry into Patient Outcome and Death (2012) *Cardiac Arrest Procedures: Time to Intervene?* London: National Confidential Enquiry into Patient Outcome and Death.

National Health Service Improvement (2018) *Patient Safety Alert. Risk of Death and Severe Harm from Failure to Obtain and Continue Flow from Oxygen Cylinders.* Available at: https://improvement.nhs.uk/news-alerts/failure-to-obtain-and-continue-flow-from-oxygen-cylinders/; accessed 9 December 2019.

National Patient Safety Agency (2007) Safer care for the acutely ill patient: Learning from serious incidents. The fifth report from the Patient Safety Observatory, London: NPSA.

NICE (2007) *Acutely Ill Patients in Hospital: Recognition of and Response to Acute Illness in Adults in Hospital* CG50. London: National Institute for Health and Care Excellence.

Pumphrey, R.S., Gowland, M.H. (2007) Further fatal allergic reactions to food in the United Kingdom 1999–2006. *J Allergy Clin Immunol*, 119(4):1018–19.

Resuscitation Council (UK) (2015) *Adult Basic Life Support and Automated External Defibrillator.* London: Resuscitation Council (UK).

Resuscitation Council (UK) (2016a) *Immediate Life Support* 4th edn. London: Resuscitation Council (UK).

Resuscitation Council (UK) (2016b) *Advanced Life Support* 7th edn. London: Resuscitation Council (UK).

Resuscitation Council (UK) (2008) *Emergency Treatment of Anaphylactic Reactions: Guidelines for Healthcare Providers*. London: Resuscitation Council (UK).

RCP (2017) *National Early Warning Scores 2: Standardizing the assessment of acute illness severity in the NHS.* London: Royal College of Physicians.

Schwartz, L.B. (2006) Diagnostic value of tryptase in anaphylaxis and mastocytes *Immunol Allergy Clin N Am*, 26(3):451–63.

Smith, G.B. (2000) Assessment and stabilisation of the critically ill outside the ICU. *Anaesth Int Care Med*, 1(3):88–90.

Smith, G.B. (2003) *ALERT: Acute Life—Threatening Events Recognition and Treatment* 2nd edn. Portsmouth: University of Portsmouth.

Thygesen, K., Alpert, J.S., Jaffe, A.S., *et al.* (2018) Fourth universal definition of myocardial infarction. *Eur Heart J.* Available at: https://doi.org/10.1093/eurheartj/ehy462; accessed 9 December 2019.

Waldie, J., Day, T., Tee, S., *et al.* 2016 Patient safety in acute care: are we going around in circles? *Br J Nurs*, 2 (3):747–51.

12 Transfer of acutely ill patients

Emma Gardner

Chapter contents

Transfers are undertaken to improve the management of the patient and therefore play a crucial part within a patient's journey. It is essential to have an understanding of the effects that transfers have on the acutely ill patient and the associated risks. This chapter will examine:

- intra- and inter-hospital transfer
- physiological changes during transfer
- pre-transfer preparation and clinical assessment
- clinical skills required during transfer
- transfer equipment
- handover
- medical and legal issues related to transfer

Learning outcomes

This chapter will enable you to:

- understand the rationale and challenges in patient transfer
- understand the decision-making process and nursing responsibilities during transfer
- analyse the risk of transferring acutely ill patients
- recognize the need for good communication processes
- analyse the skills required for escorting personnel
- evaluate the equipment that may be required to support the patient transfer

Introduction

The acutely ill patient is at an increased risk of haemodynamic instability during a transfer. This is because the body's ability to compensate the effects of movement is compromised by its acute pathology and additional drug therapy. The transfer of the patient is therefore not without risk. The decision to transfer must be based on the benefits of the move to the patient verses potential risk it may cause.

The transfer of acutely ill patient occurs for many reasons and can be either intra-hospital or inter-hospital. Intra-hospital transfers occur within the hospital, for example the admission of a patient from the Emergency Department (ED) to the ward, moving to and from an area of higher care (e.g. critical care), or taking a patient for specialist imaging or intervention (X-ray, computerized tomography (CT) scanner, operating theatre) (Kulshrestha and Singh 2016). Inter-hospital transfers however involve moving a patient to another location outside the hospital, for example to a tertiary centre, different hospital sites within a trust, and repatriation (Wilcox *et al.* 2016). Logistically inter-hospital transfers require more organization because they require the use of the ambulance service combined with the transfer of patient information.

The decision to transfer a patient to another environment should be taken by a Senior Clinician (Consultant), ideally following a discussion with the patient and their relatives. Transfers may be elective: facilitating advanced planning and preparation, or if urgent or an emergency, will have reduced preparation time, potentially increasing risk. Regardless of the reason for transferring a patient, a comprehensive assessment must be carried out to reduce harm. A disorganized transfer can significantly contribute to morbidity and mortality (Kulshrestha and Singh 2016).

Although this chapter will focus on the needs of the acutely ill patient, the principles of assessment must be applied to all patients being transferred. It may be challenging to balance the clinical priorities and needs of the patient group but, as with the deteriorating patient, staff should seek advice if unsure how to manage the situation.

The Intensive Care Society states that for the inter-hospital transfer of critically ill patients, the 'standard of care should be at least as good as that at the referring hospital or base unit' and that it must include written documentation of patient status, monitored values, and treatment given during transfer (Intensive Care Society 2011). The Faculty of Intensive Care Medicine provides further guidance with specific standards and recommendations for the transfer of critically ill patients (Johnston and Tulloch 2016).

Changes on physiology during transfer (movement)

The physical process of transfer (i.e. motion) may cause the patient to deteriorate. This is the result of inertial forces created from acceleration and deceleration which can create significant alterations in blood pressure, heart rate, gastric and intracranial pressure. Inertia is the result of the opposite reaction caused by an action (Newton's Third Law). As an ambulance accelerates the external force causing acceleration is towards the patient's head. The inertia force is in the opposite direction (i.e. towards the feet) causing displacement of blood to the feet. The opposite happens during deceleration: blood is displaced towards the head.

The consequences of acceleration (blood pooling in the feet) is decreased venous return and cardiac output causing hypotension. This occurs because an acutely patient may not be able to compensate for the shift in fluid. Acute illness can reduce or block the baroreceptor receptor reflex which in normal circumstances would be triggered to increase vascular tone. Cerebral perfusion will also be reduced in response to the hypotension thus potentially altering a patient's conscious level. For the patient in respiratory failure who is spontaneously breathing, sitting in an upright position, and on high-flow oxygen, the physical exertion and any ensuing changes of position (e.g. bed to bed) may alter ventilation/perfusion, which could be enough to cause a physiological deterioration (Beard *et al.* 2016).

Deceleration has the opposite effect because the inertial forces push blood towards the head. The increased blood volume entering the right ventricle can lead to heart failure, pulmonary oedema, and arrhythmia. It is important that the transfer team are aware of any pre-existing cardiac problems such as arrhythmia or ischaemic heart disease because these heighten the risk of haemodynamic instability (Knight *et al.* 2015).

The neurological system may be affected because the intra-cranial pressure (ICP) increases during movement which subsequently lowers cerebral perfusion pressure (Trofimov *et al.* 2016).

The gastrointestinal system can also be affected by inertial forces which may cause displacement of the stomach contents. This in turn increases the risk of aspiration. There may also be a change in ventilation status (reduced tidal volumes) because any shift in abdominal contents places additional pressure on the diaphragm. The motion of an ambulance, trolley, or wheelchair can also evoke travel sickness therefore an anti-emetic should be considered pre-transfer (Beard *et al.* 2016).

To minimize the effect of acceleration and deceleration, the patient should be maximally stabilized. One should consider the need for a fluid challenge prior to transfer because this will increase the circulating volume, improving cardiac output

Another physical effect which may occur is the displacement of unstable spinal fractures.

As well as the dynamic effects of motion one must consider the effects of noise and vibration caused by the movement of the trolleys. The noise from monitor alarms and communication of the team can also heighten anxiety. Vibration can cause nausea, discomfort, headache, and visual disturbance (Sethi and Subramanian 2014). Minimizing the effects of temperature variation as the patient travels between different environments will also reduce potential stress.

In summary, although the patient transfer may be urgent, to reduce the potentially harmful haemodynamic changes to the patient caused by acceleration/deceleration, the transferring team should be advised to proceed as quickly as possible at a constant pace avoiding any sudden changes in speed. Clearly, it is crucial that the patient is carefully monitored throughout the transfer process (Resuscitation Council (UK) 2017).

The features of a 'good' transfer to ensure that the patient arrives to the required location safely

- The patient is involved in the decision-making (if possible).
- The patient transfer should be planned, organized, and timely as a delay in the transfer of the patient may result in a delay in gaining timely treatment or a diagnosis.
- The receiving department/hospital is prepared and expecting admission.
- All relevant patient information is communicated to the receiving team.
- Team work: the appropriately trained escort staff are available, they should work together as a team and have a clear understanding of each other's role in monitoring the patient.
- Risk is assessed based on the acuity and dependency of the patient considering the potential for what could go wrong, what the consequence would be if it did go wrong, and what the likelihood is of this happening.
- No adverse events occur.

Many adverse events which occur within healthcare are related to equipment failure, inadequate preparation, and poor communication. (Achrekar *et al.* 2016). Effective communication and teamwork are particularly important non-technical skills which contribute to a safe transfer. Other human factors required for transporting patients include situational awareness, decision-making, leadership/followership, task/time management, and the ability to cope with stress (Hulme and Low 2014).

Reason (2016) discusses the use of foresight training to enable staff to consider:

- the current safety level at which the practitioner is working (*self*);
- the *context* in which they are working; for example other ward activities/staffing;
- the *task* they are required to do.

Reason (2016) suggests it is the balance between these three aspects of self, context, and task that increases or decreases the risk of a clinical incident or 'near miss' occurring (see Box 12.1).

Emergency transfers of patients where rapid decision-making is required without clear leadership and clarity over roles of professionals for patient monitoring can create a high-risk environment (*context*). Again, by increased awareness, healthcare professionals involved in transfer can minimize the risk to the patient. For example, it should be clear who is monitoring the airway, adequacy of ventilation, and haemodynamic response, and who is documenting the patient's observations.

Preparation for safe transfer of the acutely ill patient

Team work and preparation are crucial to assist in minimizing this risk to the patient, even if this has to be undertaken rapidly.

The preparation should include:

- documentation regarding the patient, that is clinical assessment of the patient, past medical history, care management plan;

Box 12.1 A clinical example

Consider this scenario. You have returned to work and are in charge on shift following two days off (having just finished nights). You have found it difficult to adjust to a normal sleeping pattern and feel tired (**self**). The ward is busy and staff are dealing with a medical emergency (**context**). You are asked to prepare an intravenous antibiotic for the patient. However, you have only given this drug once previously (**task**) and are interrupted several times during its preparation to answer questions regarding other patients (**context**).

Could this happen? What is the potential for a clinical incident?

Combining all these factors, Reason (2016) would consider this to be a high-risk situation but by increasing self-awareness and others' awareness, the risk can be minimized; for example, by asking a second nurse to check the process or take over the intravenous preparation of the drug therapy.

- identification of who is/are the most appropriate healthcare professional/s to assist with the transfer and an awareness of what effect this will have on the remaining service;
- identification of the equipment required for the transfer of the patient along with confirmation of the frequency of observations for an inter-hospital transfer.

Clinical assessment before transfer

This should include a comprehensive assessment as outlined in previous chapters. The ABCDE is a system orientated approach to patient management. This model facilitates a rapid assessment and reassessment if any changes occur in the patient's parameters before and/or during transfer (Resuscitation Council (UK) 2017). To prevent adverse risk and limit the physiological changes which may occur during the transfer, one must stabilize the patient and prepare for any potential problems.

Airway: Mouth, endotracheal tube, tracheostomies, or permanent tracheal stomas

Throughout the transfer the patient's airway should be checked for patency and the patient's position optimized. As most transfers require the patient to be supine for the journey, any patient who has a lowered level of consciousness is at increased risk of airway obstruction. The transfer team must therefore be skilled in simple airway manoeuvers such as head tilt or chin lift as well as having access to airway adjuncts such a nasopharyngeal or oral airway (depending on the patient's degree of consciousness).

If the patient has a tracheostomy, backup safety equipment, for example spare inner tube, tracheal dilators, portable suction, and oxygen, must accompany the patient in case the airway becomes blocked (see Chapter 2 for further details). A recent NHS Improvement Safety Alert (2018) identifies the potential for risk of death or severe harm from failure of healthcare practitioners to understand how to utilize portable oxygen cylinders. All healthcare practitioners have responsibility to ensure that they have regular opportunities to practice operating oxygen cylinder controls and NHS Trusts must prioritize training for staff groups and clinical areas where this equipment is used.

A patient with a Glasgow Coma Scale of less than 9 will require intubating to maintain and protect their airway and ensure adequate oxygenation and ventilation. The patient will also need a nasogastric tube to prevent aspiration of gastric fluid.

Breathing: Adequate oxygenation and ventilation

The work of breathing should be assessed by visual inspection of chest movement and observing the respiratory rate, and depth of breathing. Oxygen saturation should be assessed and recorded using pulse oximetry. A target saturation should be identified for the individual patient by their medical team. Recent guidance from the British Thoracic Society recommends a target saturation of 94–98% for most patients or 88–92% for those at risk of hypercapnic respiratory failure (British Thoracic Society 2017). Oxygen saturation is extremely useful in aiding the clinical assessment the transfer motion can affect the accuracy of the signal. An ear rather than finger probe may provide increased accuracy (Resuscitation Council Guidelines (UK) 2017).

Depending on the inspired oxygen required (which should be recorded on the prescription chart), the appropriate device for administering the oxygen should be obtained: nasal cannulae, simple face mask, venturi mask, or reservoir mask (British Thoracic Society 2017). If a patient is requiring non-invasive ventilation, such as Biphasic Positive airway Pressure (BiPAP) therapy, the battery backup for the machine should be established as this may impose limitations on transporting the patient. If the patient requires intubation, a portable mechanical ventilator (with portable oxygen supply) will be required.

The distance and time for travel should be estimated to calculate the amount of oxygen required for journey. As a guide, this figure should be doubled for the journey to allow for any unforeseen delays. The equation to determine how long a cylinder will last is:

$$\text{Cylinder Time (minutes)} = \frac{\text{Cylinder Volume (L)}}{\text{Flow Rate (L / min)}}$$

For example, calculating the amount of time a D-size cylinder (340 L) will last for a patient receiving oxygen via nasal cannulae at 4 L/min would be as follows:

$$\text{Cylinder time} = 340\,\text{L} \div 4\ \text{L/min} = 85\,\text{min} = 1.4\,\text{hours}$$

For a ventilated patient, the oxygen flow rate needs to be calculated which is dependent on the FiO_2 (expressed as a fraction, not percentage), bias flow (continuous background gas flow), and minute volume (tidal volume in litres multiplied by respiratory rate). The equation to use for a ventilated patient is then:

$$O_2\ \text{Flow Rate ventilated patient} = FiO_2 \times (\text{Minute Volume} + \text{Bias Flow})$$

This example is for a portable ventilator with a bias flow of 0.5 L/min, tidal volume of 500 mL, respiratory rate of 16 breaths/min, and 50% oxygen (FiO_2 of 0.5). An E-size oxygen cylinder (680 L) is used.

$$\text{Minute volume} = 0.5\,\text{L} \times 16\,\text{breaths/min} = 8\,\text{L/min}$$

$$O_2\ \text{flow rate} = 0.5 \times (8\ \text{L/min} + 0.5\ \text{L/min}) = 0.5 \times 8.5\ \text{L/min} = 4.25\ \text{L/min}$$

$$\text{Cylinder time} = 680\,\text{L} \div 4.25\,\text{L/min} = 160\ \text{min} = 2.7\,\text{hours}$$

Medical oxygen cylinders are stored with the valve closed to reduce the risk of fire. Some cylinders require a key to open the valve while others have an integral valve to be keyless. It is crucial to know the valve opening procedure, otherwise oxygen therapy could be delayed during an emergency or not delivered at all despite staff believing the oxygen flow is on. NHS Improvement (2018) issued a safety alert about the risk of significant harm and death from failure to correctly use an integral valve cylinder. The steps for preparing an integral valve cylinder from BOC Healthcare (2013) are listed in Box 12.2.

Circulation: Adequate perfusion

Simple physical assessment techniques reflect the patient's haemodynamic status, such as skin colour, core temperature, limb temperature, capillary refill time, signs of sweating, and evidence of peripheral oedema. The blood pressure and pulse (rate, regularity, and strength) should be assessed and compared to previous data for monitoring trends. The frequency of observations must be confirmed and reviewed in accordance to the patient's condition.

The patient must have an assessment of fluid balance: input (fluids, blood, drugs) and output (urine, vomit/gastric blood from drains). This information will allow the team to assess the patient's overall haemodynamic status and response to any fluid interventions. In general, the critically ill patient should have two patent large-bore intravenous (IV) cannulae *in situ* to ensure a constant availability of IV access as well as the administration of multiple infusions.

Box 12.2 Oxygen cylinder preparation with integral valve

1. Check medical gas in cylinder is oxygen and expiry date
2. Check volume gauge is in green area to have sufficient amount
3. Remove the tamper-evident hand-wheel cover (pull the tear ring)
4. Pull down valve outlet cover
5. Check flow rate is set at zero (0) and hand-wheel turned off

Firtree outlet—nasal cannulae or mask tubing	Schrader outlet—portable ventilator
6. Connect tubing from facemask or nasal cannulae to firtree outlet	6. Open the valve to turn on cylinder by fully rotating hand wheel anti-clockwise until it stops
7. Open the valve to turn on cylinder by fully rotating hand wheel anti-clockwise until it stops	7. Put oxygen probe into Schrader outlet
8. Set the prescribed flow rate of oxygen using the dial flow selector	8. Check there is no leak indicated by a hissing sound
9. Check oxygen is being delivered and not leaking	

Adapted from Medical oxygen. Integral valve cylinders (CD, ZD, HX, ZX). BOC: Living healthcare. 2019: 2–3. https://www.bochealthcare.co.uk/en/legacy/attachment?files=tcm:6409-54069,tcm:409-54069,tcm:09-54069. Accessed 7 June 2019.

Disability: Neurological assessment

This can be undertaken initially using the patient's response as indicated on the ACVPU scale (Alert, Confused, Voice, Pain, Unconscious/Unarousable). A more detailed assessment (Glasgow Coma Score) should be undertaken for patients who are not registering as alert or are showing signs of confusion or disorientation (see Chapter 4 for more detailed neurological assessment). Pupils should be assessed: are they equal and reacting to light? A blood sugar should also be checked to eliminate hypoglycaemia as a cause of a change in the level of consciousness. Pain assessment (on movement) is important to ensure that the patient receives adequate analgesia before transfer.

Exposure: Examination from head to toe

This is an opportunity to assess the patient's skin integrity, inspect wounds, and observe for signs of rash, skin discoloration, or anatomical abnormality.

The checking of intravenous lines, invasive monitoring sites, drains, and catheters is essential to reduce infection as well as ensure that any tubing is secure and maintains patency. The catheter bag should also be emptied before transfer, kept below the level of the bladder, to avoid reflux or contamination, and hung on the side of the patient's bed (Department of Health 2014). Chest drains are a closed system that should be positioned upright and unobstructed to allow drainage. The patient with a bubbling chest drain or a patient on mechanical ventilation should not have the drain clamped because of the risk of developing a tension pneumothorax (Senanayake *et al.* 2017). Chest drains must have their collection vessel below the level of the chest at all times and the vessel should have a one-way mechanism to prevent the aspiration of air (this is created by an underwater seal or a flutter valve). Not all patients require suction attached to the drain.

Equipment should not be placed on top of the patient. A transfer table can be used and positioned at the foot of the bed or equipment hung on the side of the bed to avoid disconnection.

Health records

Other information should be gathered, including the demographic data, relevant patient information, including nursing care, history, drug prescription, allergies, next of kin information, religion, and number contacts checked. The patient must have an identity band *in situ* and this should be checked against current health records. Many NHS Trusts have a patient transfer checklist which should record this information and ensure SBAR (Situation, Background, Assessment, and Recommendation) handover of the patient at the beginning and end of the transfer. Information regarding infection control status must be forwarded to the receiving unit before transfer as this may affect their preferred location of the patient on admission.

If the patient is being transferred between organizations X-rays/scan results will need to be digitally transferred.

Box 12.3 A guide to decision-making regarding patient escort for the transfer of adult patients

1 clinical competence—the ability to perform physical assessment and undertake skills
2 clinical knowledge of the illness and individual patient
3 knowledge of the effect of transfer on patient's condition
4 the ability to utilize transfer equipment and plan equipment/drugs required for safe transfer
5 the ability to communicate between a range of healthcare professionals, patient, and family.

Clinical skills required for patient transfer

The skills required of the health professional will be dependent on the condition of the individual patient (see Box 12.3). The transferring team should be qualified to anticipate and manage any complications that may arise during the transfer process. The skills may be provided through a combination of escorting personnel and will include the following.

1. Clinical competence

Clinical competence is required in a range of clinical activities depending on the clinical assessment and requirements of the patient. The practitioner should be aware of their own limitations and practice in accordance with their professional role. If the practitioner feels unable to carry out the transfer, then they should escalate their concerns (NMC 2015).

The transfer team's skills should include:

- airway and ventilation management
- cardiovascular management
- neurological management

2. Clinical knowledge of illness and the individual patient

The transferring staff should be familiar with the patient's history, illness, current and future management plan, and any potential complications (foreseeable risk).

3. Knowledge of effect of transfer on patients' condition

All staff involved should be aware of the effect of movement on the unstable patient and be able to manage changes in the patient's condition.

4. Ability to utilize transfer equipment

The transfer of a patient should be a continuation of the care provided in an acute area but as a mobile one. The transferring staff should therefore have a comprehensive knowledge of the monitoring equipment, mechanical ventilator, defibrillator, suction, infusion devices, and any drugs required in the transfer. They should also be aware of transfer specific equipment (gas supply batteries, oxygen cylinders) and incident management (defibrillator, intubation kit) (Droogh *et al.* 2015).

The amount of equipment required will depend on the dependency of the patient along with duration, distance, and mode of transfer (road, sea, air). Even within hospital sites there may be considerable distance to move the patient, involving several lifts. Healthcare professionals must be adequately equipped to manage any reasonable foreseeable situations.

Equipment failure or technical problems are common. Battery life of all electronic devices should be checked before commencing the transfer.

5. Ability to communicate with the patient, their family, and personnel involved in the transfer process

The escorting staff should be able to give concise, accurate information, and know the handover plan regarding the patient. Communication also includes documentation of any care given during the transfer process.

The escort staff who can potentially be available to transfer the patient are outlined in Table 12.1, each providing a different skill set.

Personal care

If leaving the hospital site for inter-hospital transfer, the escort team should consider their own personal requirements (warm clothing, money, refreshments, mobile phone, essential contact numbers). The ambulance service will endeavour to return escorting staff to their base, but when in their locality they may be required to respond to other emergency calls, necessitating the team to travel back by alternative means (with their equipment). Vehicles can occasionally break down, therefore escort staff should have personal protective equipment such as high-visibility jackets.

Moving and handling

The principles of safe patient moving and handling should always be adhered to within the transfer process. Additional devices such as slide sheets/pat slides and hoists must be available to assist the process moving of patient between beds/trolleys. This is governed by the Health and Safety at Work Act 1974 (Health and Safety Executive 1974).

Table 12.1 Potential escorting personnel

Hospital staff	Ambulance staff
Anaesthetist	Technician
Intensive care doctor	Paramedic (able to intubate in cardiac arrest situations and give intravenous drugs)
A&E doctor	
Doctor	Emergency care practitioner
Operating department practitioner	Critical care paramedic (air ambulance)
A&E nurse	
ICU nurse	
Trained nurse (ward based)	
Healthcare assistant	
Clinical site practitioner	
Critical care outreach practitioner	

Escorting staff should have training in safe patient transfer.

The specialist needs of the bariatric patient require consideration to ensure the use of appropriately designed trolley/beds in the transfer process. The weight of any equipment attached to trolleys must also be assessed.

Patient handover

The communication between healthcare professionals plays a major part in the acutely ill patient's journey.

Clinical handover has been identified as one of the nine areas that could be improved to make a significant difference to patient safety (World Health Organization 2007). Every time there is a handover between personnel, there is a potential for key information to be omitted or poorly communicated; such errors could potentially increase morbidity and mortality. Indeed, handover is highlighted as a point at which errors may occur and the Royal College of Physicians (2011) identifies that preventable harm is principally related to human factors.

A structured approach to the handover has proven to improve the quality of the transfer (Achrekar *et al.* 2016). A communication tool which has gained popularity within health care is SBAR. This tool is used to facilitate organized, prompt, and appropriate communication between healthcare practitioners.

Using the SBAR headings allows information regarding the patient's current medical status, recent changes in condition, potential changes to watch for, resuscitation status/advance care planning documents/Gold Standard Framework status, test results, allergies, and a medical plan to be provided.

A transfer checklist can aid in the gathering of information required within SBAR, acting as an aide memoir and reduce the risk during transfer (Van Sluisveld *et al.* 2015), including the following:

- patient demographics, key contact next of kin (and any communications)
- relevant past medical history
- patient's response to treatment to date, major changes
- care given during transfer
- drug therapy—drugs given/due to be given
- infection control status
- any specific aspects of care that require ongoing assessment and management on admission, for example wound, pressure care, nutrition, mobility
- patient's property.

Clinical link activities

The purposes of the following link activities are to encourage the reader to consider how they would manage different situations. They are not exhaustive but reflect some of the varied reasons an acute patient may require transfer. You may reflect on your own experience of a 'good' patient transfer and the features of this.

Clinical link 12.1 (see Appendix for answers)

You are caring for a 65-year-old post-operative patient following over-sewing of bleeding duodenal ulcer. She has become acutely breathless, respiratory rate 36, now requiring 10 L oxygen via a reservoir mask, SpO_2 98% (previously SpO_2 88%). Medical staff suspect a pulmonary embolus (PE) and require the patient to be transferred to CT for a CT pulmonary angiogram to confirm the diagnosis.

Consider:

- Patient escort—who should go?
- What are the risks—what could happen during transfer?
- What equipment do you require?
- What monitoring should the patient have during the transfer?
- How should this be documented?

Medico-legal issues regarding transfer

In inter-hospital transfer the patient remains the responsibility of the parent team until the handover is complete within the receiving hospital/department. If a clinical incident should occur, then it must be reported and investigated. Whether or not the incident involves a medico-legal claim will depend on the individual case.

Clinical negligence may allege that there has been a breach of duty of care where there has been a failure to meet the standard of the ordinary skilled person (exercising and professing to have that special skill). It is therefore crucial that individual healthcare professionals are aware of their own limitations and skills. The action of the healthcare professional must be an accepted practice that would withstand logical analysis.

Clinical link 12.2 (see Appendix for answers)

You are working the night shift in an elective hospital site and are caring for a 70-year-old male patient following routine orthopaedic surgery (hip replacement). He has had one episode of fresh vomiting blood earlier in the evening and was uncompromised, but he has a further episode of vomiting blood. The medical team would like to transfer the patient for an emergency oesophogastroduodenoscopy, which can only be undertaken at the main hospital site (16 km away). The patient must be prepared for immediate transfer. He is currently on 4 L oxygen via nasal cannulae, respiratory rate 24, SpO_2 95%, blood pressure 105/60, pulse 110, temperature 36.0°C. His Hb is 8.0 g/dL, and he has had one unit of blood. He has one IV cannula *in situ* and an infusion of colloid 500 mL in progress over 1 h.

Consider:

- Patient escort—who should go?
- What are the risks—what could happen during transfer?
- What equipment do you require?
- What monitoring should the patient have during the transfer?
- How should this be documented?

Emergency situations

Q: You are escorting a patient on an inter-hospital transfer. The ambulance you are travelling in is also the first on scene to a serious road traffic accident (RTA). Do you have a duty of care to anyone injured in the RTA?

A: Your duty of care is to the patient already entrusted in your care. However, the ambulance personnel may stop and instigate emergency care (radioing for additional help and support) and when that help arrives continue on the inter-hospital transfer.

Q: You are returning from an inter-hospital transfer and the ambulance is required to attend an emergency. Do you have a duty of care to the patient they are attending?

A: Duty of care does not begin until you touch the patient. However, it should be noted that the ambulance personnel are now in their 'normal environment' and will have more skills and experience of working in this scenario. As an escort team you may offer help and be prepared to help if required.

Incident reporting

Incidents are any unintended or unexpected events which may have or did cause harm to a patient (NHS Improvement 2017).

Measures to ensure that NHS staff are free to speak up about patient safety concerns have been implemented since the Francis Report published in 2013. Reporting safety incidents or near misses allows the NHS to learn from mistakes which will promote a patient safety culture.

End of chapter test

It is important that you understand both the theory related to transfer of the acutely ill adult and the practice of transfer skills to safely care for patients whose condition may be deteriorating. In order to test your knowledge and apply this knowledge to clinical practice you should undertake the following assessment with an appropriately trained member of staff in clinical practice. If you are unable to answer any questions it may be helpful to revisit the section in this chapter.

Knowledge assessment

Work with your mentor/supervisor in practice and ask them to test your knowledge in relation to the following. Incorrect answers/lack of knowledge will require further revision/ re-reading of this chapter.

- Discuss your organization's policy on patient transfer.
- Discuss situations that may necessitate intra-hospital or inter-hospital transfer.
- Discuss the differences between intra-hospital transfer and inter-hospital transfer.
- Identify the groups of patients who may require inter-hospital transfer and analyse the particular risks of this group of patients.
- Describe the process of risk assessment related to transfer of the patient.
- Discuss which groups of patients may require intubation before transfer and analyse the associated risks.
- Analyse which groups of patients may have additional risk associated with transfer.
- Describe the characteristics of a 'good hospital transfer'.
- Discuss the changes in physiology that may be noted during hospital transfer.
- Describe the assessment of the patient that is required before transfer.
- Discuss the role of personnel who may be involved in the transfer.
- Discuss equipment that may be required before transfer.
- Analyse health and safety issues associated with transfer, including:
  - manual handling;
  - equipment;
  - electrical safety;
  - transport of gases;

    - appropriate training to use equipment.
- Analyse infection control issues that may occur during transfer.
- Analyse situations where transfer may not be appropriate.
- Discuss how appropriate communication and documentation can enhance transfer.
- Discuss the organization processes involved in inter-hospital transfer (e.g. coordination of ambulance staff).

Skills assessment

Work with your mentor/supervisor in practice and ask her to assess your ability to care for patients who require transfer using the following criteria where appropriate. Note: you may not be able to demonstrate all these skills. Ask your mentor/supervisor to give you feedback on areas that you did well and areas that may require improving.

Intra-hospital transfer

- Identifies patient requiring transfer to another area and communicates with other multidisciplinary team members.
- Considers which personnel are required to ensure safe patient transfer and ensures that all members are available for a safe transfer.
- Conducts an appropriate assessment of the patient's condition and ensures that patient is sufficiently stable to transfer (unless extenuating circumstances, e.g. ruptured aortic aneurysm).
- Considers the risks associated with the transfer of the patient and identifies how these risks may be reduced.
- Explains the need to transfer to another area to the patient and gains their consent where appropriate.
- Reassures patient and tries to reduce any anxiety related to transfer.
- Communicates effectively with patient and their family throughout the transfer process.
- Contacts patient's relatives and explains need to transfer, giving details of relocated area.
- Considers suitability of transferring patient on their bed or the need to move the patient to a transfer trolley.
- Considers manual handling risks associated with patient transfer.
- Ensures that patient has sufficient IV access and liaises with doctor/senior nurse if more access required.
- Ensures appropriate monitoring for transfer is available and attached to patient.
- Secures monitoring equipment to reduce risk of injury to the patient or transferring personnel.
- Ensures monitoring equipment is charged, has sufficient battery life for transfer, and does not pose safety hazard to patient/accompanying personnel.
- Ensures that portable oxygen is available and has sufficient gas for transfer.
- Ensures oxygen is secure in oxygen holder and does not pose a health and safety risk.
- Ensures that there is sufficient oxygen for duration of transfer.
- Ensures that portable suction is available and has sufficient battery life for transfer.

- Checks that there is appropriate suction equipment, for example emergency suction catheters.
- Provides appropriate IV equipment, for example syringe drives/pumps, and ensures that equipment is charged and has sufficient battery life for transfer.
- Gives special consideration to the following:
  - patient with deteriorating levels of consciousness.
  - patient with unprotected airway (requires intubation).
  - intubated patient (anaesthetist required, portable ventilator, re-breath bag, appropriate oxygen source, end-tidal carbon dioxide monitoring, emergency reintubation equipment).
  - patient who is haemorrhaging (sufficient fluid replacement).
  - patient with cardiac arrhythmias (portable defibrillator).
  - confused patients (may require sedation, bed rails).
- Checks that appropriate emergency equipment and drugs are available during transfer.
- Ensures that adequate infection control is in place during transfer and all personnel have appropriate personal protective equipment.
- Considers additional risks if patient has known infection control risks, for example methicillin-resistant *Staphylococcus aureus* (MRSA), and follows hospital's infection control procedure.
- Liaises with receiving area to confirm timing for transfer.
- Communicates effectively with receiving area, providing details of:
  - patient history/reason for admission to hospital;
  - reason for transfer;
  - patient's medical team;
  - who has taken decision to transfer patient;
  - whether patient is intubated;
  - patient's current condition;
  - current medication;
  - ongoing treatment;
  - any allergies;
  - current monitoring required;
  - details of next of kin;
  - details of infectious status;
  - any religious considerations if transfusion likely (Jehovah witness, etc.);
  - time frame of transfer;
  - who will be accompanying patient;
  - any particular concerns that you have.
- Documents the need for transfer in patient's notes and provides a brief account of patient's condition during transfer.
- Documents staff involved in transfer and any adverse events that may occur during transfer.
- Works well as a team member during transfer and only acts within own level of competence.
- Ensures that a senior person is responsible for coordinating the transfer.
- Ensures that any accompanying relatives travel to new area separately from the rest of the transfer team.

- Introduces patient to new staff and ensures that patient has understood why transfer was required (where appropriate).

Inter-hospital transfer

Inter-hospital transfer carries additional risk for the patient and should only be carried out by staff who are competent and skilled at inter-hospital transfer. Consideration should be given to all the criteria above and in addition to this the practitioner will need to:

- explain the need to transfer to another hospital to the patient and their family.
- liaise with receiving hospital about availability of appropriate bed.
- liaise with receiving hospital about timing issues.
- liaise with ambulance staff over timing of transfer and requirements of accompanying ambulance personnel.
- consider the condition of the patient and liaise with medical team about suitable accompanying personnel.
- ensure that there are sufficient staff available to accompany patient.
- ensure that accompanying staff are competent to transfer patient.
- ensure that the patient's comfort is maintained throughout transfer and temperature is maintained with sufficient clothing/blankets.
- provide the next of kin with geographical details of the new hospital and directions for getting to it.
- ensure that the receiving hospital is informed when the patient leaves and the estimated time of arrival provided.
- handover and documentation (recommended by the Intensive Care Society 2011) should include:
  - transfer details of patient (patient's name, date of birth, next of kin, previous hospital, ward, medical staff, referring doctor, name and status of accompanying personnel);
  - a medical summary (to include reason for admission, past medical history, ongoing procedures and care, patient assessment, medications and fluids, IV access, any recent blood results, MRSA status);
  - nursing summary (to include nursing care, nursing assessment of current status, ongoing care plan);
  - patients status during transfer (vital signs during transfer, medication, fluid status, condition during transfer, any adverse events).

References

Achrekar, M., Murthy V., Kanan S., *et al.* (2016) Introduction of situation, background, assessment, recommendation into nursing practice: A prospective study. *Asia-Pac J Oncol Nurs*, 3:45–50.

Association of Anaesthetists of Great Britain and Ireland Anaesthesia (2009) AAGBI Inter hospital Transfer, AAGBI Safety Guideline. Available at: http://www.aagbi.org/publications/guidelines.htm; accessed 9 December 2019.

Beard, L., Lax, P., Tindall, M. (2016) Physiological effects of transfer for the critically ill patient Basic Science Tutorial 330. Anaesthesia tutorial of the week. Available via: www.wfsahq.org; accessed on 9 December 2019.

British Thoracic Society (2017) Guideline for emergency oxygen use in adult patients. Available at: http://www.brit-thracic.org.uk/ClinicalInformation/EmergencyOxygen/; accessed on 9 December 2019.

BOC Healthcare (2019) *Medical oxygen. Integral valve cylinders (CD, ZD, HX, ZX)*. Available at: http://www.bochealthcare.co.uk/internet.lh.lh.gbr/en/images/504370-Healthcare%20Medical%20Oxygen%20Integral%20Valve%20Cylinders%20leaflet%2006409_54069.pdf; accessed on 9 December 2019.

Department of Health (2014) Quality Standard QS61: Infection prevention and control. Available via: http://www.dh.gov.uk; accessed on 9 December 2019.

Droogh, J.M., Smit, M., Absalom, A.R, *et al.* (2015) Transferring the critically ill patient: Are we there yet? *Crit Care*, 19:62.

Health and Safety Executive (1974) Health and Safety at Work Act 1974. Available at: http://www.hse.gov.uk/legislation/hswa.htm; accessed on 9 December 2019.

Hulme, J., Low, A. (2014) *ABC of Transfer and Retrieval Medicine*. Chichester: Wiley-Blackwell.

Intensive Care Society (2011) Guidelines for Transport of the Critically Ill Adult 3rd edn. Available at: http://www.ics.ac.uk/ics-homepage/guidelines-and-standards; accessed on 9 December 2019.

Johnston, A., Tulloch, L. (2016) Transfer medicine. Guidelines for the provision of Intensive Care Services. Faculty of Intensive Care Medicine and Intensive Care Society. Available at: https://www.ficm.ac.uk/sites/default/files/gpics_ed.1.1_-_2016_-_final_with_covers.pdf; accessed on 9 December 2019.

Knight, P.H., Maheshwari, N., Hussain, J., *et al.* (2015) Complications during intrahospital transport of critically ill patients: Focus on risk identification and prevention. *Int J Crit Illn Inj Sci*, 5(4):256–64.

Kulshrestha, A., Singh, J. (2016) Inter-hospital and intra-hospital patient transfer: Recent concepts. *Indian Journal of Anaesthesia*, 60(7):451–7.

National Health Service Improvement (2017). Report a patient safety incident. Available at: http://improvement.nhs.uk; accessed on 9 December 2019.

National Health Service Improvement (2018) Patient Safety Alert—oxygen cylinders. Available at: https://improvement.nhs.uk/uploads/documents/Patient_Safety_Alert_-Failure_to_open_oxygen_cylinders.pdf; accessed on 9 December 2019.

National Patient Safety Agency (2005) Seven steps to patient safety in primary care. Available at: http://www.nrls.npsa. nhs.uk/resources/collections/seven-steps-to-patient-safety/; accessed on 9 December 2019.

National Patient Safety Agency (2008) Improving patient safety. Available at: http://www,npsa.nhs.uk/nrls/improvingpatientsafety; accessed on 9 December 2019.

NMC (2015) *The Code: Professional Standards of Practice and Behavior for Nurses and Midwives*. London: Nursing and Midwifery Council.

Newton, I. Newton's 3rd Law. Newton's Laws of Motion. Available at: www.britannica.com/science/Newton; accessed 9 December 2019.

Reason, J. (2016) *Organisational Accidents Revisited*. Boca Raton, FL: CRC Press.

Resuscitation Council (UK) (2017) Adult Advanced Life Support Guidelines. London: Resuscitation Council UK. Available at: https://www.resus.org.uk/resuscitation-guidelines/adult-advanced-life-support/; accessed on 9 December 2019.

Royal College of Physicians (2011) *Acute Care Toolkit 1: Handover*. London: Royal College of Physicians. Available at: https://www.rcplondon.ac.uk/guidelines-policy/acute-care-toolkit-1-handover; accessed on 9 December 2019.

Sethi, D., Subramanian, S. (2014) When place and time matter: How to conduct safe inter-hospital transfer of patients. *Saudi J Anaesth*, 8(1):104–13.

Senanayake, E.L., Smith, G.D., Rooney, S.J., *et al.* (2017) Chest drains—an overview. *Trauma*, 19(2):86–93.

Trofimov, A., Kalentiev, G., Yuriev, M., *et al.* (2016) Intra hospital transfer of patients with traumatic brain injury: Increase in intracranial pressure. *Acta Neurochir Suppl*, 122:125–7.

Van Sluisveld, N., Hesselink, G., van der Hoeven, J., *et al.* (2015) Improving clinical handover between intensive care unit and general ward professionals at intensive care unit discharge. *Intensive Care Med*, Apr; 41:589–604.

Wilcox, S., Saia, M., Waden, H., *et al.* (2016) Mechanical ventilation in critical care transport. *Air Medical J*, 35:161–5.

World Health Organization (2007) Nine safety solutions. Available at: http://www.who.int/mediacentre/news/releases/2007/pr22/en/index.html; accessed on 9 December 2019.

World Health Organization, Collaborating Centre for Patient Safety Solutions (2007). Communication during patient hand-overs. Available at: http://www.who.int/patientsafety/ solutions/patientsafety/PSSolution3.pdf; accessed on 9 December 2019.

13
Planning for emergency care and treatment when recovery is uncertain

Kate Kemsley

Chapter contents

Nurses working in the acute hospital setting will often care for a patient with multimorbidity and/or frailty that can be managed but cannot be cured. Managing patients with chronic and frailty conditions is complex and planning their goals of care and treatment may need adapting, particularly for an acute deterioration.

This chapter will:

- discuss the identification of a patient who may be or is at risk of becoming clinically unstable with uncertain recovery
- illustrate the more complex process of advanced assessment, planning, and communication skills that may be required.
- consider ethical dilemmas, where treatment is withdrawn or withheld
- discuss role of the acute care nurse as an essential member of the healthcare team (HCT) the as an advocate for the patient and family.[1]

Learning outcomes

This chapter will enable you to:

- understand the history, politics, and economics of healthcare and the impact these have on planning emergency care and treatment in the acute hospital setting
- understand the treatment options available in level 2 and 3 areas in the context of decision-making
- identify and assess a patient who needs a plan for emergency care and treatment
- understand how the nurse advocacy role can support a patient and their family in the decision-making and communication aspects of the planning process
- discuss how to call for support in the planning process and in the event of deterioration when recovery is uncertain

[1] Family refers to a person significant to the adult patient.

- explore the nurse's role within the team and gain insight into the perspectives of others in the HCT when assessing and planning emergency care and treatment
- evaluate what is required in the documentation of a plan for emergency care and treatment
- understand the ethical and medico-legal framework within which decisions in healthcare are made
- appreciate the religious and spiritual elements of a patient and their family's care

What is a Plan for Emergency Care and Treatment?

A Plan for Emergency Care and Treatment (PECT) is a guide for healthcare professionals (HCPs) to manage a patient in the event of clinical deterioration. These plans are often referred to as treatment escalation plans (Devon Treatment Escalation Plan 2012; Paes and O'Neill 2012), goals of care (Thomas *et al.* 2014), limitations of medical treatment (Jaderling *et al.* 2013) and ceilings of treatment (Taylor 2011; Taylor 2014) plans. The United Kingdom has a standardized Do Not Attempt Cardio-Pulmonary Resuscitation (DNACPR) form (UK Resuscitation Council 2015) with guidelines (UK Resuscitation Council 2014) that have been adapted by National Health Service (NHS) Trusts across the country. More recently the UK Resuscitation Council has developed the national ReSPECT for use in primary and secondary healthcare settings (Pitcher 2017).

PECTs and Advance Care Plans (ACPs) made in community and hospital settings do exist across the United Kingdom and internationally. ACPs differ from PECT as they are often completed by a patient during periods of stable health in a community setting. However, a PECT is a record of decisions around cardio pulmonary resuscitation (CPR) and other aspects of a person's care and treatment to be referred to in an emergency, (UK Resuscitation Council 2016; Pitcher *et al.* 2017) and is usually completed by a member of the HCT.

There are events that can be unpredictable and sudden, however; deterioration in a chronic condition, for example, an infective exacerbation of chronic obstructive pulmonary disease (COPD), can often be predicted before a patient requires the medical emergency or cardiac arrest team.

The ideal time to make an anticipatory plan is around the time of a new diagnosis or when increasing frailty is recognized. Exploring the potential path of a condition to enable an awareness of benchmarks of deterioration can pre-empt decisions in an emergency. When everyone in the team, including the patient and their family, is aware of these benchmarks of illness, this can significantly prevent stress and anxiety for all and can manage healthcare resources better (Detering *et al.* 2010; Beaussant *et al.* 2015).

Planning requires time and engagement from the HCT to discuss treatment options with the patient and their family. However, often the reality is that plans are made when a patient is unstable and is often addressed by the critical care outreach (CCOT), the medical emergency team (MET), and intensive care team (Jones *et al.* 2012; Pattison *et al.* 2015; Kemsley 2017;).

The complexities of emergency care and treatment planning

Improved nutrition and living conditions coupled with advances in medical treatment have led to longer life. With increased longevity comes the complexity of caring for patients with chronic health conditions (Nolte and McKee 2008) and frailty (World Health Organization 2011).

The political focus over the last 20 years, particularly within acute hospital care, has been about patient safety and improved quality of patient care (McQuillan *et al.* 1998; NICE 2007; Francis, 2013). The development of national early warning scores (NEWS), the widespread use of advanced communication techniques like SBAR, CCOTs, and METs, and human factors training have all contributed to the support of the deteriorating patient. The result of these patient safety measures may have contributed to the reduction in avoidable hospital deaths, estimated to be as low as 5% (Hogan *et al.* 2015).

There is, however, a growing population of people with chronic and frailty conditions and an emerging condition: chronic critical illness (CCI). In the United States, it is recognized that CCI has now reached epidemic proportions (Nelson *et al.* 2010). As new treatment options are developed, the political debate is often how the NHS can afford to fund them (Campbell, 2016). An ageing population, frail and with complex disease is expensive and requires extensive resources but with it comes the responsibility of individual patient-centred treatment plans.

Chronic disease and frailty is managed predominantly in the community. When a patient experiences an exacerbation requiring hospital treatment their disease or condition is potentially at an advanced stage (Thomas 2011). Decisions to withhold or withdraw treatment are often made in the middle of a busy emergency department or during a MET or cardiac arrest call with little information to hand. Gathering information about a patient takes time.

The main business of acute hospitals is active life-saving treatment. This culture is further reinforced when death is considered a failure by society and preservation of life is sometimes sought at high costs. Disease management is divided into specialisms and rather than a patient being treated holistically, a culture exists of treating the disease rather than the patient (Nolte and McKee 2008). This culture is further reinforced as hospital Trusts are assessed in terms of mortality and morbidity. However, measuring hospital standards using mortality rates is a controversial (Lilford and Pronovost 2010; Francis 2013) and arguably inaccurate measure of quality of care (McCormick *et al.* 2015). More people now are dying at home by choice (Merrifield 2015) but for others hospital can also be an appropriate place in which to die (Office for National Statistics (ONS) 2015).

Dementia and Alzheimer's are now the leading cause of death in the United Kingdom, followed by ischaemic heart disease, cerebro-vascular disease, COPD, and lung cancer (ONS 2015). In the final years of life, 90% of the UK population spend time in hospital and 55% of deaths occur in acute hospitals (Nuffield Trust 2013). The prognosis of frailty and non-cancer disease is often difficult to predict and thus creates uncertainty. This uncertainty leads to a reluctance to discuss prognosis and PECT. The unpredictable nature of exacerbations of chronic disease and resulting death is demonstrated in Figure 13.1.

Healthcare policy presents a conflict for hospital healthcare professionals (HCPs). Failure to rescue patients who would have survived is a problem that exists and must be addressed within acute hospitals. There is, however, a significant group of patients that are aggressively treated due to a lack of recognition of the end of their disease process (Jones *et al.* 2012; National Confidential Enquiry Patient Outcome and Death (NCEPOD) 2012). The extent of patients in the last year of life in acute NHS hospitals is illustrated by Clark and colleagues' large retrospective study (2014).

There has been a recent shift in policy that impresses the need for HCPs to recognize that group of patients who are in the last year of their life and adapt their treatment plan and care accordingly,

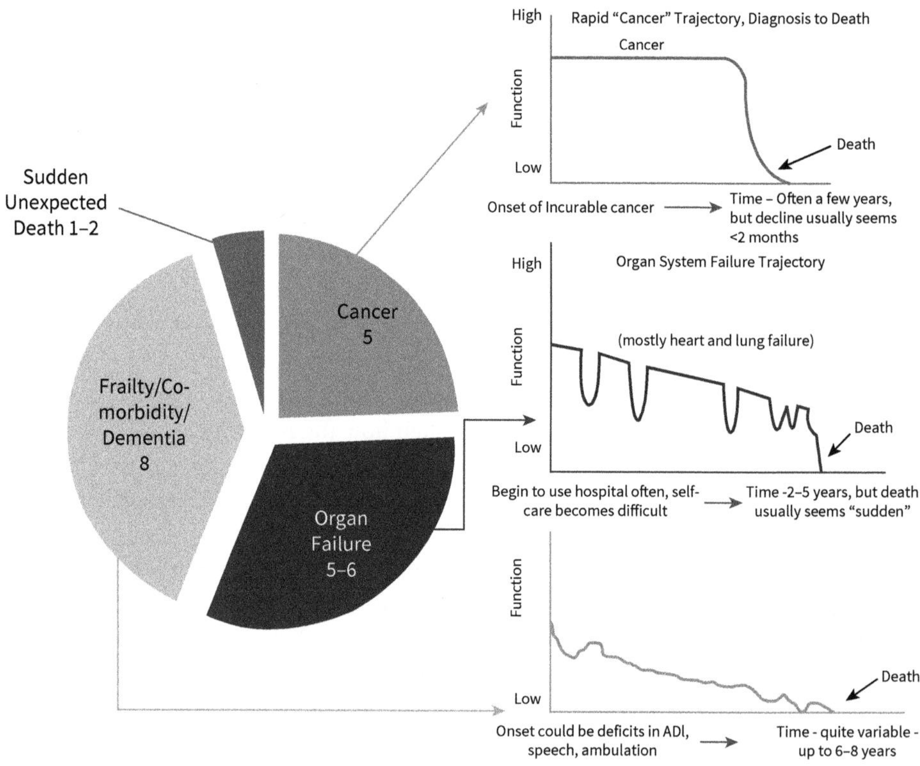

Figure 13.1 Dying trajectories.

Reproduced from Principles and materials for The Gold Standards Framework © K Thomas, the National GSF Centre 2003 - 2019. Used with permission from the National GSF Centre in End of Life Care. http://www.goldstandardsframework.org.uk/.

(NCEPOD 2009, 2012; National Partnership for Palliative and End of Life Care (NPPEoLC) 2015). However, much more needs to be done to protect this vulnerable group of patients.

The complexity of making a PECT in acute hospitals

Barriers to decision-making around PECT in hospital settings have been highlighted by many nursing and medical studies over the last 15–20 years. Patients and families can lack awareness or understanding of disease or prognosis either due to health illiteracy or a lack of information giving from HCPs, (Micallaf *et al.* 2011; Watts 2012). This leads to differing expectations between patients, families, and HCPs, (Barclay and Mayer 2010; Watts 2012; Kemsley 2017). Lack of capacity due to acute illness or longer-term disease or frailty also prevents discussion, (Kemsley 2017). The Human Rights Act (HRA) (1998) and the Mental Capacity Act (MCA) (2005) have led to a shift of power, giving patients more autonomy in their healthcare choices (Bowker 2009), but have also led to confusion and sometimes a reluctance in HCPs to approach the topic with patients and families.

HCPs experience significant lack of resources daily, where competing priorities between caring for acutely unwell patients and other work exist (Beaussant *et al.* 2015; Kemsley 2017).

Information giving and managing patients and family's expectations requires time to build rapport (Watts 2012; McCourt *et al.* 2013; Beaussant *et al.* 2015; Kemsley 2017). Assessing a patient often requires access to information from community and specialist healthcare providers and IT systems, particularly out of hours (Kemsley 2017). A lack of knowledge, experience, and training further compounds the problem, (NCEPOD 2009).

Nurses and medical staff, including consultants, report lack of confidence in information giving to patients and each other especially when prognosis and diagnosis is uncertain, (Beaussant *et al.* 2015; Kemsley 2017). Perceived hierarchies in hospital teams mean junior staff are often reluctant to raise concerns with senior clinicians in time to make plans (Kemsley 2017). A lack of training also leads to a lack of confidence managing anger, distress, and denial of patients and family members (Beaussant *et al.* 2015; Kemsley 2017).

Lack of knowledge of a medico-ethical-legal framework can also prevent decision-making amongst HCPs (Kemsley 2017). Lack of patient exposure of medical and surgical staff due to working time directives has also reduced clinical exposure to unwell patients (Chikwe *et al.* 2004). This all leads to a culture of avoiding advanced decision-making with patients and eventually this can devolve responsibility in an emergency to critical care and other specialist teams (Kemsley 2017).

Communication is the foundation to the process of decision-making. Often patients and families are left to fend for themselves following initial diagnosis (Watts 2012; Beaussant *et al.* 2015). A perceived inability of HCPs to build rapport with patients and family as well as reports of poor intra-professional relationships, particularly between medical and nursing staff, affects the process (Barclay and Mayer 2010; Micallaf *et al.* 2011; McCourt *et al.* 2013; Kemsley 2017). Inadequate documentation of conversations between patient and HCPs and amongst HCP teams further exacerbates this (McCourt *et al.* 2013; Kemsley, 2017).

Organizationally, poor management of ward rounds and multidisciplinary team (MDT) meetings is also reported (Kemsley 2017). This can be attributed to short staffing and a lack of senior, experienced supernumerary nursing staff which prevents good inter-professional communication and planning. There is also a lack of continuity of patient care across all acute care areas due to shift and working patterns (Barclay and Mayer 2010). Busyness of acute hospitals leads to more focus on treating the immediate symptoms with little or no emphasis into long-term planning (Watts 2012).

There is also evidence that colleagues in primary and secondary care cannot always prioritize advance care planning also due to lack of confidence, time, and overwhelming workload (Age UK 2013). The culture of nursing, medical, and allied health professional (AHP) cultures also differ in their ideologies of patient care which can lead to a lack of consensus in patient care (McCourt *et al.* 2013).

Planning for emergency care and treatment is often perceived to be someone else's role. In the acute setting, research has found that decision-making and communicating decisions lie firmly with the senior doctor (Kemsley 2017). Junior nurse and medical team members assume decision-making to be a hierarchical role and therefore often do not get involved in gathering information or decision-making. Junior members of the team will often leave responsibility with a more senior team member, (McCourt *et al.* 2013; Kemsley 2017). Recent research has also highlighted a reluctance of senior medical staff in hospitals to make Do Not Attempt Cardio-Pulmonary Resuscitation (DNACPR) decisions for fear of reduced monitoring and quality of treatment for patients (Fritz *et al.* 2013).

However, the PECT is a process. Identification of a patient who requires a PECT is complex but the bedside nurse has skills and tools to identify and raise concerns about a patient. Nurses have a recognized advocacy role and good communication skills that can support their medical colleagues in decision-making and communicating that decision (Adams *et al.* 2011; Watts 2012; Kemsley 2017). However, it is essential for nurses to understand the process of assessment and planning for patients to become part of the decision-making process, (Muller-Joge *et al.* 2013).

Treatment available within acute hospitals

Acute hospitals can provide a wide range of treatments for patients between the hospital ward, high dependency, and intensive care units. Rather than view a patient as either for or not for CPR, patient treatment including CPR and defibrillation would be better viewed at one end of a treatment continuum.

The Intensive Care Society (ICS 2009) has outlined levels of care according to the organ support a hospital inpatient may require depending on their acuity of illness. The levels range from 0, 1, 2, and 3.

Treatment at level 2 could involve inotropic drugs to support blood pressure via a central line or non-invasive ventilation. Treatment at level 3 supports the respiratory system through invasive ventilation requiring sedation, opiates, and sometimes paralysing agents. If ventilation continues longer than a few days, the patient may undergo a tracheostomy. Other examples of treatment given in level 2 and 3 care areas are slow dialysis or continuous veno-venous haemofiltration to support failing kidneys, invasive and non-invasive monitoring of intracranial pressure to manage brain injury. Both areas of care will also involve continuous monitoring of observations and response to treatment via an arterial line and regular repositioning and intense physiotherapy.

To tolerate and survive higher dependency care, it is vital the patient has a certain level of physical and psychological fitness. The decision to admit to level 2 and 3 care facilities is not taken lightly. A patient who survives treatment may find the physical and psychological effects of that treatment can remain with them long after they leave hospital. These are exhibited as symptoms of post-traumatic stress disorder and CCI (Nelson *et al.* 2010; ICU Steps 2016).

Identifying a patient who needs a PECT

It is important to recognize when a patient's care needs may be transitioning from an active to a palliative phase. There are two well-recognized tools that are easy to use in the identification of the patient who may be moving from an active management to a more supportive phase of their disease. It is often an acute deterioration that can help highlight this and acute care nurses are in prime position to identify that patient and support them and the medical team to enable this.

The supportive and palliative indicators care tool or SPICT (2016) allows early identification of a patient who is potentially in their last year of life (Highet *et al.* 2013). It can be used in any healthcare setting as part of an initial or ongoing assessment of a patient by any member of the HCT. The Gold Standards Framework (Thomas 2011) has also developed prognostic

Box 13.1 Patient Example

Situation: Sarah is a 72-year-old retired teacher. She was admitted to hospital two days ago, to the acute medical unit via the emergency department with a right-sided pneumonia. She has received 36 hours' worth of IV antibiotics and IV fluid. She continues to receive the ACE inhibitor she takes long term for her heart failure but has stopped her diuretic and beta blocker since admission.

Background: Sarah has a history of biventricular heart failure and has chronic kidney disease (CKD) with an eGFR normally of 32–35.

Assessment: Her breathing is worsening and her NEWS score is now 11. Her respiratory rate is 26, her oxygen saturations are 93–94%, on 60% humidified oxygen her effort to breathe is increasing. Her heart rate is 110–120 and is irregular and faint peripherally. Her blood pressure is 100–110 systolic but her urine output is 5–10 mL an hour and she is in a positive fluid balance. Her temperature is normal. She is awake and alert but fidgety.

Recommendations: You are concerned and feel Sarah is deteriorating fast and needs a senior review now. You are giving her the maximum treatment she has been prescribed. The medical registrar assesses Sarah with you and requests an intensive care review.

indicator guidance like the SPICT. This tool is more comprehensive and may be more suitable to situations that are not as time dependent. However, assessing burden of chronic disease can come from a simple question, 'how are you coping?'

Following identification of the patient, assessment is the next part of the decision-making process. To explore this further a patient example is outlined in Box 13.1 and discussed through the chapter to illustrate the process of assessment, planning and communicating the PECT.

The information here is not enough to decide how to manage this situation further. The patient described has two comorbidities, biventricular heart failure, and chronic kidney disease (CKD), and is displaying signs of acute respiratory, heart, and kidney failure due to sepsis. The HCT needs to understand the bigger picture before deciding whether level 2 and 3 treatment is appropriate.

Information to make a PECT is complex but the guide in Box 13.2 and Box 13.4 can assist in the process. Note what information the nurse can collect to assist this process.

Assessment of acute illness

This requires assessment of the patient's acute physiology and is explained in detail in the various specific chapters throughout this book. In addition, laboratory tests, for example full blood count, urea and electrolytes, liver function, and arterial blood gases will monitor the acute and chronic effects of illness on organ function and cell perfusion.

Imaging such as CT, X-ray, or ultrasound can add to the picture of the progress of chronic disease or the effect the acute illness is having on organ function. Other tests, for example

Box 13.2 Information required to make a PECT

- Patient wishes (including religious and cultural concerns) *
- Patients cognition/mental capacity—discuss with relative/next of kin/independent mental capacity advocate if patient lacks capacity*
- Diagnosis of acute condition and treatment options available
- Level of acuity from assessment of observations*/blood tests*/imaging, etc.
- Prognosis of acute condition—is it reversible?
- Prognosis of existing conditions
- Treatment options available
- Response to treatment, e.g. IV fluids/IV antibiotics*
- Patients ability to manage activities of daily living*
- Other relevant medical, surgical, drug, social, family, allergy history*
- Recent hospital admissions*
- Quality of life as per patient's opinion* (not the judgement of the HCP)
- Team opinion, including nurse, AHP, and specialty team input needed.

*Denotes where the nurse can contribute to the assessment of the patient.

Reproduced from Kemsley, K. (2017) A Study of the Process of Treatment Escalation Planning in the Acute Hospital Setting: A Pilot Study. University of Brighton (Unpublished Masters Research).

angiogram, spirometry, endoscopy, and biopsy, will all contribute to the assessment of the acute illness. However, tests can take minutes, hours, or longer but the ability for a patient to tolerate them should be part of the assessment.

Assessment of chronic health

To assess whether a patient is suitable for further treatment it is important to ascertain the extent of their chronic health conditions and prognosis. Included in this is an assessment of general physical and psychological health.

Heart failure can be assessed or graded using the New York Heart Association and an echocardiogram may show whether left ventricular failure is present (NICE, 2010). CKD can be measured using trends in estimated glomerular filtration rate (eGFR) and albumin to creatinine ratio (NICE 2014). Other common chronic health disease indicators include the Medical Research Council dyspnoea scale (NICE 2011) for COPD; the Model for End-stage Liver Disease (MELD) and Child–Pugh's Classification (NICE 2016a) measures stages of liver disease; severity of pancreatitis is measured using the Modified Glasgow Score (NICE 2016b). The extent of disability due to dementia can be measured using an activities of daily living tool such as the Barthel Index (NICE 2006; Sheehan 2012).

Prognosis

Prognosis can be a difficult concept for patients, their families, and HCPs, particularly when chronic health exacerbations and worsening frailty is seemingly unpredictable. Medical professionals can be overly optimistic in their prognosis of terminally ill patients to avoid taking away hope from a patient (Christakis and Lamont, 2000). Often prognosis is based on statistics, and crude calculations which, when faced with an acute condition like a pneumonia and comorbidities are then very difficult to employ. Many chronic disease classifications contain within them a mortality rate dependent on severity of illness. It is not always possible to diagnose and prognosticate despite the wide array of tests and investigations which can be performed. In the preoccupation to diagnose and give a prognosis it is easy to lose sight of easier and earlier means of assessing the mental and physical decline of a patient (Boyd and Murray, 2010). However, research suggests in a situation of uncertainty, patients when asked will ultimately favour honest open conversations, (Tan *et al.* 2013).

Assessment of baseline function or frailty of a patient

There are many means of assessing frailty, the Barthel Index (Mahoney and Barthel 1965) or more recently developed tools such as the Clinical Frailty Scale (Dalehouse University 2007) and the FRAIL questionnaire screening tool (Morley *et al.* 2013). It is important to get a clear picture of what the patient could and could not do before this acute phase of illness. Included in this is information about washing, dressing, cooking, cleaning, leaving the house, managing stairs, and walking on flat ground without getting out of breath. Information about the number of recent hospital admissions, particularly within the last 12 months and the length of stay is also useful (Soong *et al.* 2015). All information gathered will help to indicate the patient's potential response to treatment and the rehabilitation potential required following treatment.

What is reversible?

This is related to the current acute illness and how the chronic health condition is impacting on the physiology of the person. Often the reversibility of the acute illness requires a 'watch and wait' philosophy. If a patient has symptoms of multiple organ failure, the aim would be to support those organs whilst the cause of acute illness; dehydration, bleeding, electrolyte imbalance, fluid overload, infection, or tumour, for example, is treated or removed. To illustrate an example in practice how chronic illness impacts on daily activities, see Box 13.3.

Support for the healthcare team

When a patient is deteriorating fast and there is no time to coordinate an in-depth MDT meeting, often opinions must be gathered by phone calls or brief reviews. In an urgent situation or an emergency, the following support can be called on:

- The consultant, consultant's registrar, or on-call medical registrar out of hours.
- A specialist doctor or nurse who have cared for the patient in the past, for example a cardiologist, a respiratory nurse, or an oncologist.
- The palliative care team can give advice about symptom management alongside active treatment, end of life care, or support with difficult conversations.

Box 13.3 Example of the effect of chronic health condition on ADLs

Sarah's biventricular failure limits her when walking distances longer than 45 metres or when climbing the stairs. In both instances, she must stop for a minute or two to catch her breath. She also requires three pillows to sleep at night.

Sarah's CKD is stage 3 but the blood tests you have taken to assess her organ dysfunction show worsening acute on chronic kidney injury, her eGFR is 15, her potassium is 5.6.

It is also noted that Sarah has had one previous hospital admission six months ago, with a right-sided pneumonia. She reports that since then, she feels less inclined to leave the house and takes less care of her appearance. She will leave the house with her son for shopping, can get up and down stairs, and manages cooking, housework, toileting, washing, and dressing, but with some effort. She feels less inclined to eat recently and is often low in mood. When asked, she reports perhaps needing more help around the house.

- The CCOT/MET nurse, doctor, physiotherapist, or intensive care unit (ICU) doctor can support the ward team and help diagnose and stabilize the patient's current acute symptoms as well as contribute to the communication of the PECT to the patient and family in complex situations.
- The on-call anaesthetist may also be able to support the management of the deteriorating patient especially with regard to advanced respiratory management.
- The physiotherapist who can offer advice about acute treatment options available for the patient.
- Within the community and secondary care services, the GP, community nurse, nursing home, community Macmillan or palliative care nurse, as well as hospice team can offer advice as to the patient's recent health status and symptom advice.
- In less urgent but complex situations the chaplaincy can be contacted when the patient and family are faced with religious or spiritual distress over a decision.
- A medico-legal or ethics advisor that works directly with the NHS trust or within a local university can also be useful for complex, ethically challenging decisions.
- After gathering information from the team a plan can be made. An example of a plan can be seen in Boxes 13.5 and 13.6 with the framework outlined in Box 13.8.

Box 13.4 Results of further investigations for Sarah

Sarah has sepsis related to a pneumonia that is causing her cardiovascular system to vasodilate which is dropping her blood pressure and causing hypo-perfusion of her kidneys leading to an acute on chronic kidney injury.

Her recent arterial blood gas shows a pH of 7.21, PO_2 of 7.5kPa on 60% humidified oxygen, PCO_2 of 4kPa, HCO_3 17, lactate of 4.

Chest auscultation demonstrates bronchial right basal breathing and wheeze throughout. A repeat chest X-ray confirms worsening pneumonia and moderate pulmonary oedema.

She is cool to her peripheries and her peripheral pulse is weak, fast, and irregular. She is conscious but unsettled. Her mucous membranes are dry and her capillary refill time is 5 seconds.

In terms of her organ dysfunction, Sarah has type 1 respiratory failure, acute on chronic cardiac and renal failure, cardiovascular system failure that is causing exacerbation of chronic organ dysfunction and impacting negatively on her cerebral function.

Box 13.5 What is the likely outcome for Sarah?

The team are running out of time and need to decide with Sarah as to the best course of action. You have called in Sarah's son and family to join the discussion. The discussion is held at the bedside. Present is the intensive care registrar, the medical registrar, you as the bedside nurse, the CCOT nurse, and Sarah's son.

The HCT have decided the best course of action is to offer Sarah a change in antibiotics and the support of inotropes and non-invasive ventilation (CPAP: continuous positive airway pressure) in high dependency unit (HDU). The team are reluctant to offer more invasive treatment as they feel it would not be in her best interests as it could do more harm than good. This includes CPR.

The team will discuss with Sarah and her son that they will record this as her goal of care. In the event of deterioration, the team feel that keeping her comfortable and not providing any further invasive monitoring or support as they feel this is in her best interests. They expect to see improvement in two days if the antibiotics work. However, if Sarah deteriorates or changes her mind about treatment options, the discussion can be revisited.

Box 13.6 What is the plan for emergency care and treatment?

Sarah needs a change in antibiotics to try to fight her worsening infection. Her breathing, and type 1 respiratory failure caused by pulmonary oedema need the support of CPAP.

Despite having a low blood pressure, she cannot have any more IV fluid as she is showing signs of fluid moving into the third or interstitial space. In this case, she needs support of an inotrope to aid vasoconstriction that will increase her blood pressure and improve blood supply to tissues and organs, particularly the kidneys. If her kidneys continue to fail she may need the support of renal replacement therapy.

If the CPAP fails, she may need the support of invasive ventilation via an endo-tracheal tube. This may cause worsening heart and renal failure as the positive pressure in her chest squeezes her heart and prevents venous return, leading to reduced cardiac output. Invasive ventilation could cause further ventilator associated infections which will put more pressure on her organs, particularly her heart. She may require a tracheostomy if she requires ventilation for longer than a few days.

Overall, her stay in ICU could lead to global neuropathy and impact on her psychological state. The longer she requires intensive care the more likely she will fail to make a full recovery and could need the support of homecare or have a prolonged stay in hospital or transfer to a nursing home. She may not even survive to discharge from hospital due to further hospital-acquired infections or worsening organ failure.

Communication of the plan for emergency care and treatment (PECT)

If a patient is losing capacity that prevents discussion, best efforts should be made to contact family and include them in communication of decision-making. However, where this is not possible a patient should be treated in their best interests (MCA 2005). There are no written rules as to who has the conversation or how it should play out. Best practice would be to include the patient and a family member for support, and a medical practitioner and nurse who know the patient. Content of the discussion should be agreed between medical and nursing staff beforehand. The nurse's role as advocate for the patient and family can encourage questions and discussion and to clarify any information given.

Anyone can have a conversation; the most important thing to note is that communication must be honest, free of jargon, and involve listening to the patient. There should be avoidance of giving negative descriptions of CPR and other invasive treatment, quoting chances of survival, and talking about 'limiting' and 'setting ceilings' of treatment. Emphasis instead should be on hearing what the patient's priorities and values are and giving the patient the best treatment for their condition. Some important points to remember when talking with patients are outlined in Box 13.7.

Palliative care

Once the domain of oncology, palliative care is now regarded as essential for those with chronic disease and increasingly frailty (Thomas 2011). The benefits of palliative care both

Box 13.7 Communication prompt

Before talking with the patient and family

- Make time, turn off/hand over bleep, hand over any urgent workload.
- Has the patient got support and have you got support?
- Start with first-name introductions of all people present.
- Give the person time to hear what you say and respond.
- Avoid technical language.

During the conversation

- **Opening conversation:** *What do you understand about your illness?*
- **Fears/Worries:** *What are your biggest fears and worries about the future with your health?*
- **Information preferences:** *How much information about what is likely to happen with your illness would you like from the team caring for you?*
- **Goals:** *If your health worsens, what are your most important goals?*
- **Prognosis and Treatment:** *Be honest with uncertainty and focus on what can be done.*

economically and from a healthcare perspective are becoming recognised by research and UK government policy (Department of Health 2008; Leadership Alliance for the Care of Dying People 2014; Smith *et al.* 2014).

The goal of palliative care is to maximize a patient's quality of life. Palliative care supports psychological, physical, and spiritual symptom relief for a patient, whose disease is being managed rather than cured. An acceptance that the patient is at this phase of their disease must come from the HCT, patient, and family, and the earlier it is recognized the easier the transition for all.

Palliative care, however, is not just a specialist role. It is something all members of the HCT can engage and lead in. The National Palliative and End of Life Care Partnership (2015), however, is calling for better education and training for all members of the healthcare sector to enable earlier palliative care and more honest, open communication.

Documentation of plans for emergency care and treatment (PECT)

DNACPR documentation is no longer sufficient to guide the team and record a plan should the patient deteriorate. Written communication in the form of a PECT that incorporates a CPR decision is long overdue. There is now an array of PECTs available across the NHS that allow the team to document for the benefit of the patient, family, and HCT discussions had, aims of treatment, and treatment limitations.

Examples of current good practice of both process and documentation of PECTs are:

- The Devon Treatment Escalation Plan (Devon TEP, 2014).
- The AMBER Care Bundle (Guys & St Thomas' NHS Foundation Trust, 2013).
- Recommended Summary Plan for Emergency Care and Treatment (ReSPECT) form (Pitcher *et al.* 2017).

The importance demonstrated by all documents is that the process of decision-making is a team approach, can be initiated by anyone, and is patient centred. However, it is vital that with the introduction of any new process or documentation it comes with a comprehensive training package for all healthcare staff. There is also a call for a recognized competence framework for all practitioners likely to be involved in PECT and ACP (NCPC, 2016b). This requires training in assessment of the patient, knowledge of the risks and benefits of treatment and CPR, and advanced communication skills.

As is the case with DNACPR documentation, a PECT is not legally binding. The PECT should be reviewed regularly and revised if necessary. A PECT is only workable if everyone involved in a patient's care knows about it. If your patient has a PECT documented, moves ward, goes home or into a nursing/care home, the form must be communicated and go with the patient. Where available the information should ideally be stored on the electronic palliative care coordination systems.

HCPs need a PECT that contains the technical aspects of a patient's care, and a patient needs a PECT that will treat them as an individual, preserve their dignity, and maintain their trust (Oblensky *et al.* 2010). PECT guidelines for nursing and medical staff are outlined in Box 13.8.

Box 13.8 PECT: Guidance for nursing and medical staff

-**Ward** based treatment +/– IV antibiotics/IV fluid/non-invasive ventilation (NIV)/nasogastric feed/dialysis
-**HDU** or cardiac care unit for NIV/inotropic support/antiarrhythmic drugs/external pacing
-**ICU** for Intubation and invasive ventilation/Inotropic support/haemofiltration
In the event of further deterioration:
-NEWS trigger for medical review
-MET call
-CPR and defibrillation
-Keep comfortable/stop routine observations/administer symptom relief

Communicate and check understanding of the plan with the healthcare team and patient/family and ensure content of conversations and treatment plan is clearly documented

Source data from Kemsley, K. (2017) A Study of the Process of Treatment Escalation Planning in the Acute Hospital Setting: A Pilot Study University of Brighton (Unpublished Masters Research).

The ethics of withholding and withdrawing treatment

Ethics is a system of values and principles moral decisions are based on, it is not a set of rules. Healthcare decisions also require common sense, professional judgement, and are guided by principles of duty, respect, and honesty due to the position of responsibility HCPs hold. Due to the scope of this chapter, this section is an introduction to the ethical framework used to explore common situations when making PECTs and when withdrawing treatment.

The framework used in medico-ethical problem solving and decision-making is based on Beauchamp and Childress's (2009) four principles:

- **Autonomy**—the right of the patient to make his or her own choice, thereby allowing a patient to decline treatment, even if it may be lifesaving. Respect for a person's own belief and value system is held here.
- **Beneficence**—making a judgement that is in the best interests of a patient.
- **Non-maleficence**—not doing anything that will harm a patient.
- **Justice**—or more specifically, distributive justice, means that everyone is entitled to equal access to healthcare resources. The risk/benefit of receiving that resource is also weighed here.

If a patient has expressed a wish for CPR and treatment in the intensive care unit against the agreement of the HCT, this represents an ethical and legal dilemma. In the example in Box 13.9, concern has been expressed that delivering CPR in the event of a cardio-respiratory arrest would cause more harm than benefit. A patient has a right to express their autonomy and HCPs should respect this. A decision to deliver treatment is ultimately a clinical one, however reaching a common understanding through careful communication can prevent dispute between the HCT and a patient and family. If there is still disagreement with the

Box 13.9 Patient example: treatment decision

The team have discussed with Sarah and her son her condition, her prognosis, and her treatment options, presenting their concerns that she is deteriorating and that HDU treatment is possible to reverse the acute situation. However, the concern has been raised that she is very unwell and her heart is struggling and if it continued to fail CPR would not be appropriate. The team's decision is based on the clinical and ethical judgement that to perform CPR would not be in her best interests. Giving CPR could cause more harm requiring intubation and invasive ventilation which would have a further negative effect on her heart, and rather than extend her life would more likely hasten her death.

decision after exploring a patient's values and understanding with a patient or in the absence of mental capacity, their family, then a second opinion from a senior clinician, should be sought, (General Medical Council 2013). In a situation where dispute arises, communication needs time and support from a senior trusted and experienced clinician.

Despite thorough exchange of discussion and information a patient may insist on CPR when the HCT disagrees because they believe it is not in the patient's best interests. It may be that the patient needs more time to come to terms with their disease process. Nurses can sometimes find themselves delivering treatment they do not always believe is right and like other members of the HCT may struggle to deliver CPR if it goes against the ethical principle of 'do no harm'. However, not to start CPR in this situation goes against the ethical principle of a patient's autonomy.

The failure to escalate concerns, initiate a prescribed treatment or CPR when there is no documentation to the contrary would be considered negligent and go against Article 2, the right to life, of the Human Rights Act (1998). With regards the Nursing and Midwifery Council's (NMC) code of conduct (2015), not delivering CPR or escalating concerns goes against section 1.4 that requires us to 'deliver treatment, assistance and care without undue delay' and section 1.5 that requires us to 'respect and uphold people's human rights'.

If a patient was offered higher level treatment but refused, the HCT should ensure the patient is making an informed decision. The principle of patient autonomy is applied here again, ensuring the patient has mental capacity. It would then be necessary to clarify what treatment if any the patient is willing to receive and where. However, a patient may want to decide on symptom relief and nursing care only, in which case all active medical interventions including observations should be stopped. However, this decision should be reviewed regularly with the patient to assess if this is still their wish.

Sometimes ethical principles are not enough to inform decision-making, and the law must be consulted. There has been a significant shift towards patient centred decision-making in recent years supported by the Human Rights Act (1998) and the Mental Capacity Act (2005) which are often used as a guide for decision-making around withholding and withdrawing treatment. This chapter does not have the scope to discuss further the legalities of decision-making. Exploring the legal cases of *Airedale NHS Trust v Bland* (1993), *Ms B v an NHS Trust* (FD 22 March 2002), *Tracey v Cambridge* (2014 EWCA Civ 822), and *Winspear v Sunderland* (2015, EWHC 3250 QB) may provide some insight into the impact of the law on withholding and withdrawing medical treatment.

When exploring a PECT it is important to discuss with a patient and their family what is important to them both with regards their beliefs and their healthcare. If there is likely to be any conflict or confusion between treatment options and an established faith it would be prudent to ask the advice of a religious advocate or to request their mediation via the chaplaincy of the hospital trust.

In summary, it is the objective of the HCT with the support and guidance of the nurse caring for a patient when making a PECT to:

- Gather the facts—acute, chronic, and issues of frailty as well as psycho-social, religious, and spiritual.
- Assess the patient's mental capacity, and if absent consult family, or an independent mental capacity advocate (IMCA). However, in an emergency, the ethical and legal guidance is to treat in the patient in their best interests.
- Ascertain who are the key stakeholders in decision-making. Consider the patient, their family, and members of HCT and ensure they are included from the start of the process.
- Clarify any ethical or clinical dilemma/s that may exist. Seek advice from a medico-legal/ethical specialist, chaplain, or a medical second opinion if required.
- Clarify pre-existing wishes communicated via Lasting Power of Attorney (LPA), Advance Decision to Refuse Treatment, or Advanced Care Plan.
- Apply ethical principles and legal precedent to the decision-making process.
- Optimize communication and documentation, ensure you have a clear leader to aid continuity where required.
- Re-evaluate the process and give yourself, the team, and the patient and their family time for reflection and discussion.

End of chapter test

The learning you gained from this chapter can be assessed by working through an evaluation of your knowledge and skill in assessing a patient with chronic comorbidity or frailty who might require a Plan for Emergency Care and Treatment in acute care situations.

Knowledge assessment

Evaluate your understanding of these aspects of the chapter:

- Provide a definition of a 'Plan for Emergency Care and Treatment' (PECT).
- Discuss what barriers might exist to the development of a PECT.
- Consider some of the information which might be required to develop a PECT.
- Discuss common health indicators/scales which might be used to assess/grade the patient's chronic illness.
- Consider the factors which might be used to assess the baseline function or frailty of a patient.
- Discuss a framework for medico-ethical problem solving and decision-making.
- Describe the legal frameworks required to assess whether a patient has mental capacity.

Skills assessment

- Under the guidance of your practice mentor/supervisor, undertake an assessment of a patient with chronic comorbidity or frailty who might require a PECT.
- Consider methods of documenting this information.
- Communicate the findings within an MDT meeting or ward round.

References

Adams, J.A., Bailey, D.E., Anderson, R.A., *et al.* (2011) Nursing roles and strategies in end-of-life decision making in acute care: A systematic review of the literature. *Nursing Research and Practice.* Available at: http://dx.doi.org/10.1155/2011/527834; accessed 10 December 2019.

Age UK (2013) *End of Life Care Evidence Review.* Available at: http://www.ageuk.org.uk/Documents/EN-GB/For-professionals/Research/Age%20UK%20End%20of%20Life%20Evidence%20Review%202013.pdf?dtrk=true; accessed 10 December 2019.

Airedale NHS Trust v Bland (1993) 80 A.C. 789 Online http://hillsborough.independent.gov.uk/repository/docs/WYC000000600001.pdf; accessed 10 December 2019.

Barclay, S. and Mayer, J. (2010) Having the difficult conversations about the end of life. *Br Med J.* Available at: http://www.bmj.com/content/341/bmj.c4862.full.print; accessed 10 December 2019.

Beauchamp, T.L., Childress, J.F. (2009) *Principles of Biomedical Ethics* 6th edn. Oxford: Oxford University Press.

Beaussant, Y., Mathieu-Nicot, F., Pazart, L., *et al.* (2015) Is shared decision-making vanishing at the end-of-life? A descriptive and qualitative study of advanced cancer patients' involvement in specific therapies decision-making. *BMC Palliative Care.* Available at: http://bmcpalliatcare.biomedcentral.com/articles/10.1186/s12904-015-0057-4; accessed 10 December 2019.

Bowker, L. (2009) A doctor's experience of resuscitation decision making for older patients: Coping with change. *Postgrad Med J.* Available at: http://pmj.bmj.com/content/85/1009/569; accessed 10 December 2019.

Boyd, K., Murray, S.A. (2010) Recognising and managing key transitions in end of life care. *Br Med J*, 314:649–52.

Campbell, D. (2016) How much is the government really privatising the NHS? *Guardian.* Available at: https://www.theguardian.com/society/2016/aug/15/creeping-privatisation-nhs-official-data-owen-smith-outsourcing; accessed 10 December 2019.

Clark, D., Armstrong, M., Allan, A., *et al.* (2014) Imminence of death among a national cohort of hospital inpatients. *Palliat Med*, 28(6):474–9.

Chikwe, J., de Souza, A.C., Pepper, J.R. (2004) No time to train the surgeons. *Br Med J.* Available at: http://www.bmj.com/content/328/7437/418; accessed 10 December 2019.

Christakis, N.A., Lamont, E.B. (2000) Extent and determinants of error in doctors' prognoses in terminally ill patients: A prospective cohort study. *Br Med J*, 320:469–73.

Dalehouse University, (2007) *The Clinical Frailty Scale.* Available at: http://geriatricresearch.medicine.dal.ca/pdf/Clinical%20Faily%20Scale.pdf; accessed 10 December 2019.

Department of Health (DoH, 2008) *End of Life Care Strategy: Promoting High Quality Care for Adults at the End of Life.* Available at: www.gov.uk/government/uploads/system/uploads/attachment_data/file136431/End_of_life_strategy.pdf; accessed 10 December 2019.

Detering, K.M., Hancock, A.D., Reade, M.C., *et al.* (2010): The impact of advance care planning on end of life care in elderly patients: a randomized controlled trial. *Br Med J*, 340:c1345 doi:10.1136/bmj.c1345.

Devon Treatment Escalation Plan (2014). Available at: http://www.devontep.co.uk; accessed 10 December 2019.

Francis, R. (2013) *The Mid Staffordshire NHS Foundation Trust Public Inquiry.* Available at: http://webarchive.nationalarchives.gov.uk/20150407084003/http://www.midstaffspublicinquiry.com/; accessed 10 December 2019.

Fritz, Z., Malyon, A., Frankau, J.M., *et al.* (2013) The Universal Form of Treatment Options (UFTO) as an Alternative to Do Not Attempt Cardiopulmonary Resuscitation (DNACPR) Orders: A mixed methods evaluation of the effects on clinical practice and patient care. *PLoS One.* Available at: http://journals.plos.org/plosone/article?id=10.1371/journal.pone.0070977; accessed 10 December 2019.

General Medical Council (2013) *Good Medical Practice.* Available at:: http://www.gmc-uk.org/Good_medical_practice English_1215.pdf_51527435.pdf; accessed 10 December 2019.

Guys and St Thomas' NHS Foundation Trust (2013) *The AMBER Care Bundle.* Available at: http://www.ambercarebundle.org/homepage.aspx; accessed 10 December 2019.

Highet, G., Crawford, D., Murray, S.A. *et al.* (2013) Development and evaluation of the Supportive and Palliative Care Indicators Tool (SPICT): A mixed-methods study *BMJ Support PalliatCare*, 0:1–6. doi:10.1136/bmjspcare-2013-000488

Hogan, H., Zipfel, R., Neuburger, J., *et al.* (2015) Avoidability of hospital deaths and association with hospital-wide mortality ratios: Retrospective case record review and regression analysis. *Br Med J*, 351:h3239. Available at: http://www.bmj.com/content/351/bmj.h3239; accessed 10 December 2019.

Human Rights Act (1998). Available at: https://www.health-ni.gov.uk/articles/human-rights-act-1998; accessed 10 December 2019.

Intensive Care Society (2009) Levels of Critical Care for Adult Patients. Available at: file:///C:/Users/Main%20User/Downloads/Levels%20of%20Critical%20Care%20for%20Adult%20Patients%20(revise%20(3).pdf; accessed 10 December 2019.

ICU Steps (2016) *ICU Intensive Care a Guide for Patients and Carers.* Available at: https://icusteps.org/assets/files/IntensiveCareGuide.pdf; accessed 10 December 2019.

Jaderling, G., Bell, M., Martling, C.R., *et al.* (2013) Limitations of medical treatment among patients attended by the rapid response team. *Acta Anaesthes Scandi*, 57:1268–74.

Jones, D.A., Bagshaw, S.M., Barrett J., *et al.* (2012) The role of the medical emergency team in end-of-life care: A multicentre, prospective, observational study *Crit Care Med*, 40(1):98–103.

Kemsley, K. (2017) *A Study of the Process of Treatment Escalation Planning in the Acute Hospital Setting: A Pilot Study.* University of Brighton (Unpublished Masters Research).

Leadership Alliance for the Care of Dying People (2014) *One Chance to Get It Right: Improving People's Experience of Care in the Last Few Days and Hours of Life.* London: Department of Health.

Lilford, R., Pronovost, P. (2010) Using hospital mortality rates to judge hospital performance: A bad idea that just won't go away *Br Med J.* Available at: http://www.bmj.com/content/340/bmj.c2016?rss=1; accessed 10 December 2019.

McCormick B., Pearson M., White, J. (2015) Hospital mortality rates and place of death. *J Public Health.* Available at: https://academic.oup.com/jpubhealth/redirect-unavailable?url=jpubhealth.oxfordjournals.org/lookup/doi/10.1093/pubmed/fdv188; accessed 10 December 2019.

McCourt, R., Power, J.J., Glacklin, M. (2013) General nurses' experiences of end-of-life care in the acute hospital setting: A literature review. *Int J Palliat Nurs*, 2013, 19:10.

McPhail, S.M. (2016) Multimorbidity in chronic disease: impact on health care resources and costs. *Risk Manag Healthc Policy*, 9:143–56. Available at: https://www.ncbi.nlm.nih.gov/pmc/articles/PMC4939994/; accessed 10 December 2019.

McQuillan, P., Pilkington, S., Allan, A., *et al.* (1998) Confidential enquiry into quality of care before admission to intensive care. *Br Med J*, 316:1853–8.

Mahoney, F.I., Barthel, D. (1965) Functional evaluation: The Barthel Index. *Md Med J*, 14:56–61.

Mental Capacity Act (2005) Available at: http://www.legislation.gov.uk/ukpga/2005/9/contents; accessed 10 December 2019.

Merrifield, N. (2015) Deaths at home increase as hospital mortality rates drop. *Nursing Times.* Available at: https://www.nursingtimes.net/clinical-archive/end-of-life-and-palliative-care/deaths-at-home-increase-as-hospital-mortality-rates-drop/5087219.article; accessed 10 December 2019.

Micallaf, S., Skrifars, M.B., Pass, M.J.A. (2011) Level of agreement on resuscitation decisions among hospital specialists and barriers to documenting do not attempt resuscitation (DNAR) orders in ward patients. *Resuscitation.* Available at: http://www.resuscitationjournal.com/article/S0300-9572(11)00199-7/fulltext; accessed 10 December 2019.

Morley, J.E., Vellas, B., van Khan, G.A., *et al.* (2013) Frailty consensus: A Call to action. *JAMDA*, 14:392–7.

Ms B v an NHS Hospital Trust (2002) EWHC 429 (Fam) Online: https://www.ncbi.nlm.nih.gov/pubmed/12242880; accessed 10 December 2019.

Muller-Joge, V., Cullati, S., Blondon, K.S., *et al.* (2013) Interprofessional collaboration on an internal medicine ward: Role perceptions and expectations among nurses and residents.

National Confidential Enquiry into Patient Outcome and Death (NCEPOD) (2009) *Death in Acute Hospitals: Caring to the End?* London: NCEPOD. Available at: http://www.ncepod.org.uk/2009report2/Downloads/DAH_report.pdf; accessed 10 December 2019.

National Confidential Enquiry into Patient Outcome and Death (NCEPOD) (2012) Time to Intervene? A Review of Patients who Underwent Cardiopulmonary Resuscitation as a Result of an In-Hospital Cardiopulmonary Arrest. Available at: http://www.ncepod.org.uk/2012report1/downloads/CAP_fullreport.pdf; accessed 10 December 2019.

National Council for Palliative Care (NCPC, 2016a) *The End of Life Care Strategy.* London: NCPC.

National Council for Palliative Care, (NCPC, 2016b) Planning and Capacity. Available at: http://www.ncpc.org.uk/planning-and-capacity; accessed 10 December 2019.

National Institute for Clinical Excellence (2011) Chronic Obstructive Pulmonary Disease in Over 16's: Diagnosis and Management. Available at: https://www.nice.org.uk/guidance/cg101; accessed 10 December 2019.

National Institute for Clinical Excellence (NICE) (2014) Chronic Kidney Disease: Assessment and Management. Available at: https://www.nice.org.uk/guidance/cg182; accessed 10 December 2019.

National Institute for Clinical Excellence (NICE) (2016a) Cirrhosis in Over 16s: Assessment and Management. Available at: https://www.nice.org.uk/guidance/ng50; accessed 10 December 2019.

National Institute for Clinical Excellence (NICE) (2016b) Pancreatitis: Acute. Available at: https://cks.nice.org.uk/pancreatitis-acute; accessed 10 December 2019.

National Partnership for Palliative and End of Life Care (NPPEoLC) (2015) Ambitions for Palliative and End of Life Care: A National Framework for Local Action: 2015–2020. Available at: http://endoflifecareambitions.org.uk/; accessed 10 December 2019.

Nelson, J., Cox, C.E., Hope, A.A., et al. (2010) Chronic critical illness. *Am J Respir Crit Care Med*, 182(4):446–54.

Nolte, E., McKee, M. (eds) (2008) *Caring for People with Chronic Health Conditions* Berkshire: Open University Press.

Nursing and Midwifery Council (NMC) (2015) The Code Online. Available at: https://www.nmc.org.uk/globalassets/sitedocuments/nmc-publications/nmc-code.pdf; accessed 10 December 2019.

Nuffield Trust (2013) Understanding patterns of health and social care at the end of life. Available at: https://www.mariecurie.org.uk/globalassets/archive/www2/pdf/patient-choice-v-cost_graphics.pdf; accessed 10 December 2019.

Oblensky, L, Clark, T., Matthew, G., *et al.* (2010) A patient and relative centred evaluation of treatment escalation plans: A replacement for the do-not-resuscitate process. *Journal of Medical Ethics.* Available at: http://jme.bmj.com/content/36/9/518.long; accessed 10 December 2019.

Office for National Statistics (ONS) (2015) *VOICES Survey.* Available at: https://www.ons.gov.uk/peoplepopulationandcommunity/healthandsocialcare/healthcaresystem/bulletins/nationalsurveyofbereavedpeoplevoices/england2015; accessed 10 December 2019.

Paes, P., O'Neill, C. (2012) Treatment escalation plans—a tool to aid end of life decision making? *BMJ Support Palliat Care*, doi:10.1136/bmjspcare-2012-000196.174.

Pattison, N., O'Gara, G., Wigmore, T. (2015) Negotiating transitions: Involvement of critical care outreach teams in end of life care decision making. *Am J Crit Care.* Available at: http://ajcc.aacnjournals.org/content/24/3/232.full.pdf+html; accessed 10 December 2019.

Pitcher, D., Fritz, Z., Wang, M., *et al.* (2017) Emergency care and resuscitation plans. *Br Med J.* doi:10.1136/bmj.j876.

Sheehan, B. (2012) Assessment scales in dementia, *Ther Adv Neurol Disord*, 5(6):349–58. Available at: http://doi.org/10.1177/1756285612455733; accessed 10 December 2019.

Smith, S., Brick, A. O'Hara, S., *et al.* (2014) Evidence on the cost and cost effectiveness of palliative care: A literature review. *Palliat Med*, 28(2) 130–50.

Soong, J., Poots, A.J., Scott, S., *et al.* (2015) Developing and validating a risk prediction model for acute care based on frailty syndromes. *Br Med J.* Available at: doi:10.1136/bmjopen-2015-008457.

Supportive and Palliative Indicators Care Tool (SPICT) (2016). Available at: file:///C:/Users/Main%20 User/Downloads/SPICT_April2016.pdf; accessed 10 December 2019.

Tan, H.M., Lee, S.F., O'Connor, M.M., *et al.* (2013) A case study approach to investigating end-of-life decision making in an acute health service. *AustHealth Rev.* Available at: http://www.publish.csiro.au/ah/AH11125; accessed 10 December 2019.

Taylor, D.R. (2011) End-of-life care for patients with chronic disease: The need for a paradigm shift. *Best Practice Journal New Zealand.* Available at: http://www.bpac.org.nz/BPJ/2011/november/docs/bpj_40_end-of-life_pages_9-13.pdf; accessed 10 December 2019.

Taylor, D.R. (2014) COPD, end of life and ceiling of treatment. *Thorax*, 69:497–9.

Thomas K. (2011) *Prognostic Indicator Guidance* 4th edn. Available at: http://www.goldstandardsframework.org.uk/PIG; accessed 10 December 2019.

Thomas, R.L. Zubalr, M.Y. Hayes, B., *et al.* (2014) Goals of care: A clinical framework for limitation of medical treatment. *Med J Aust*, 201(8):452–5.

Tracey v Cambridge University Hospitals NHS Foundation Trust (2014) EWCA Civ 822. Available at: https://www.judiciary.gov.uk/wp-content/uploads/2014/06/tracey-approved.pdf; accessed 10 December 2019.

UK Resuscitation Council (2014) Decisions Related to Cardiopulmonary Resuscitation 3rd edn. Available at: file:///C:/Users/Main%20User/Downloads/DecisionsRelatingToCPR.pdf; accessed 10 December 2019.

UK Resuscitation Council (2015) *DNACPR form Adult.* Available at: https://www.resus.org.uk/dnacpr/do-not-attempt-cpr-model-forms/; accessed 10 December 2019.

UK Resuscitation Council (2016) *ReSPECT.* Available at: https://www.resus.org.uk/consultations/re-spect/; accessed 10 December 2019.

Watts, T. (2012) Initiating end-of-life care pathways: A discussion paper. *Journal of Advanced Nursing* 68(10):2359–70.

Winspear v City Hospitals Sunderland NHS Foundation Trust (2015) EWHC 3250 (QB). Available at: http://www.mentalhealthlaw.co.uk/Winspear_v_City_Hospitals_Sunderland_NHSFT_(2015) EWHC_3250_(QB),_(2015)_MHLO_104; accessed 10 December 2019.

World Health Organization (2011) *Global Health and Aging.* Available at: http://www.who.int/ageing/publications/global_health.pdf; accessed 10 December 2019.

APPENDIX

Clinical link answers

This section contains suggested answers to the clinical link activities for each chapter. These are not exhaustive; you may have additional considerations depending on your own role and organization. You are reminded that you must always adhere to local policy and national guidance, and act within the Nursing and Midwifery Council (NMC) code of professional conduct whenever patient care is being delivered.

Chapter 2

Clinical link 2.1a

This patient has a respiratory acidosis, with a pH of 7.3 and an increased $PaCO_2$. She also has a lower than normal oxygen level (hypoxia) and there are no signs of compensation. The treatment would include:

- Ensuring airway is maintained.
- Increasing the FiO_2 in line with the British Thoracic Society guidelines (O'Driscoll 2017) and titrate to saturations of 94–98% with a fixed-performance face mask.
- Conducting a neurological assessment (AVCPU).
- Considering reducing analgesia until patient is more awake and reviewing analgesia with your medical colleagues.
- Encouraging the patient to cough and change position to reduce atelectasis.

Clinical link 2.1b

This patient has type II respiratory failure. Her blood gas indicates respiratory acidosis with some partial compensation. The patient is hypoxic and has CO_2 retention. This requires:

- Adequate positioning of the patient.
- Increased oxygen in line with the British Thoracic Society guidelines (O'Driscoll 2017) to maintain saturations at 88–92% with a fixed performance face mask.
- Regular vital signs.
- Repeat blood gases.
- Urgent medical review is required and the following may be requested:
    - urgent chest X-ray.
    - intravenous antibiotics.
    - non-invasive ventilation.
    - nebulizers.
    - physiotherapy.

Clinical link 2.2

This patient has type I respiratory failure with a low oxygen but a normal pH and carbon dioxide as indicative of her obstructive lung disease. Her carbon dioxide is a little low because her respiratory rate is high but the metabolic parameters are within normal limits. She has acute asthma and her vital signs indicate that she is critically ill because she is still wheezing and still desaturated on supplemental oxygen.

The main priorities are:

- calculate a risk score using a track-and-trigger system if available and follow the recommended escalation process as indicated.
- carry out an urgent medical review because of failure to improve.
- repeat nebulized bronchodilators according to prescription.
- increase her oxygen saturation.
- close observation of her respiratory function to ensure early detection of any deterioration. She has a high respiratory rate and is already using her accessory muscles but is desaturated on 35% oxygen. If she becomes tired, she will move to type II respiratory failure and alveolar hypoventilation. A rising carbon dioxide is a cause for concern and an indication of deterioration in an asthmatic patient but this is not detectable by pulse oximetry. Frequent observations of vital signs every 30 min should be initiated and clinical signs to watch for an increase in respiratory rate, more shallow apical breathing, and decreasing ability to manage speech. Peak expiratory flow rates before and after nebulizers should be rigorously recorded.
- Ensure that this patient receives the prescribed nebulizers to relieve the bronchospasm. This is the treatment required to alleviate her symptoms and should not be delayed.
- Reassure the patient so that she keeps the mask on long enough for her nebulizers to work. This means phoning her husband to ensure that her children are safely collected from school. She will not settle until she knows that this has been arranged. Do not leave the patient behind closed curtains; reassure her that you will watch her closely.

The following actions are required:

- Request urgent medical review giving clear indication of the patient's respiratory condition. State clearly the respiratory rate, use of accessory muscles, and desaturation to explain why you are concerned. An increase in inspired oxygen to 50–60% is needed to bring the saturations up and request repeat arterial blood gas analysis to monitor the carbon dioxide.
- Ensure that a treatment plan is in place and discuss this with senior medical staff. If this patient does not improve, admission to the intensive therapy unit (ITU) for intubation and ventilation is likely. Close liaison between nursing and medical staff is needed.
- Ensure that the patient's family is aware of her admission and the severity of her illness. Remain calm and reassuring and position the patient with enough pillows to maintain a comfortable sitting position to facilitate ventilation.

Clinical link 2.3

This patient has type II respiratory failure with a low oxygen and a high carbon dioxide and a low pH. His arterial blood gas analysis indicates a respiratory acidosis with metabolic compensation because the metabolic parameters indicate alkalosis but the pH is still low. The pyrexia and expectoration of thick green sputum indicate that he has an infective exacerbation of chronic obstructive pulmonary disease (COPD).

The main priorities are:

- ensure that nebulizer and antibiotic medication is given as prescribed to treat this infective exacerbation of his COPD.
- change the FiO_2 in line with the British Thoracic Society guidelines (O'Driscoll 2017) starting with a fixed performance face mask delivering oxygen at 28% to achieve saturations of 88–92%.
- Reposition the patient to facilitate ventilation.
- Encourage oral intake of fluid and maintain a strict fluid balance chart. He is dehydrated (as shown by urine colour, dry mouth, and viscous sputum). This will make it more difficult for him to expectorate.

The following actions are required:

- Contact medical team to discuss oxygen prescription.

- Sit the patient up in a comfortable position well supported with pillows and tilt the foot of the bed up a little to prevent him slipping back down.
- Oral fluids must be increased to maintain oral hygiene and increase urine output. Find out what he likes to drink and ask his daughter to bring it in. Ensure that the nursing team are aware of the need to increase his oral intake and provide drinks that are acceptable to the patient.
- Ensure that physiotherapists visit the patient to assist with expectoration and mobility if necessary.
- Ensure that the patient is well supported with pillows in a sitting position to facilitate ventilation.
- Encourage diet and refer to dietician for food supplements to prevent further weight loss. Discuss diet with the patient and his daughter, who does the shopping.
  - This patient may be depressed as he has recently been bereaved and may be feeling lonely and isolated. Discuss this with the patient and his daughter and try to encourage a positive outlook.
  - Discharge planning should ensure that the community team, for example the community matron, is contacted with regard to case management to prevent repeated admissions and improve the patient's ability to manage his disease.

Chapter 3

Clinical link 3.1

Systematic analysis of the arrhythmia, including diagnosis:

- rate—fast, variable: using RR interval method, rate varies from 125/min to 214/min
- rhythm—irregularly irregular
- P–QRS ratio—no p-waves are discernible
- P–R interval—impossible to measure P–R interval as no p-waves evident
- QRS complex—narrow, normal duration
- ST segment—ST segment is deviated 2 mm below the isoelectric line, indicative of myocardial ischaemia
- T waves—positive, normal
- Diagnosis: This arrhythmia is a fast, irregularly irregular rhythm indicative of atrial fibrillation. The patient appears to have some degree of myocardial ischaemia secondary to the atrial fibrillation and the tachycardia indicated by the ST segment depression.
- Nursing actions for the next 10 min:
  - Reassure Mrs Jones. Sudden onset of atrial fibrillation is a very frightening experience as the patient is often aware of the fast, irregular palpitations in their chest. In addition, extreme anxiety will exacerbate her breathlessness and potentially make the tachycardia faster. Assure Mrs Jones that you will stay with her.
  - Alert medical staff and senior nurse on the ward that assistance is required.
  - Check Mrs Jones' vital signs.
    - Establish continuous ECG monitoring.
    - Record and compare radial and apical heart rate.
    - Record blood pressure in both arms.
    - Record respiratory rate.
    - Attach oxygen saturation probe and monitor O_2 saturation.
    - Establish baseline and record 15-min recordings as above.
  - Position patient appropriately—if blood pressure will tolerate, sit patient in upright position, and administer oxygen if prescribed.
  - Record a 12-lead ECG to check for evidence of myocardial ischaemia/infarction.
  - Prepare emergency equipment at bedside. Ensure that patient has an intravenous line *in situ* for administration of emergency drugs.
- Potential medical interventions:
  - Sudden onset of atrial fibrillation with haemodynamic compromise requires urgent medical treatment. The most likely option is to aim to restore sinus rhythm as quickly as possible by electrical cardioversion under anaesthetic.

- Direct current cardioversion is performed under general anaesthetic.
- Intravenous heparin will be commenced before cardioversion to protect against potential thromboembolism.
- 12-lead ECG should be examined for any indication of myocardial infarction or ischaemia.

Clinical link 3.2

- Immediate actions and why?
  - Reassure the lady, but explain that you need to record some more investigations.
  - You suspect sudden onset of atrial fibrillation as the pulse rate is fast and irregular. Record a synchronized radial and apex beat and record a 12-lead ECG.
  - You suspect sudden onset left ventricular failure as she is hypoxic and breathless, her capillary refill is prolonged. Ask for medical staff to attend to review this lady, but in the meantime administer oxygen if prescribed to achieve an oxygen saturation of 92–94%.
  - It is possible that she has re-infarcted—review 12-lead ECG against last recording.
- Other investigations by doctor and why?
  - Check medications—some drugs in combination can cause hypotension (β-blockers and ACE inhibitors). Similarly, β-blockers can cause left ventricular failure, especially immediately post-myocardial infarction.
  - Review 12-lead ECG as above.
  - Conduct a thorough cardiac and respiratory physical examination; sudden onset heart failure may present with bilateral crackles at both lung bases and the addition of a third heart sound (S3) to the normal heart sounds S1 and S2.
  - Request U&Es, cardiac markers (troponins, CK), FBC.
  - Request a chest X-ray to review for possible pulmonary oedema.
- Potential problems.
  - Atrial fibrillation secondary to recent acute myocardial infarction (AMI).
  - Left ventricular failure secondary to recent AMI and possible atrial fibrillation.
  - Possible further myocardial infarction.

Chapter 4

Clinical link 4.1

Part 1

Assessment of this patient will be difficult due to his aggression. However, assessment is vital and needs to be undertaken. Assessment will also be made difficult by the presence of alcohol (although it is vital not to assume that this man is drunk, his aggression and agitation could be as a result of head injury). Assessment during the initial period following head injury (6 hours) is very important (NICE 2007).

It may be helpful to explain quietly and carefully to this man the need for neurological observation. His aggression and agitation may be worsened by pain so adequate pain assessment and pain control is vital. Observations should be recorded at least half hourly as his GCS is below 15 (NICE 2014). Any changes should be reported and acted on immediately. Care should be taken by the nurse to ensure that he/she is not harmed whilst recording observations. Increasing aggression/agitation may be a sign of worsening head injury and should be dealt with immediately.

Care should be taken to maintain the safety of this patient.

Part 2

His GCS is now 12 (E2, V4, M6). Although he is less agitated it is worrying that he now needs painful stimuli to awaken him. His ovoid sluggish pupils are also a worrying sign as this may indicate a raising intracranial pressure. In accordance with the NICE (2014) guidance immediate help should be sought as he:

- has new neurological symptoms (pupil changes);
- has a drop in GCS.

Whilst awaiting assistance, neurological observation frequency should be increased to quarter-hourly. It may be of benefit to check a blood glucose level. If further deterioration occurs whilst awaiting medical review urgent assistance should be sought.

This patient will require medical examination, a more in-depth neurological assessment by the doctor, and possibly a CT scan.

Clinical link 4.2

Your immediate action would be to ensure that the patient cannot be harmed during this seizure. Any optical glasses should be removed from the patient. Any objects/furniture that may hurt the patient should be removed and the area around the patient should be cleared as much as possible.

You will need to time and observe the seizure so an accurate estimation of how long the seizure lasted and what occurred during the seizure should be noted. Things to observe include:

- any aura or warning (not likely in this case);
- which parts of the body are moving, what sort of movement, the spread of movement, and the amount of time in the tonic and clonic phases;
- whether patient becomes cyanosed;
- whether patient stops breathing;
- whether there is any incontinence (urinary and faecal);
- pupil changes (once seizure stopped);
- post ictal state.

Seizures will normally limit themselves but this patient's seizure appears to be progressing into status epilepticus (a series of seizures with little or no recovery of consciousness between seizures). This is a *medical emergency* and immediate help is required. You should ensure that someone stays with patient and intubation equipment and monitoring is bought to the patient (crash trolley). Drugs should be available for the doctors arrival (this includes benzodiazepines—these may be given rectally or intravenously if access is available). Oxygen via a non-re-breathe mask should be applied (10–15 L) until the anaesthetist arrives and assesses need for intubation.

Should this patient require an ITU bed then hospital policy for transfer of level 2/3 patient should be followed. This usually necessitates the need for a trained nurse and doctor to accompany the patient (see Chapter 12).

Chapter 5

Clinical link 5.1

Mr T has a variety of problems that need to be prioritized. He should be recovering from musculoskeletal pain but instead his condition is aggravating quickly. His early warning score would suggest that he has become acutely ill with pyrexia, possible acute kidney injury, and possible bowel obstruction. He needs an urgent medical review; if that is not possible you should contact the outreach team. Mr T should be catheterized for hourly monitoring of urinary output, be asked to fast, and have a peripheral cannula inserted to commence intravenous fluids, with possible addition of potassium to correct hypokalaemia. An urgent blood sample for urea and electrolytes should be taken as soon as possible, together with a blood culture sample. Intravenous antibiotics will be needed as Mr T has a urinary infection, as suggested by the presence of leucocytes at the urinalysis. A mid-stream urine sample should be taken after catheterization for microbiology culture. You should monitor urinary output hourly, maintain a fluid balance chart, and consider nasogastric intubation for gastric drainage. In Mr T's case acute kidney injury may be caused by urinary sepsis, prostatic obstruction, or cancer metastasis.

Clinical link 5.2

- Lydia may be developing pulmonary oedema. You should sit Lydia upright to encourage ventilation, you should also commence prescribed oxygen therapy
- Pulmonary oedema is present; this is evident in Lydia's sense of impending doom, her fast respiratory rate and 'bubbly' breathing.
- The medical team need to be contacted urgently and taking an electrocardiogram prior to their arrival is necessary. The medical team prescribe furosemide intravenously which initially improves her breathing. She is catheterized and fluid balance carefully monitored.

Clinical link 5.3

- For Lydia, sepsis may have caused acute kidney injury, or it may be the result of the nephrotoxicity of vancomycin on silent chronic kidney failure (Lydia has had long-standing hypertension). Lydia is now acutely ill and needs urgent medical attention. She has incipient pulmonary oedema and acute kidney failure.
- The high potassium is due to acute kidney failure and this may exacerbate cardiac dysfunction and cause cardiac arrhythmias.
- The medical team need to take cognizance of the incipient heart failure whilst managing the acute kidney failure. The most pressing problem is the hyperkalaemia and Lydia will have glucose 5% intravenous fluid infusion prescribed. The glucose triggers a surge in insulin release, which in turn pushes potassium molecules back into the intracellular space. The medical staff also need to replace fluid, but in the presence of incipient pulmonary oedema, this is dangerous and they will therefore insert a central venous catheter prior to commencing fluid replacement therapy and you will be advised to monitor the central venous pressure regularly, maintaining it within prescribed limits. If Lydia does not respond to the fluid replacement management, the hyperkalaemia may worsen, causing cardiac arrhythmias, and in addition the pulmonary oedema may escalate. You need to maintain regular monitoring of Lydia's vital signs and seek assistance from the nurse in charge and from the outreach team.

Clinical link 5.4

Calcium gluconate given intravenously increases the arrhythmia threshold and has a cardiac protective effect against hyperkalaemia. Insulin changes cell permeability to potassium and causes a shift to the intracellular space, immediately improving the hyperkalaemia risk to the cardiac muscle. However, if you give Lydia insulin, she needs glucose to prevent hypoglycaemia. Please note that only human insulin can be given intravenously.

Once the hyperkalaemia emergency is averted, the focus changes to address the life-threatening pulmonary oedema. Urgent fluid reduction is needed, but this cannot be too sudden as blood pressure is low and therefore haemodiafiltration is the optimal choice for solute and fluid removal.

Chapter 6

Clinical link 6.1

- Priorities for this patient are:
  - Check to see if dysphagia is due to airway obstruction: observe for obstruction.

- Evaluate swallowing reflex (if you are competent to do so) by placing your fingers along the thyroid notch and instructing the patient to swallow. If you feel the larynx rise, the reflex is functioning. If uncertain, follow local protocol and refer to SALT for swallowing assessment.
- Ask patient to cough to assess the cough reflex.
- If certain that both the swallowing and the cough reflex are present assess the gag reflex.
- Look at the face and listen to the speech for signs of muscle weakness.
- Ask whether solids or liquids are more difficult to swallow.
- Ask whether the symptoms disappear after trying to swallow a few times. Is the swallow affected by the position in bed or chair?

- What actions will you take to ensure her nutritional and fluid needs are met?
  - Ensure that patient is sitting up and able to reach food.
  - Ensure that patient has a clean, moist mouth and if present, correctly fitting dentures. This will aid the formation of a bolus which will assist swallowing.
  - Ensure that patient has a soft diet avoiding use of mixed foods such as soup and breakfast cereals. Foods that contain both liquids and solids are more difficult to swallow.
  - If patient is unable to consume large volumes of food offer supplements or snacks between meals.
  - Monitor intake of food and fluids, recording amount consumed on a food and fluid chart.
  - Repeat nutritional screening tool according to local protocol.
  - Refer to dietician in accordance with local policy.
  - Refer to SALT in accordance with local policy.
- What signs might indicate that she has a problem with swallowing?
  - Drooling of saliva from the mouth.
  - Inability of the patient to poke her tongue out.
  - Drooping to left side of face and mouth.
  - Patient has aphasia or dysarthria.
  - When attempting to speak voice sounds 'wet'.

Clinical link 6.2

- What actions will you take to plan the nutritional support for Eva during the acute phase of her illness?
  - Complete the MUST screening tool.
    Eva is elderly and has multiple fractures, both these factors increase her risk of being malnourished before and during this period of hospitalization.
  - Using a pragmatic approach, calculate her energy requirement: 59 × 1.25 × 30 = 2,655 calories.
    Although dieticians would normally calculate the energy requirements of a patient, using a pragmatic approach nurses can have some idea as to how much energy should be consumed.
  - Monitor how long Eva is nil by mouth. If it exceeds 6 h ensure a plan is in place for when eating and drinking can resume.
    Evidence has indicated that elderly orthopaedic patients can be nil by mouth for excessive periods of time. They are often malnourished and under-hydrated before surgery and as a result their recovery from the operation could be further compromised.
- What actions will you take to ensure that Eva's nutritional status is not compromised during this period?

  - Review intravenous regimen.

Eva is having an intravenous infusion of normal saline but is having no calories. Discuss with the medical team about reviewing the intravenous regimen. Intravenous 5% dextrose contains 5 g/100 mL fluid, 20 kcal/100 mL fluid. A volume of 1 L of 5% dextrose will supply 200 kcal, which may help to conserve skeletal muscle.

- Record intake of food and fluids.

  - Encourage small frequent intakes of liquid such as water; milk-based drinks.

- Encourage small, easily digested, energy-dense meals.
  If Eva is still not able to consume an adequate intake consider complete liquid supplementation.
- Monitor fluid output.

Increased fluid intake will replace fluid loss associated with the operation and filtration by the kidney. As fluid loss is replaced urine output will increase. Elderly patients are susceptible to fluid overload due to reduced kidney function.

Clinical link 6.3

- Critically discuss the actions you will take before commencing the feed.
  - Ensure George is in a position to facilitate gastric emptying.
    Although George is on traction he is able to be positioned at an angle no less than 30° and no greater than 45°. This will facilitate gastric emptying by gravity and reduce the risk of reflux occurring.
  - Check position of feeding tube using pH indicator paper.
    The position of a feeding tube must be checked after insertion and before commencing each feed using pH indicator paper. The HCl released from the oxyntic cells reduces the pH to between 1 and 3. The use of proton pump inhibitors and histamine-2 receptor antagonists reduces the amount of HCL present in the stomach. The gold standard for checking position of a feeding tube is an X-ray.
  - Flush nasogastric tube with a minimum of 20 mL of clean water or sterile water (according to local protocol).
    Feeding tubes must be flushed before and after each feed. The volume of water used must be recorded on a fluid chart.
  - Ensure that giving set has been in place no longer than 24 h.
    Formula feed provides an ideal environment for bacteria, and although tubes are flushed before and after a feed they are at high risk of being contaminated.
  - Ensure that a clean procedure is adopted in the preparation of the formula feed and connection to the feeding tube.
    Washing hands before and after connecting the formula feed, and ensuring that the tip of the feeding tube and the formula feed container are not touched will reduce the risk of contamination of the feed by bacteria.
  - Ensure that feeding rate is correctly set.
    The formula feed is prescribed to ensure that George receives adequate nutrition and fluids over each period of 24 h. Ensuring that the feed rate is correct will ensure that the correct volume of feed is administered and reduce the risk of complications associated with incorrect feeding.
- After 8 h George complains of feeling sick and nauseous. What actions will you take?
  - Check that George is in the correct position.
  - Check the feed rate.
    If these checks are satisfactory it may be of benefit to administer anti-emetics (if they are prescribed).

Chapter 7

Clinical link 7.1

- What would be your next immediate actions and why?
  - Look for signs of external bleeding (dressing, drains, and nasogastric drainage) because clinical signs are indicating post-operative bleeding.

- Call for the doctor to come and assess the patient immediately in order to confirm post-operative bleeding or another cause for the abnormal clinical findings.
- Apply pressure to site of bleeding if this becomes obvious.
- Inform the nurse in charge because you may need more support to care for this patient or other patients you are responsible for that shift.

- What other signs and symptoms would indicate that post-operative bleeding is occurring?
  - Abdominal distension, drop in haemoglobin, reduced urine output, increased lactate.
  - If active bleeding was ruled out, what other reasons could be causing these abnormalities?
  - Sepsis, hypotension from epidural infusion, or cardiogenic shock.
  - If active bleeding was confirmed, how would you coordinate care of the patient, including interaction with the nurse in charge and surgical team?
  - Pass on to the nurse in charge and another nurse colleague key information about other patients you are for caring that will need to be delegated to another nurse while you are busy with this patient.
  - Liaise with surgical team about if/when patient will return to theatres and make suitable arrangements with porters and attach patient to monitoring equipment.
  - Administer blood products as prescribed.
  - Continue to monitor vital signs and level of consciousness.

Clinical link 7.2

- Identify all the potential causes for fluid and electrolyte deficit with this patient.
  - Confusion, which may be impairing his oral intake of food and fluids.
  - Large amounts of watery stools.
  - Urine output may be low from poor oral intake of fluids or from renal failure, which could be altering sodium and water excretion.
- How would you manage the diarrhoea?
  - Faecal collection bag to protect skin, promote dignity for the patient, and prevent patient from having to be cleaned and moved as frequently.
  - Skin care, including barrier cream/sprays after cleaning patient for diarrhoea if faecal collection bag becomes detached.
  - Monitor colour, amount, frequency, and consistency of stool.
- How would you manage improving the fluid input?
  - Encourage oral intake.
  - If oral intake insufficient, liaise with doctor regarding the need for an intravenous infusion.
- What investigations and treatments does this patient appear to need?
  - Blood tests: full blood count, urea, creatinine, electrolytes.
  - Stool sample for culture and sensitivity to identify any infection.
  - Urine sample for culture and sensitivity to rule out urine infection.
  - Full physical assessment to identify potential causes for confusion besides infection.

Clinical link 7.3

- Explain why hypotension due to hypovolaemia may occur with this patient, who has both peripheral oedema and ascites.
  - There is an excess amount of fluid in the body but this is in the interstitial space rather than intravascular.
  - Low albumin from liver failure reduces the oncotic pressure within the blood, which then causes fluid to leak out of vessels into interstitum.
  - Low intravascular volume (hypovolaemia) then occurs, although excess fluid rests in the interstitial space.

- What impact does the excessive fluid in the peritoneal space have on other body systems?
  - Abdominal distension may prevent normal expansion of the lungs because the larger abdomen pushes up into diaphragm restricting ventilation.
  - Ascites may cause discomfort and prevent normal mobility due to the excessively large abdomen.
- Why was an albumin infusion prescribed?
  - If a large amount of ascitic fluid is removed, there can be clinically significant fluid shifts resulting in a drop in intravascular volume.
  - The aim of the albumin infusion is to prevent hypovolaemia and to increase the oncotic pressure from the large albumin molecules to prevent further movement of fluid into the interstitial space.
  - Although the use of albumin as a colloid for fluid resuscitation has not been supported by research, there remains debate on the value of albumin following drainage of a large amount of ascites.

Chapter 8

Clinical link 8.1

Septic shock is sometimes defined as a 'distributive' shock because it is the distribution of circulating plasma fluid between the cellular, interstitial, and intravascular compartments that becomes problematical in sepsis. A disproportionate amount of fluid moves from the intravascular space into the interstitium due to endothelial 'leakiness'. This fluid normally stays in the vasculature and helps maintain blood pressure—without it, the patient experiences shock.

Septic hypovolaemia is referred to as 'relative' because unlike situations where blood losses are 'absolute', such as haemorrhage, the volume of fluid is still in one of the fluid compartments, albeit in the wrong one.

Clinical link 8.2

Early sepsis is sometimes called 'hot' or 'warm' sepsis because of vasodilation and increased cardiac output states bringing a lot of blood and therefore metabolic warmth to the skin surface. Also because of the presence of pyrexia in response to invading organisms.

Later sepsis is sometimes called 'cold' or 'cool' sepsis because these states are when the compensation mechanisms have failed, but also because there is frequently the development of oedema globally, resulting in 'waterlogged' skin, which often feels cold to touch.

Clinical link 8.3

- Which risk factors for developing sepsis does John have?

John is somewhat elderly and may have a weaker immune system than a younger person. He has had recent surgery and we know his gut has been perforated by an ulcer. He has a peripheral cannula still in use and a urinary catheter *in situ*. These are both invasive devices and may be a route for infection.

- What suggests to you that John is possibly developing sepsis? How advanced is this development?

The increase in respiratory rate is nearly always a sign of deterioration. His temperature and falling blood pressure are actually quite developed signs of sepsis—John is moving noticeably into severe sepsis. Note that it is the diastolic pressure especially that is falling. The increasing heart rate is a compensatory mechanism and, again, is a fairly advanced sign that John is being compromised by the developing sepsis. The fact that his urine output has been poor for several hours will be indicative of poor perfusion pressure and this will all need to be relayed to the surgeons. John's complaint of queasiness is non-specific but often the patient will only identify rather general symptoms before becoming extremely unwell.

- What possible sources for the infective agent might there be that are identified in the scenario?

The cannula or the catheter. John has had recent surgery. Signs of inflammation would be apparent on the cannula site. Urine may be discoloured in appearance or offensive in odour, urinalysis may be abnormal.

- What other possible causes of infection might you follow up to find the cause of a possible infection?

John's wound site and the state of his dressings need reviewing. There is no mention of John's respiratory function besides the tachypnoea—as a smoker he is more liable to a chest infection than a non-smoker.

- Which of John's recent laboratory results will the surgical team be particularly interested in, in relation to your findings?

The white cell count—a rise would indicate infection. Any MC&S sample results that have come back as positive would also be important in terms of treating the source of infection. The doctors would also review the CRP and lactate.

- What would your course of action be in response to your findings for John?

John requires an urgent review by his doctors. It would be important to handover the key physiological findings and also alert them to positive MC&S results and white cell results if they have been received on the ward or hospital information system after the ward round, for example. Generally, the sepsis six guidelines are the ones to follow:

- Oxygen to maintain saturations above 94%.
- Blood cultures: even if you are not able to perform venepuncture, the necessary equipment can be ready to expedite this.
- Intravenous antibiotics: these will probably be 'broad-spectrum' antibiotics at this point unless a sample has been positive from MC&S.
- Intravenous fluids: John already has some 0.9% saline running but will need more fluid as he is becoming cardiovascularly compromised. These fluids will need to be prescribed: is his cannula patent? Does he need a new cannula?
- It may be useful to insert an additional cannula.
- Lactate and haemoglobin levels: lactate can be measured using a blood gas analyser or handheld device. Failing this, a sample may be sent to the laboratory, as can a full blood count if haemoglobin levels have not been taken recently.
- Measure and improve urine output. John has a catheter so monitoring is easier—his observations show inadequate renal function which will need to be prioritized.

The HCA would need to be encouraged to report these findings earlier but also explanation as to what the signs of deterioration were.

Chapter 9

Clinical link 9.1

This gentleman is describing both nociceptive and neuropathic pain. From reading the medical notes, this is pain which has never been managed by a pain expert in the past.

- He has no contraindications for continuing his paracetamol at the current dose, provided his weight stays above 50 kg.
- Although potentially effective, he is unable to have NSAIDs because his eGFR is 4 and NSAIDs are contraindicated in renal failure.

- For the nociceptive pain morphine should been administered with caution because of the presence of the active metabolite M-6-glucuronide which will accumulate in renal failure. Oxycodone in low doses with long time spans between doses may be effective as the metabolites are not clinically significant, but ideally fentanyl would be the safest opioid to use for this patient as it has no active metabolites and it is not removed during dialysis when used transdermally (and therefore continues effective analgesia). If a fentanyl patch is used the daily opioid requirements for oxycodone should be used to calculate the size of the fentanyl patch required starting at 12 mcg (equivalent to 30 mg oxycodone daily).
- For the neuropathic pain he states that gabapentin was effective but he felt awful, so trying pregabalin instead follows local guidelines for neuropathic pain and could be increased if tolerated but monitoring for sedation or other unwanted side effects.

Due to the presence of infection, invasive regional procedures are not an option

Chapter 10

Clinical link 10.1

Significant findings

Your ABCDE findings highlight that the patient's airway is intact, but her respiratory rate is above 130: this is a sepsis RED FLAG. Her breathing pattern does not suggest respiratory distress and she is not requiring supplemental oxygen and her saturations are normal. Her heart rate is above 130 and this is a sepsis RED FLAG. It is also bounding, indicative of a high cardiac output state, seen in the early signs of sepsis. Her CRT is also low, and her blood pressure has a widening pulse pressure (70) indicating vasodilation which can be attributed to mediators of sepsis. She is currently alert but is tiring, this is a concerning sign. Her temperature is elevated at 39.2°C indicating that sepsis is the likely cause of deterioration. In addition, she is experiencing a rigour and care must be taken to avoid overheating this patient with excessive blankets.
On exposure she has a red wound indicative of infection (AMBER FLAG) and her history of recent surgery is also another AMBER FLAG.

SEPSIS Is the likely cause of her deterioration.

Changes to Care Following sepsis.org, the GIVE 3/ TAKE 3 protocol should be considered

GIVE

- **Antibiotics**
  - She will require a senior medical review within an hour (sepsis golden hour) and she should commence IV antibiotics within 1 hour. Guidance can be sought from the Microguide APP in relation to antibiotic protocols for your own Trust if you work in the United Kingdom (useful site to guide junior doctors to if you cannot get immediate senior review).
- **Oxygen**
  - Oxygen may be administered with caution. Current evidence from the International consensus paper recommends only giving supplemental oxygen if target saturations are not met. It is important to note that excessive oxygen may be detrimental to the patient BUT you are advised to follow your own hospital policy.
- **Fluids**
  - Fluid should be administered to maintain hydration. Discussion with senior medical staff will determine if aggressive fluid resuscitation is required, this should be administered at a rate of 30 mL/ kg. The patient should have a repeat medical review during periods of fluid resuscitation.
  - At the direction of the doctor if hypotension worsens.

TAKE

- **Blood lactate measurement**
  - This is the most sensitive indicator and studies have identified the prognostic value of lactate. Serial lactate measurements should be taken, especially during periods of fluid resuscitation to evaluate response to treatment. Worsening lactate is a poor prognostic indicator.
- **Urine measurements**
  - Check when the patient last passed urine. A urinary catheter with urometer may be required. Urine output should be 0.5 mL/kg/hour.
- **The patient should be monitored for signs of AKI**
- **Blood cultures**
  - The source of the infection needs to be identified but this MUST NOT delay the administration of antibiotics. Blood cultures should be taken percutaneously and it is useful to do this whilst inserting an additional venflon as this may be required for fluid resuscitation. Other sources of infection should also be excluded and other specimens may be required (urine, sputum, wound swabs, line swabs if VIP is elevated).

Reassure patient throughout and explain all actions and gain consent.

NEWS2 Score

This is 9 and the NEWS2 escalation policy identifies that this requires AN URGENT/EMERGENCY RESPONSE. It would be wise to contact the MET and CCOT.

Handover using SBAR

Remember key phrases when handing over and convey a SENSE OF URGENCY.

Commence the conversation by stating:

- **Situation**
  - When the MET arrive, state that you are concerned that the patient is SEPTIC and rapidly deteriorating. State that the NEWS2 score is 9.
- **Background**
  - Relevant history and state that patient has had recent abdominal surgery.
- **Assessment**
  - Use ABCDE and highlight deranged observations:
  - Breathing is rapid and shallow at 28 breaths. She is tachycardic with a decreasing blood pressure (110/70) and increasing pulse pressure, her CRT is 1 second. She is alert but tiring. Her temperature is 39.2°C and she feels hot to touch but is shivering and appears to be having a rigour. Her last blood gas shows a metabolic acidosis and her blood lactate is 3 mmol/l. Her wound is red and inflamed.
  - Other observations are in a normal range currently.
- **Recommendation**
  - Review and commence the sepsis protocol

Chapter 11

Clinical link 11.1

Part A

- Immediate actions
  - Call for help—senior nurse on ward initially for support.
  - Reassess **A—Airway**: look, listen, and feel. This is important to ensure that she is still maintaining her own airway (the sedative agents she had been given for her endoscopy have made her very sleepy).
  - Administer high-flow oxygen via non rebreathe mask with reservoir at 15 L as O_2 saturations are only 86%. Call 2222 (or appropriate local number) for medical emergency call if senior nurse help is not immediately available. When O_2 saturations are this low they are inadequate and are unable to supply enough oxygen to the tissues, and this is a sign of critical illness and a potential for cardiorespiratory arrest.
  - It is important to turn her onto her side because if she vomits this will help to protect her airway and prevent choking and/or aspiration.
  - Reassess **B—Breathing**: look, listen, and feel. This is important to see if O_2 saturations are improving with high-flow oxygen. Also assess if there is a problem identified with breathing as a cause for inadequate O_2 saturations. Are both sides of the chest moving equally? Check rate and depth of breathing as well.
  - O_2 saturations improve to 100% and then are maintained at 95% on 3 L O_2 via nasal specs. Your colleague leaves you but will be available if needed.
- Other assessments
  - After **A** & **B** reassessment, check **C—Circulation**: colour, pulse, blood pressure, 12-lead ECG, check adequate intravenous access. If so check it is patent with a 5 mL saline flush. If not, a cannula will be required. Check recent blood results.
  - **D—Disability** (neurological) assessment: ACVPU. Are pupils equal and reactive to light (PEARL)? Blood sugar check. Can she move all four limbs? Obey commands? GCS score?
  - E—**Exposure** to perform a quick top to toe assessment. Check abdomen is soft, check calves for signs of deep vein thrombosis and perfusion to limbs and feet. Check for any evidence of bleeding. Check for rashes. Record central temperature.
  - It is also important to check fluid balance charts. Check all prescription charts, especially looking at the endoscopy procedure information, to see what she had been given for sedation and how much.

Part B You go to get help so she can be turned onto her side. She is cyanosed and noises are radiating from her airway.

- Priorities:
  - Call for help! Pull bedside buzzer.
  - Assess **ABC**—look, listen, feel for 10 s only.

Patient is breathing regular respirations and noise and cyanosis disappears with head tilt chin lift. Colour improves. She has a rapid regular central pulse. She is not moving and does not resist head tilt, chin lift.

- Other actions/interventions
  - Call 2222 medical emergency number (or appropriate local number).
  - Maintain airway opening manoeuvre. Reapply high-flow O_2 with non-rebreathe and reservoir at 15 L. Check O_2 saturations and colour. Remember: *simple manoeuvres will almost always open an obstructed airway.*
  - Ask for suction (bedside) to be turned on and ensure yankauer suction available.

- Call for resuscitation trolley so equipment is near to hand for you and for when the team arrive.
- With A being maintained, reassess B and C. (Because of the patient's deterioration it is vital a repeat of ABCDE is carried out so nothing is missed.) Remember: *Even though the tubing has been attached to the O_2 cylinder confirm it HAS been turned on and the reservoir bag is moving in and out with the patient's breathing.* Then reassess D and E again.
- Anticipate the need for simple and advanced airway equipment so ensure that your colleague is preparing this when the trolley arrives.
- Consider obtaining antidotes (if known) to sedatives given to patient, such as naloxone for morphine overdose. This will save important time for when the doctors arrive.

- Signs of airway obstruction.

Complete:

- Absent breath sounds at mouth/nose.
- Use of accessory muscles.
- Paradoxical chest movements ('see-saw' breathing).
- Central cyanosis may not be evident initially as it can be a late sign.

Partial:

- Air entry diminished.
- Noisy breathing depending on cause of obstruction, that is gurgling may be blood or vomit, snoring noise due to tongue partially occluding the airway.

Clinical link 11.2

Rate and depth

The sternum must be compressed hard and fast. The depth should be 5–6 cm (2 inches) and the rate of 100–120 a minute (almost two compressions every second). Try not to allow your fingers to press on the chest wall over the ribs. The heels of your hands are much stronger. With the wrists bent and fingers up, it allows better force to be applied. After each compression the pressure must be released to allow full recoil of the chest but without taking away the hand position. This allows for better cardiac filling and blood flow to the myocardium

For a list of reversible causes of cardiac arrest, see Table A.

Treatment

In PEA or asystole as soon as chest compressions are underway administer 1 mg adrenaline. Ensure that the leads are attached in asystole to confirm the rhythm. If only p-waves are visible, attempt to externally pace

The reversible causes should be considered treated whilst CPR is continued and reversible causes treated as indicated in the chapter.

As the likely diagnosis is PE, immediate thrombolysis IV is usually provided for known or high suspicion pulmonary embolism. This often requires a prolonged resuscitation attempt to enable the thrombolysis to take effect. A full resuscitation commitment of ALS up to 1 hour is required once the decision to commence thrombolysis has been made

Mechanical devices for continuous chest compressions are available in most acute hospital trusts and can be considered for use in prolonged resuscitations.

Consideration should be given to notifying the patient's family about the patient's deterioration and notifying ITU in the event that a critical care level 3 bed may be required

Table A 1.1 Reversible causes of cardiac arrest

Hypoxia	Airway obstruction Respiratory failure Sepsis
Hypovolaemia	Haemorrhage Trauma Sepsis Gastrointestinal bleed Ruptured aortic aneurysm
Hypothermia (< 35°C, severe < 30°C)	Exposure—collapse outside Immersion in water Ingestion of drugs/alcohol
Hyper/hypokalaemia and metabolic disorders	Renal disease Calcium channel blocker overdose Documented electrolyte imbalance
Tamponade	Penetrating chest trauma Myocardial infarction Cardiac surgery
Tension pneumothorax	History of chest trauma Asthma CVP line insertion Missed pneumothorax plus positive pressure ventilation
Toxic/therapeutic disorders	Drug overdose A good history Industrial exposure
Thrombo-embolic	Pulmonary embolism (surgery/pregnancy/DVT/long haul travel)

Chapter 12

Clinical link 12.1

- Patient escort—who should go?

At least one healthcare professional with advanced life support skills, for example experienced trained nurse, doctor.

- What are the risks—what could happen during transfer?

This is an acute event, the patient is already symptomatic before any movement and at this stage diagnosis not confirmed. Due to the requirement for the patient to change position, to lie horizontal for transfer to imaging table and for CT itself, they are at high risk of becoming more hypoxic and therefore breathless and anxious. If the patient has a pulmonary embolus and the embolus large enough it could potentially lead to cardiopulmonary arrest. Escorting staff need to be prepared for complications and ensure adequate intravenous access before transfer. It is also imperative that any movement is carefully controlled and patient lies flat for the least amount of time possible. Escorting staff also should provide continual reassurance to the patient explaining each stage of movement. During the actual CT scan the patient is usually left alone (to reduce risk of radiation to healthcare staff) therefore monitoring needs to be positioned to allow staff to view both visual and audible alarms. It is important that the patient understands that they are still being monitored, that the time in the CT will be brief and that they can still communicate with staff in the control room.

- What equipment do you require?

Oxygen (adequate supply consider oxygen may need to be increased to 15 L/min), cardiac monitor, 'emergency bag' with access to intubation equipment, bag/valve/mask, emergency cardiac drugs, intravenous administration equipment, ABG syringe.

- What monitoring should the patient have during the transfer?

Respiratory rate, work of breathing, cardiac monitor, including pulse oximetry (SpO_2), continuous ECG, non-invasive blood pressure and alarms set appropriately, level of consciousness (any signs of increasing respiratory distress or confusion). CT scanner will usually have CCTV to allow vision of patient and communication with patient. The screen should be closely observed to monitor during procedure.

- How should this be documented?

Take observation charts (useful to trend patient response and in addition facilitate documentation at regular intervals (every 15 min). Trend of track-and-trigger score.

Clinical link 12.2

- Patient escort—who should go?

As an unplanned inter-hospital transfer the decision should be made by the consultant responsible for the patient. At least one healthcare professional with advanced life support skills, ability to prescribe fluids, manage the changing patient haemodynamics, for example doctor/anaesthetist.

- What are the risks—what could happen during transfer?

This is an acute event and the patient is at high risk of further bleeding. Vomiting blood could cause a compromised airway through aspiration particularly if there is a reduction in conscious level due to haemodynmic instability (consider anti-emetic). Hypovolaemia (due to blood loss) and ensuing haemodynamic instability (if not adequately fluid resuscitated) could potentially lead to cardiopulmonary arrest. The patient must have adequate intravenous access before transfer with two large cannulae and be optimized with fluid replacement, consider urinary catheterization to assess response to fluid resuscitation.

If the patient has a distended abdomen this could cause pressure on diaphragm, reduced lung expansion.

- What equipment do you require?

Oxygen, cardiac monitor (adequate battery life), 'emergency bag' with access to intubation equipment, bag/valve/mask, emergency cardiac drugs, intravenous fluids administration, ABG syringe. Portable suction. Blood and crossmatch information. All health records, including recent blood results.

- What monitoring should the patient have during the transfer?

Respiratory rate and evaluation of work of breathing. Cardiac monitor, including pulse oximetry, continuous ECG, non-invasive blood pressure, and alarms set appropriately, level of consciousness (any signs of increasing respiratory distress or confusion). Response to intravenous fluids. Trend of track-and-trigger score.

- How should this be documented?

Use hospital transfer, document at regular intervals (every 15 min).

Index

Note: Subjects are indexed under their non-abbreviated form. A list of abbreviations appears on pp. xiii–xvii. Tables, figures, and boxes are indicated by *t*, *f*, and *b* following the page number.